LIPPINCOTT MANUAL
of NURSING PRACTICE
Series

DOCUMENTATION

◆

 Wolters Kluwer | Lippincott Williams & Wilkins
Health

Philadelphia • Baltimore • New York • London
Buenos Aires • Hong Kong • Sydney • Tokyo

STAFF

Executive Publisher
Judith A. Schilling McCann, RN, MSN

Editorial Director
H. Nancy Holmes

Clinical Director
Joan M. Robinson, RN, MSN

Art Director
Mary Ludwicki

Editorial Project Manager
Jennifer Kowalak

Clinical Project Manager
Beverly Ann Tscheschlog, RN, BS

Editor
Julie Munden

Copy Editors
Kimberly Bilotta, Linda Hager

Designers
Debra Moloshak (book design)

Digital Composition Services
Diane Paluba (manager),
Joyce Rossi Biletz, Donna S. Morris
(project manager)

Manufacturing
Beth J. Welsh

Editorial Assistants
Megan L. Aldinger, Karen J. Kirk,
Linda K. Ruhf

Indexer
Barbara Hodgson

Printed in China.

LMNPDOC010207

Library of Congress
Cataloging-in-Publication Data
Documentation.
    p. ; cm. — (Lippincott manual of nursing practice series)
    Includes bibliographical references and index.
    1. Nursing records—Handbooks, manuals, etc. 2. Nursing—Documentation—Handbooks, manuals, etc. I. Lippincott Williams & Wilkins. II. Series.
    [DNLM: 1. Nursing Records—Handbooks. 2. Documentation—methods—Handbooks. 3. Forms and Records Control—methods—Handbooks. 4. Specialties, Nursing—organization & administration—Handbooks.   WY 49 D637 2008]
    RT50.D612 2008
    651.5'04261—dc22
ISBN-13: 978-1-58255-699-4 (alk. paper)
ISBN-10: 1-58255-699-7 (alk. paper)
                                    2006037407

CONTENTS

CONTRIBUTORS
AND CONSULTANTS

◆

Joyce Bedoian, MBE, MSN, CRNP
Coordinator Nursing Learning Resource
   Center
Widener University School of Nursing
Chester, Pa.

Susan Boggs, RN, BSN
Director of Professional Services
Complete Home Health Care
Clarksville, Tenn.

Kevin Giordano, JD
Attorney
Keyes and Donnellan, PC
Springfield, Mass.

Ginny Wacker Guido, RN, MSN, JD, FAAN
Associate Dean and Director, Graduate
   Studies
University of North Dakota, School of
   Nursing
Grand Forks

Kenneth W. Hazell, ARNP, MSN
Professor of Nursing
Palm Beach Community College
Lake Worth, Fla.

Joy L. Herzog, RN
Assistant Director of Nursing Services
Beverly Healthcare of Doylestown (Pa.)

Roseanne Hanlon Rafter, APRN, BC, MSN
Director of Nursing Professional Practice
Pottstown (Pa.) Memorial Medical Center

Donna Scemons, RN, MSN, FNP-C, CNS, CWOCN
Family Nurse Practitioner
Healthcare Systems, Inc.
Castaic, Calif.

Leslie Stevenson-Johnson, BSN
Tenured Faculty Practical Nursing Program
Lake Washington Technical College
Kirkland, Wash.

Jacqueline Walus-Wigle, RN, JD, CPHQ
Auditor
UCSD Audit & Management Advisory
   Services
University of California, San Diego
La Jolla, Calif.

DOCUMENTING EVERYDAY EVENTS

The patient's chart communicates important information about his condition and course of treatment. To avoid serious documentation problems, always follow these cardinal rules:

• Take time to document accurately, objectively, and thoroughly.
• Be consistent and document legibly.

Routine nursing procedures

Nursing notes about routine nursing procedures should appear in the patient's chart and include:

• the type of procedure performed
• who performed it
• how it was performed
• how the patient tolerated it
• adverse effects, if applicable.

Other documentation for routine nursing procedures typically includes documentation on:

• medication administration and I.V. therapy
• supportive care and assistive procedures
• infection control

• diagnostic tests
• pain control
• codes
• changes in the patient's condition
• intake and output monitoring
• wound and skin care
• patient's personal property
• shift reports
• patient teaching.

MEDICATION ADMINISTRATION

Most facilities include a medication administration record (MAR) in their documentation systems. It serves as the central record of medication orders and their execution, and it's part of the patient's permanent record. (See *The medication administration record,* pages 2 to 5.) When using an MAR, follow these guidelines:

• Know and follow your facility's policies and procedures for recording medication orders and documenting medication administration.
• Sign your full name and licensure status, and place your initials in the space provided.
• Make sure that all medication orders include the patient's full name, the date, and the medication's name,

(Text continues on page 4.)

THE MEDICATION
ADMINISTRATION RECORD

The medication administration record contains a permanent record of the patient's medications. It may also include the patient's diagnosis and information about allergies and diet. A sample form is shown below.

NURSE'S FULL SIGNATURE, STATUS AND INITIALS

	INIT.
Roy Charles, RN	RC
Theresa Hopkins, RN	TH
Carol Slane, RN	CS
Marie Keller, RN	MK

DIAGNOSIS: Heart failure, Atrial flutter

ALLERGIES: ASA

ROUTINE/DAILY ORDERS/FINGERSTICKS/ INSULIN COVERAGE			DATE: 1/4/07	DATE: 1/5/07	[

ORDER DATE	MEDICATIONS DOSE, ROUTE, FREQUENCY	TIME	SITE	INIT.	SITE	INIT.
1/4/07	digoxin 0.125 mg	0900		RC		RC
RC	I.V. every day	HR		68		70
1/4/07	furosemide 40 mg	0900		RC		RC
RC	I.V. q12h	2100		TH		TH
1/4/07	enalapril 1.25 mg	0500		TH		TH
RC	I.V. q6h	1100		RC		RC
		1700		RC		RC
		2300		TH		TH

	INIT.			INIT.

DIET: *Low sodium*

DATE: 1/6/07		DATE:		DATE:		DATE:		DATE:		DATE:		DATE:	
SITE	INIT.	SITE	INIT.	SITE	INIT.	SITE	INIT.	SITE	INIT.	SITE	INIT.	SITE	INIT.
CG													
72													
CG													
MK													
MK													
CG													
CG													
MK													

(continued)

Addressograph

INITIAL	SIGNATURE & STATUS	INITIAL	SIGNATURE & STATUS	ITIAL
RC	Roy Charles, RN			
TH	Theresa Hopkins, RN			

YEAR 2007

ORDER DATE: 1/4/07	RENEWAL DATE: /	DISCONTINUED DATE: /	DATE	1/4/07	
MEDICATION: acetaminophen		DOSE 650 mg	TIME GIVEN	0930	
DIRECTION: p.r.n. mild pain		ROUTE: P.O.	SITE	P.O.	
			INIT.	RC	

ORDER DATE: 1/4/07	RENEWAL DATE: 1/6/07	DISCONTINUED DATE: /	DATE	1/4/07	
MEDICATION: Morphine sulfate		DOSE 2 mg	TIME GIVEN	0930	
DIRECTION: 15 minutes prior to changing ® heel dressing		ROUTE: I.V.	SITE		
			INIT.	RC	

ORDER DATE: 1/4/07	RENEWAL DATE: /	DISCONTINUED DATE: /	DATE	1/4/07	
MEDICATION: Milk of Magnesia		DOSE 30ml	TIME GIVEN	2115	
DIRECTION: q6h p.r.n.		ROUTE: P.O.	SITE	P.O.	
			INIT.	TH	

ORDER DATE: 1/5/07	RENEWAL DATE: /	DISCONTINUED DATE: /	DATE	1/5/07	1/5/07
MEDICATION: prochlorperazine		DOSE 5 mg	TIME GIVEN	1100	2230
DIRECTION: q8h p.r.n.		ROUTE: I.M.	SITE	®glut.	®glut.
prn nausea and vomiting			INIT.	RC	TH

ORDER DATE: /	RENEWAL DATE: /	DISCONTINUED DATE: /	DATE		
MEDICATION:		DOSE	TIME GIVEN		
DIRECTION:		ROUTE:	SITE		

dose, administration route or method, and frequency. Include the specific number of doses given or the medication stop date.

● Record medication administration and the time of the administration immediately.

PRN MEDICATION

ALLERGIES:

INITIAL	SIGNATURE & STATUS	INITIAL	SIGNATURE & STATUS

P.R.N. MEDICATIONS								

● If you can't administer a medication as scheduled, document the reason.

● Make sure that the patient's known drug allergies, if any, are included on his chart.

REPORTING ADVERSE EVENTS
AND PRODUCT PROBLEMS TO THE FDA

Even large, well-designed clinical trials can't guarantee that adverse reactions will never arise after a drug or medical device is approved for use. An adverse reaction that occurs in only 1 in 5,000 patients could easily be missed in clinical trials. The drug could also interact with other drugs in ways unrevealed during clinical trials.

As a nurse, you play a key role in reporting adverse events and product problems. Reporting such problems helps ensure the safety of products that the U.S. Food and Drug Administration (FDA) regulates. The FDA's Medical Products Reporting Program supplies health care professionals with Med-Watch forms on which they can report adverse events and product problems.

WHAT TO REPORT
Complete a MedWatch form when you suspect that a drug, medical device, special nutritional product, or other product regulated by the FDA is responsible for:
- congenital anomaly
- death
- disability
- initial or prolonged hospitalization
- life-threatening illness
- the need for any medical or surgical intervention to prevent a permanent impairment or an injury.

Also, promptly inform the FDA of product quality problems, such as:
- defective devices
- inaccurate or unreadable product labels
- intrinsic or extrinsic contamination or stability problems
- packaging or product mix-ups
- particulates in injectable drugs
- product damage.

YOUR RESPONSIBILITY IN REPORTING
When filing a MedWatch form, keep in mind that you aren't expected to establish a connection between the product and the problem. You don't have to include a lot of details; you only have to report the adverse event or the problem with the drug or the product.

Additionally, you don't even have to wait until the evidence seems compelling. FDA regulations protect your identity and the identities of your patient and employer.

FURTHER GUIDELINES
The MedWatch form merges the individual forms used in the past to report adverse drug reactions, drug quality product problems, device quality product problems, and adverse reactions to medical devices. Send completed forms to the FDA by using the fax number or mailing address on the form.

File a separate MedWatch form for each patient, and attach additional pages if needed. If appropriate, report product problems to the manufacturer as well as to the FDA. Also, remember to comply with your health care facility's protocols for reporting adverse events associated with drugs and medical devices.

Product lot numbers are used in product identification, tracking, and product recall; therefore, the lot number should be retained and a copy of the report should be kept on file by your supervisor.

FDA RESPONSE
The FDA will report back to you on the actions it takes and will continue to work to instruct health care professionals about adverse events.

- If you suspect a connection between a patient's medication and an adverse event, such as illness, injury, or even death:
  - Follow your facility's policy on reporting adverse drug events.
  - Use a MedWatch form to report the information to the Food and Drug Administration (FDA). (See *Reporting adverse events and product problems to the FDA.*)

  Patient safety *Write legibly, and use only standard abbreviations approved by your facility. Remember that the Joint Commission on Accreditation of Healthcare Organizations (JCAHO) pro-*

A. Patient information

1. Patient identifier	2. Age at time of event: _____ or Date of birth: _____	3. Sex ☑ female ☐ male	4. Weight _____ lbs or _59_ kgs

In confidence

B. Adverse event or product problem

1. ☐ Adverse event and/or ☐ Product problem (e.g., defects/malfunctions)

2. Outcomes attributed to adverse event (check all that apply)
- ☐ death (mo/day/yr)
- ☐ life-threatening
- ☐ hospitalization – initial or prolonged
- ☐ disability
- ☐ congenital anomaly
- ☐ required intervention to prevent permanent impairment/damage
- ☐ other: _____

3. Date of event (mo/day/yr) 1/8/07	4. Date of this report (mo/day/yr) 1/8/07

5. Describe event or problem

After reconstituting 100 mg vial with
10 ml of bacteriostatic water, the drug
crystallized and turned yellow.

Drug was not given.

6. Relevant tests/laboratory data, including dates

7. Other relevant history, including preexisting medical conditions (e.g., allergies, race, pregnancy, smoking and alcohol use, hepatic/renal dysfunction, etc.)

(side text, vertical) PLEASE TYPE OR USE BLACK INK

C. Suspect medication(s)

1. Name (give labeled strength & mfr/labeler, if known)
#1 Leucovorin Calcium for injection — 100 mg vial
#2

2. Dose, frequency & route used	3. Therapy dates (if unknown, give duration) from/to (or best estimate)
#1 100 mg. IV X 1	#1 1/8/07
#2	#2

4. Diagnosis for use (indication)
#1 Megaloblastic Anemia
#2

5. Event abated after use stopped or dose reduced
#1 ☐ yes ☐ no ☑ doesn't apply
#2 ☐ yes ☐ no ☐ doesn't apply

6. Lot # (if known)	7. Exp. date (if known)
#1 #891	#1
#2	#2

8. Event reappeared after reintroduction
#1 ☐ yes ☐ no ☐ doesn't apply
#2 ☐ yes ☐ no ☐ doesn't apply

9. NDC # (for product problems only)
– –

10. Concomitant medical products and therapy dates (exclude treatment of event)

D. Suspect medical device

1. Brand name

2. Type of device

3. Manufacturer name & address	4. Operator of device ☐ health professional ☐ lay user/patient ☐ other: _____

5. Expiration date (mo/day/yr)

6. model # _____
catalog # _____
serial # _____
lot # _____
other # _____

7. If implanted, give date (mo/day/yr)

8. If explanted, give date (mo/day/yr)

9. Device available for evaluation? (Do not send to FDA)
☐ yes ☐ no ☐ returned to manufacturer on _____ (mo/day/yr)

10. Concomitant medical products and therapy dates (exclude treatment of event)

E. Reporter (see confidentiality section on back)

1. Name & address | phone #
Patricia Cohen
987 Elm Ave
Cincinnati, Ohio

2. Health professional? ☑ yes ☐ no	3. Occupation RN	4. Also reported to ☐ manufacturer ☐ user facility ☑ distributor

5. If you do NOT want your identity disclosed to the manufacturer, place an "X" in this box. ☐

---

hibits the use of certain abbreviations (those that appear on the "do not use" list). When in doubt, write out the word or phrase.

● Communicate one-time orders to be given on another shift to the next shift, or use a medication alert sticker to flag the order.

Medications given "as needed"
● Document all medications administered "as needed."
● For eye, ear, or nose drops, document the number of drops and where they were inserted.

- For suppositories, document the type (rectal, vaginal, or urethral) as well as the patient's tolerance.
- For dermal medications, document the size, location, and condition of the site where the medication was applied.
- For dermal patches, document the location of the patch.
- Document exceptional information, such as a patient's refusal to accept prescribed medication, in your progress notes; include your nursing interventions in your charting.

Remember: Medications administered according to accepted standards don't need to include other information in the chart.

| 1/8/07 | 0900 | Pt. refused KCL elixir, stating that it makes her feel nauseated and that she can't stand the taste. Dr. Miller notified. K-Dur tabs ordered and given. Pt. tolerated K-Dur well. ——— Betty Griffin, RN |

Single-dose medications

Single-dose medications should be documented in the patient's MAR as well as in his progress notes. Documentation of these medications should include:
- who gave the order
- why the order was given

Chart right

CONTROLLED SUBSTANCE INVENTORY RECORD

The sample controlled substance inventory record demonstrates proper documentation of controlled substances and an end-of-shift controlled substance count.

CITY HOSPITAL

24-HOUR RECORD CONTROLLED SUBSTANCES

1900 INVENTORY			CODEINE 30 MG TAB	PERCOCET TAB	TYLENOL #3 TAB	VALIUM 2 MG TAB	VALIUM 5 MG TAB	TEMAZEPAM 15 MG TAB		
			25	20	18	15	16	10		
Time	Patient name	Patient number								
0915	Orr, Carl	555112								
1000	Davis, Donna	555161				16				
1115	McGowen, John	555111					15			

the patient's response to the medication.

For example, if you gave a one-time dose of I.V. Lasix, you would write:

1/3/07	0900	Lasix 40 mg I.V. given as per Dr. Singh's order. Pt. with SOB, crackles bilaterally, and O₂ saturation decreased to 89% on room air. ———— ———— Ann Barrow, RN
1/3/07	1000	Responded with urine output of 1500 ml, decreased SOB, and O₂ saturation increased to 97% on room air. ———— ———— Ann Barrow, RN

Controlled substances

The administration and documentation of controlled substances must adhere to strict federal, state, and facility regulations. Whenever you administer controlled substances, be sure to document that you:
● verified the amount of the medication in the container and signed out the medication on the appropriate form (See *Controlled substance inventory record*.)
● counted all controlled substances at the end of shift and verified an accurate count
● had a second nurse observe and document your activities, especially if a controlled substance or part of a dose had to be wasted

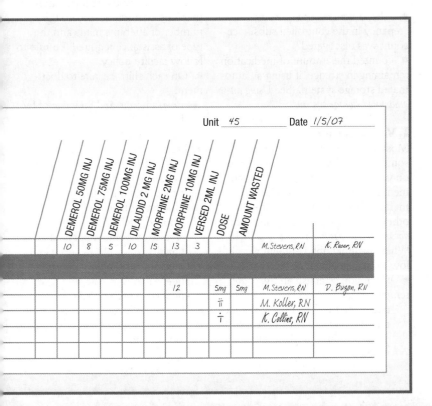

Unit __45__   Date __1/5/07__

	DEMEROL 50MG INJ	DEMEROL 75MG INJ	DEMEROL 100MG INJ	DILAUDID 2 MG INJ	MORPHINE 2MG INJ	MORPHINE 10MG INJ	VERSED 2ML INJ	DOSE	AMOUNT WASTED		
	10	8	5	10	15	13	3			M. Stevens, RN	K. Racer, RN
						12		5mg	5mg	M. Stevens, RN	D. Bugon, RN
								ii̅		M. Koller, RN	
								ī		K. Collins, RN	

– update the patient's records each time you change the insertion site or the I.V. tubing, making sure you document the reasons for the change, such as extravasation, phlebitis, occlusion, patient removal, or a routine change according to facility policy.

1/16/07	0200	Complained of pain in Ⓛ hand at I.V. site. Hand reddened from I.V. insertion site to 2" above site, tender and warm to touch. Slight swelling noted. I.V. discontinued and a warm, moist towel applied to Ⓛ hand. 20G I.V. started in Ⓡ forearm. — Kathy Costello, RN

● filled out an event report if a discrepancy in the controlled substance count was discovered
● counted the amount of medication remaining in storage, if using an automated storage system. (See *Using an automated storage system.*)

I.V. THERAPY

Most hospitalized patients receive some form of I.V. therapy. Depending on your facility's policy, you'll document I.V. therapy on a special I.V. therapy sheet, nursing flow sheet, or other format. (See *Using a flow sheet to document I.V. therapy,* pages 12 and 13.) When documenting I.V. therapy, follow these guidelines:
● When you establish an I.V. route, remember to:
– document the date, time, venipuncture site, and equipment used, such as the type and gauge of catheter or needle

● If a venipuncture requires more than one attempt, document the number of attempts made and the type of assistance required. Be sure to follow facility policy.
● On each shift, be sure to document:
– type, amount, and flow rate of I.V. fluid
– condition of the I.V. site.
● Each time that you flush the I.V. line, identify the type and amount of fluid used for each flush.
● If complications arise, make sure you document that you:
– stopped the I.V. line
– assessed the amount of fluid infiltrated
– provided other appropriate nursing interventions
– notified the practitioner.
● If a chemotherapeutic medication extravasates, follow facility procedure and document:
– appearance of the I.V. site

– type of treatment given (especially any medication used as an antidote)
– dressing applied to the site
– that you notified the practitioner.

● If an allergic reaction occurs while the patient is receiving I.V. therapy, notify the practitioner immediately and complete an adverse reaction form, making sure you include all pertinent information, including:
– type and extent of the reaction
– when the reaction was identified
– treatments and the patient's response to them.

● Document patient teaching that you perform with the patient and his family. Document that you:
– explained the purpose of I.V. therapy
– described the procedure
– discussed possible complications.

Total parental nutrition

Total parenteral nutrition (TPN) is the administration of a solution of dextrose, proteins, electrolytes, vitamins, and trace elements in amounts that exceed the patient's energy expenditure and thereby achieve anabolism. For a patient receiving TPN, follow these guidelines:

● Document the type and location of the central line, the condition of the insertion site, and the volume and rate of the solution infused.

● Monitor for adverse reactions, and document your observations and interventions.

● When you discontinue a central or peripheral I.V. line for TPN, document the date and time, the type of dressing applied, and the appearance of the administration site.

1/3/07	2020	2-L bag of TPN hung at 2000. Infusing at 65 ml/ hr via infusion pump through ® subclavian CV line. Transparent dressing intact, and site is without redness, drainage, swelling, or tenderness. Told pt. to call nurse if dressing becomes loose or soiled, site becomes tender or painful, or tubing or catheter becomes dislodged. Reviewed reasons for TPN and answered pt.'s questions about its purpose. ———————— Meg Callahan, RN

Blood transfusions

Whether you administer blood or blood components, use proper identification and cross-matching procedures to ensure that the patient receives the correct blood product for transfusion. Follow these documentation guidelines:

Patient safety *According to JCAHO's National Patient Safety Goals, the blood or blood component must be identified by two licensed health care professionals, both of whom should sign the slip that comes with the blood and verify that the information is correct.*

● Document the I.V. site, catheter gauge, and flow rate of the I.V. fluid.

● After the transfusion, document:
– date and time the transfusion was started and completed
– total amount of the transfusion
– any infusion device or blood-warming unit that was used.

● Also be sure to record the patient's vital signs before, during, and after the transfusion.

(Text continues on page 14.)

USING A FLOW SHEET
TO DOCUMENT I.V. THERAPY

This sample shows the typical features of an I.V. therapy flow sheet.

INTRAVENOUS CARE RECORD

INTRAVENOUS CARE COMMENT CODES
C = CAP F = FILTER T= TUBING D = DRESSING

START DATE/ TIME	INITIALS	I.V. VOLUME & SOLUTION	ADDITIVES	FLOW RATE	
1/3/07 1100	DS	1000 cc D$_5$W	20 meq KCL	100/hr	
1/3/07 2100	JM	1000 cc D$_5$W	20 meq KCL	100/hr	
1/5/07 0700	DS	1000 cc D$_5$W	20 meq KCL	100/hr	

SITE	STOP DATE/ TIME	TUBING CHANGE	COMMENTS
RFA	1/3/07 2100	T	
RFA	1/5/07 0700		
LFA	1/5/07	TD	

If the patient receives his own blood, be sure to document:
- amount of autologous blood retrieved and reinfused in the intake and output records
- laboratory data during and after the autotransfusion
- patient's pretransfusion and post-transfusion vital signs.

Transfusion reaction
If the patient develops a reaction during the transfusion, be sure to document:
- time and date of the reaction
- type and amount of infused blood or blood products
- time the infusion was started and stopped
- clinical signs of the reaction in order of occurrence
- patient's vital signs
- urine specimens or blood samples sent to the laboratory for analysis
- treatments given and the patient's response.

2/13/07	1400	Pt. reports nausea and chills. Cyanosis of the lips noted at 1350 hours, with PRBCs transfusing. Infusion stopped, approximately 100 ml infused. Tubing changed. I.V. of 1,000 ml D₅NSS infusing at KVO rate in ® arm. Notified Dr. Cahill. BP 168/88; P 104, RR 25; T 97.6° R. Blood sample taken from PRBCs. Two red-top tubes of blood drawn from pt. and sent to the laboratory. Urine specimen obtained from catheter. Urine specimen sent to lab for UA. Gave pt. diphenhydramine 50 mg I.M. ——— Maryann Belinsky, RN

2/13/07	1415	Pt. reports he's getting warmer and less nauseated. BP 148/80; P 96; RR 20; T 98.2° R. ——— Maryann Belinsky, RN
2/13/07	1430	Pt. no longer complaining of nausea or chills. I.V. of 1,000 ml D₅NSS infusing at 125 ml/hr in ® arm. BP 138/76; P 80; RR 18; T, 98.4° R ——— Maryann Belinsky, RN

Some health care facilities require the completion of a transfusion reaction report that must be sent to the blood bank. (See *Transfusion reaction report*.)

SUPPORTIVE CARE PROCEDURES

Daily nursing interventions constitute supportive care measures. Many of these can be documented on graphic forms and flow charts; others must be documented in progress notes or other forms. Among the most commonly documented nursing interventions are:
- those that are provided before and after a surgical procedure (for example, pacemaker insertion, peritoneal dialysis, peritoneal lavage, suture removal, or thoracic drainage)
- those provided to support the patient throughout treatment (for example, cardiac monitoring, chest physiotherapy, mechanical ventilation, nasogastric [NG] tube insertion and removal, seizure management, tube feedings, and withdrawing arterial blood for analysis).

(Text continues on page 18.)

TRANSFUSION REACTION REPORT

If your facility requires a transfusion reaction report, you'll include the following types of information.

TRANSFUSION REACTION REPORT

Nursing report

1. Stop transfusion immediately. Keep I.V. line open with saline infusion.
2. Notify responsible physician.
3. Check all identifying names and numbers on the patient's wristband, unit, and paperwork for discrepancies.
4. Record patient's post-transfusion vital signs.
5. Draw posttransfusion blood samples (clotted and anticoagulated), avoiding mechanical hemolysis.
6. Collect posttransfusion urine specimen from patient.
7. Record information as indicated below.
8. Send discontinued bag of blood, administration set, attached I.V. solutions, and all related forms and labels to the Blood Bank with this form completed.

Clerical errors
☑ None detected
☐ Detected

Vital signs

	Pre-TXN	Post-TXN
Temp.	98.4°F	98°F
B.P.	120/60	134/80
Pulse	88	80

Signs and Symptoms

☑ Urticaria	☐ Nausea	☐ Shock	☐ Hemoglobin-
☐ Fever	☑ Flushing	☐ Oozing	uria
☐ Chills	☐ Dyspnea	☐ Back pain	☐ Oliguria or
☐ Chest pain	☐ Headache	☐ Infusion site	anuria
☐ Hypotension	☐ Perspiration	pain	

Reaction occurred

During administration? ___yes___
After administration? _____
How long? _____
Medications added? _____
Previous I.V. fluids? ___1 unit FFP___
Blood warmed? ___No___

Specimen collection

Blood: ___Yes – Sent to lab___
Urine: Voided ___Yes – Sent to lab___   Catheterized _____

Comments:

Signature _Jacqueline Brown, RN_   **Date** ___1/10/07___

(continued)

BLOOD BANK REPORT

Unit #	1. Clerical errors
22FM80507	☑ None detected
Component Returned	☐ Detected
Yes	Comments:
Volume Returned	
185 ml	

2. Hemolysis:

Note: If hemolysis is present in the posttransfusion sample, a posttransfusion urine sample must be tested for free hemoglobin immediately.

	None	Slight	Moderate	Marked
Patient pre-TXN sample	☑ None	☐ Slight	☐ Moderate	☐ Marked
Patient post-TXN sample	☑ None	☐ Slight	☐ Moderate	☐ Marked
Blood Bag	☑ None	☐ Slight	☐ Moderate	☐ Marked
Urine HGB (centrifuged)	☐ None	☐ Slight	☑ Moderate	☐ Marked

3. Direct antiglobulin test

Pretransfusion _____

Posttransfusion _____

If No. 2 and No. 3 are negative, steps 4 through 6 are not required. Report results to the blood bank physician. Steps 7 and 8 or further testing will be done as ordered by blood bank physician.

4. ABO and Rh Groups

Repeat testing	Cell reaction with							
	Anti-A	Anti-B	Anti-A,B	Anti-D	Cont.	Du	Cont.	CCC
Pretransfusion								
Posttransfusion								
Unit #								
Unit #								

Repeat testing	Serum reaction with		ABO/Rh
	A₁ cells	B cells	
Pretransfusion			
Posttransfusion			
Unit #			
Unit #			

BLOOD BANK REPORT *(continued)*

5. Red cell antibody screen

Pretransfusion	Cell	Saline/AB				INT
		RT	37°C	AHG	CCC	
Date of sample	I					
	II					
By:	Auto					

Posttransfusion	Cell	Saline/AB				INT
		RT	37°C	AHG	CCC	
Date of sample	I					
	II					
By:	Auto					

Specificity of antibody detected:

6. Crossmatch compatibility testing

Use patient pre- and post-TXN serum and the suspected unit red cells obtained from inside the container or from a segment still attached to bag. Observe appearance of blood in bag and administration tubing.

Pretransfusion	Albumin				INT
	RT	37°C	AHG	CCC	
Unit #					
Unit #					

Posttransfusion	Albumin				INT
	RT	37°C	AHG	CCC	
Unit #					
Unit #					

All units on hold for future transfusion must be recrossmatched with the posttransfusion sample.

7. Bacteriologic testing

Pretransfusion _____ Posttransfusion _____

8. Other testing results

Total bilirubin	Coagulation studies	Urine output studies
Patient pre-TXN _____ mg/dl		
Patient 6 hrs. post-TXN		
_____ mg/dl		

Pathologist's conclusions:

Signature _____ Date _____

Preoperative documentation

Effective nursing documentation during the preoperative period focuses on two primary elements:

- the baseline preoperative assessment
- patient teaching.

Documenting these elements encourages accurate communication among caregivers. Most facilities use a preoperative checklist to verify that:

- required data have been collected
- preoperative teaching has occurred
- prescribed procedures and safety precautions have been executed.

Be sure to document the name of the person you notified of any abnormalities that could affect the patient's response to the surgical procedure or any deviations from facility standards. For example, if you find there isn't a completed history or physical, your note might read as follows:

1/14/07	0800	No completed history and
		physical found in pt's
		medical record. O.R. charge
		nurse, Margaret Little,
		notified. Also called Dr.
		Steven Adler's answering
		service. Message given to
		Operator 34. ————
		———— Susan Altman, RN

Preoperative surgical site identification

Patient safety To prevent wrong-site surgery and improve the overall safety of patients undergoing surgery, the Joint Commission on Accreditation of Healthcare Organizations launched the Universal Protocol for Preventing Wrong Site, Wrong Procedure, Wrong Person Surgery in 2004. This protocol encompasses three important steps:

- A preoperative verification process to ascertain that all important documents and tests are on hand before surgery and that these materials are evaluated and consistent with one another as well as with the patient's expectations and the surgical team's understanding of the patient, surgical procedure, surgical site, and any implants that may be used. All missing information and inconsistencies must be resolved before starting surgery.
- Marking the operative site by the surgeon performing the surgery and with the involvement of the awake and aware patient, if possible. The mark should be the surgeon's initials or YES.
- Taking a "time out" immediately before surgery is started, in the location where the surgery is to be performed, so that the entire surgical team can confirm the correct patient, surgical procedure, surgical site, patient position, and any implants or special equipment requirements.

Most facilities use a detailed checklist to ensure that all steps of the verification process have been completed. Each member of the intraoperative team should document the checks that they performed to ensure proper surgical site identification. All documentation on the checklist should include the date, time, and initials of the team member providing the check. When using initials on a checklist, be sure that you sign your full name and initials in the signature space provided. Any discrepancies in the verification process should be noted on the checklist with a description of actions taken to rectify the discrepancy. Include the names of any people notified and their actions. (See *Preoperative surgical identification checklist*.)

Preoperatively, document that you have identified the patient using two identifiers. Confirm that the patient understands the procedure and that he can correctly describe the surgery being performed and identify the sur-

PREOPERATIVE SURGICAL IDENTIFICATION CHECKLIST

If your facility requires a transfusion reaction report, you'll include the following types of information. A preoperative surgical identification checklist such as the one below is commonly used to ensure the safety of patients undergoing surgery.

PREOPERATIVE SURGICAL IDENTIFICATION CHECKLIST

Patient's name _Thomas Smith_   Date _1/6/07_   Time _1032_

Medical record number _123456_   Initials _MC_

	HEALTH TEAM MEMBER INITIALS	DATE	TIME
Preoperative verification			
Patient identified using two identifiers	MC	1/6/07	1032
Informed consent with surgical procedure and site (side/level) signed and in chart	MC	1/6/07	1045
History and physical complete and in chart	MC	1/6/07	1045
Laboratory studies reviewed and in chart	MC	1/6/07	1045
Radiology and ECG reports reviewed and in chart	MC	1/6/07	1045
Medications listed in chart	MC	1/6/07	1045
Patient/family member/guardian verbalizes surgical procedure and points to surgical site	MC	1/6/07	1055
Surgical site marked	HD	1/6/07	1100
Patient, surgery, and marked site verified by patient/ family/guardian	MC	1/6/07	1100
Surgical procedure and site, medical record, and tests are consistent	MC	1/6/07	1100
Proper equipment and implants available	MC	1/6/07	1100
Describe any discrepancies and actions taken:	N/A		
"Time out" verification			
Patient verification with two identifiers	BT	1/6/07	1135
Surgical site verified	BT	1/6/07	1135
Surgical procedure verified	BT	1/6/07	1135
Implants and equipment available	N/A		
Verbal verification of team obtained	BT	1/6/07	1135
Describe any discrepancies and actions taken:	N/A		

Signature _Mary Cooke, RN_ Initials _MC_   Signature _Beverly Thomas, RN_ Initials _BT_

Signature _Howard Dunn, MD_ Initials _HD_   Signature _____ Initials_____

gical site. Check that the consent form has been signed and that it includes the name of the surgery and the surgical site. The preoperative verification checklist also includes checking the medical record for the physical examination, medication record, laboratory studies, radiology and electrocardiogram (ECG) reports, and anesthesia and surgical records and confirmation that the medical record is consistent with the type of surgery planned and the identified surgical site.

In the intraoperative area, the checklist includes documenting that the patient was identified by staff as well as by the patient or his family. Documentation also includes confirmation of the surgical procedure by the staff as well as the patient or family member. The surgical site should be clearly marked and the patient or family member should verify that the marked surgical site is correct. Ideally, site marking should be completed by the surgeon performing the surgery. The checklist should also indicate that the medical record is consistent with the planned surgery and surgical site. The availability of implants and special equipment, if relevant, should also be noted.

Documentation of "time out" occurs in the operating room, before the surgical procedure starts, and includes verbal consensus by the entire surgical team of identification of the patient, surgical site, and surgical procedure and the availability of implants and special equipment, if needed. Document any discrepancies in verification during "time out" and interventions taken to correct the discrepancy.

Surgical incision care

In addition to documenting vital signs and level of consciousness (LOC) when the patient returns from surgery, pay particular attention to maintaining records pertaining to the surgical incision and drains and the care you provide. Document that you:

- reviewed the records that traveled with the patient from the postanesthesia care unit (See *Operating room and PACU records.*)
- looked for a practitioner's order directing whether you or the practitioner would perform the first dressing change.

When caring for a patient with a surgical wound, be sure to document:

- date, time, and type of wound care performed
- wound's appearance (size, condition of margins, necrotic tissue if any), odor (if any), location of any drains, and drainage characteristics (type, color, consistency, and amount)
- dressing information, such as the type and amount of new dressing or pouch applied

1/10/07	0830	Dressing removed from mid-line abd. incision; no drainage noted on dressing. Incision well approximated and intact with staples. Margins ecchymotic; dime-sized area of serosanguineous drainage noted from distal portion of wound. Dry 4" x 4" sterile gauze pad applied. JP drain in LLQ draining serosanguineous fluid. Emptied 40 ml. JP drain intact. Insertion site without redness or drainage. Split 4" x 4" gauze applied to site and taped securely. ——— Grace Fedor, RN

OPERATING ROOM AND PACU RECORDS

When your patient recovers sufficiently from the effects of anesthesia, he can be transferred from the operating room–postanesthesia care unit (OR–PACU) to his assigned unit for ongoing recovery and care. As the nurse, you should review the documentation records from the OR and PACU.

OR RECORD

The following information is recorded in the OR report:
■ procedure performed
■ type and dosage of anesthetics administered
■ length of time the patient was anesthetized
■ patient's vital signs throughout surgery
■ volume of fluid lost and replaced
■ drugs administered
■ surgical complications
■ tourniquet time
■ any drains, tubes, implants, or dressings used in surgery and removed or still in place.

POSTANESTHESIA RECORD

This record includes information about:
■ pain medications and pain control devices that the patient received and how he responded to them
■ patient's postanesthesia recovery scores on arrival and discharge in these areas: activity level, respiration, circulation, level of consciousness (LOC), and color (all recorded on a flow sheet)
■ unusual events or complications that occurred on the PACU—for instance, nausea or vomiting, shivering, hypothermia, arrhythmias, central anticholinergic syndrome, sore throat, back or neck pain, corneal abrasion, tooth loss during intubation, swollen lips or tongue, pharyngeal or laryngeal abrasion, and postspinal headache
■ interventions that should continue on the unit (For example, if the patient underwent leg surgery and had a tourniquet on for a long time, he'll need more frequent circulatory, motor, and neurologic checks. Additionally, if the anesthesiologist inserted an epidural catheter, the record should note any practitioner's orders regarding medication administration or special care procedures.)
■ patient's status at the time of transfer. (Information should include the patient's vital signs, LOC, and sensorium.)

● additional wound care procedures provided, such as drain management, irrigation, packing, or application of a topical medication
● special or detailed wound care instructions and pain management measures on the nursing care plan
● patient's tolerance of the procedure.

If the patient will need wound care after discharge, provide and document appropriate instruction. The record should show that you:
● explained aseptic technique

● described how to examine the wound for signs of infection and other complications
● demonstrated how to change the dressing
● provided written instructions for home care.

Pacemaker care

Caring for a patient undergoing pacemaker implantation requires detailed documentation practices. Be sure to document:
● type of pacemaker used
● date and time of pacemaker placement

- physician who inserted it
- reason for placement
- pacemaker settings
- patient's LOC and vital signs, noting which arm you used to obtain the blood pressure reading
- complications (such as infection, chest pain, pacemaker malfunction, or arrhythmias)
- interventions performed and their results (such as X-rays to verify correct electrode placement and information obtained from a 12-lead ECG.

Remember to obtain and include rhythm strips in the medical record at these times:
- before, during, and after pacemaker placement
- anytime pacemaker settings change
- anytime the patient receives treatment resulting from a pacemaker complication.

1/7/07	0800	Temporary transven-ous pacemaker in ℚ subclavian vein. Rate 70, mA2, mV full de-mand. 100% ventricular paced rhythm noted on monitor. ECG obtained. Pacer sensing & cap-turing correctly. Site w/o redness or swell-ing. Dressing dry & in-tact. — John Mora, RN

As ECG monitoring continues, document:
- capture
- sensing rate
- intrinsic beats
- competition of paced and intrinsic rhythms.

If the patient has a transcutaneous pacemaker, be sure to document:

- reason for this kind of pacing
- time pacing started
- locations of the electrodes.

Peritoneal dialysis

Peritoneal dialysis is indicated for patients with chronic renal failure who have cardiovascular instability, vascular access problems that prevent hemodialysis, fluid overload, and electrolyte imbalances. When caring for a patient receiving peritoneal dialysis, follow these documentation guidelines:
- During therapy, document the amount of dialysate infused and drained and any medications added.
- Monitor and document the patient's response to treatment before and after dialysis. Document his vital signs every 10 to 15 minutes for the first 1 to 2 hours of exchanges, then every 2 to 4 hours or as often as necessary.
- Document any abrupt changes in the patient's condition, making sure you notify the practitioner. Be sure to document your notification.
- Complete a peritoneal dialysis flowchart every 24 hours.
- Keep a record of the effluent's characteristics and the assessed negative or positive fluid balance at the end of each infusion-dwell-drain cycle.
- Document the patient's daily weight (immediately after the drain phase) and abdominal girth.
- Document the time of day and any variations in the weighing-measuring technique. Also document physical assessment findings and fluid status daily.

1/15/07	0700	Receiving exchanges q2hr
		of 1500 ml 4.25 % dialy-
		sate with 500 units hep-
		arin and 2 mEq KCL. Dialy-
		sate infused over 15 min.
		Dwell time 75 min. Drain
		time 30 min. Drainage clear,
		pale-yellow fluid. Weight
		235 lb, abdominal girth 40".
		Lungs clear, normal heart
		sounds, mucous membranes
		moist, good skin turgor.
		VSS (See flow sheets for
		fluid balance and frequent
		VS assessments.) Tolerating
		procedure. No c/o cramp-
		ing or discomfort. Skin
		warm, dry at RLQ catheter
		site, no redness or drain-
		age. Dry split 4" X 4" dress-
		ing applied after site
		cleaned per protocol. ——
		———— Liz Schaeffer, RN

- Document equipment problems, such as kinked tubing or mechanical malfunction, and your interventions.
- Document the condition of the patient's skin at the dialysis catheter site, the patient's reports of unusual discomfort or pain, and your interventions.

Peritoneal lavage

Used as a diagnostic procedure in a patient with blunt abdominal trauma, peritoneal lavage helps detect bleeding in the peritoneal cavity. When caring for a patient receiving peritoneal lavage, follow these documentation guidelines:

- During the procedure, frequently monitor and document the patient's vital signs, making sure you document signs or symptoms of shock (such as tachycardia, decreased blood pressure, diaphoresis, dyspnea, or vertigo).

- Keep a record of the incision site's condition.
- Document the type and size of peritoneal dialysis catheter used, the type and amount of solution instilled and withdrawn from the peritoneal cavity, and the amount and color of fluid returned.
- Document whether the fluid flowed freely into and out of the abdomen.
- Document the specimens that were obtained and sent to the laboratory.
- Document any complications that occurred and the nursing actions you took to manage them.

1/2/07	1500	NG tube inserted via Ⓛ
		nostril and connected to
		low continuous suction,
		draining small amount of
		greenish fluid, hematest
		negative #16 Fr. Foley
		catheter inserted to
		straight drainage. Drained
		200 ml clear amber
		urine, negative for blood.
		Dr. Fisher inserted #15
		peritoneal dialysis cathe-
		ter below umbilicus via
		trocar. Clear fluid with-
		drawn. 700 ml warm NSS
		instilled as ordered and
		clamped. Pt. turned from
		side to side. NSS dwell
		time of 10 min. NSS
		drained freely from
		abdomen. Fluid samples
		sent to lab, as ordered.
		Peritoneal catheter
		removed and incision
		closed by Dr. Fisher.
		4" X 4" gauze pad with
		povidone-iodine ointment
		applied to site. Tolerated
		procedure well. Prepro-
		cedure P 92, BP 110/64,
		RR 24. Postprocedure
		P 88, BP 116/66, RR 18.
		———— Angela Novack, RN

Suture removal

Although suture removal is primarily a practitioner's responsibility, this procedure may be delegated to a skilled nurse with a written medical order. When documenting this procedure, document:

- appearance of the suture line
- date and time the sutures were removed
- whether the wound site contained purulent drainage.

If you suspect infection at the site, document that you notified the practitioner and collected a specimen and sent it to the laboratory for analysis.

1/14/07	1030	Order obtained from
		MD to remove sutures
		from index finger. Su-
		ture line well approx-
		imated and healed. No
		drainage present upon
		assessment. Site clean
		and dry. No redness.
		Patient complaining of
		"a numb feeling" when
		the finger is touched.
		All three sutures re-
		moved without diffi-
		culty. Dry adhesive
		dressing applied to the
		finger.—Pauline Primas, RN

Thoracic drainage

A chest tube provides drainage of air or fluid from the pleural space. After chest tube insertion, the tube is connected to a thoracic drainage system that removes air, fluid, or both and prevents backflow into the pleural space, thus promoting lung expansion. When beginning thoracic drainage, be sure to document:

- date and time the procedure began
- type of system used
- amount of suction applied to the system
- initial presence or absence of bubbling or fluctuation in the water-seal chamber (Bubbling in the water-seal chamber may indicate an air leak.)
- initial amount and type of drainage
- patient's respiratory status.

When caring for the patient with a thoracic drainage setup, be sure to document:

- how frequently you inspected the drainage system
- presence or absence of bubbling or fluctuation in the water-seal chamber
- patient's respiratory status
- condition of the chest dressings
- name, amount, and route of any pain medication you gave
- complications that developed
- subsequent interventions that you performed.

When documenting ongoing care, following these guidelines:

- Be sure to keep a record of the time and date of each observation.
- Document the results of your respiratory assessments, including:
  - rate and quality of the patient's respirations
  - auscultation findings
  - each chest tube dressing change
  - findings related to the patient's skin condition at the chest tube site.
- Document the time and date when you notify the practitioner of serious patient conditions, such as cyanosis, rapid or shallow breathing, subcutaneous emphysema, chest pain, excessive bleeding.
- Keep a record of patient-teaching sessions and subsequent activities that the patient will perform, such as

coughing and deep-breathing exercises, sitting upright, and splinting the insertion site to minimize pain.

1/11/07	0900	① anterior chest tube
		intact to Pleur-evac
		suction system to 20 cm
		of suction. All connec-
		tions intact. 50 ml
		bright red bloody drain-
		age noted since 0800.
		No air leak noted +
		water chamber fluctu-
		ation. Chest tube site
		dressing dry and intact,
		no crepitus palpated.
		Lungs clear bilaterally.
		Chest expansion equal
		bilaterally. No SOB
		noted. RR 18-20 non-
		labored. O₂ @ 2 L/min
		via NC. ————
		———— Andrew Ortiz, RN

Cardiac monitoring

Cardiac monitoring uses electrodes placed on the patient's chest to transmit electrical signals that are converted into a tracing of cardiac rhythm on an oscilloscope. When caring for a patient undergoing cardiac monitoring, follow these documentation guidelines:
- In your notes, document the date and time that monitoring began and the monitoring leads used.
- Document rhythm strip readings to the record. Be sure to label the rhythm strip with:
  - patient's name
  - room number
  - date and time.
- Document any changes in the patient's condition.

1/8/07	0720	Placed on 5-lead
		electrode system. ECG
		strip shows NSR @ a rate
		of 80 ͡ occasional PACs.
		PR .16, QRS .08; 6-sec.
		episode of PAT – rate
		160 noted @ 0710.
		Dr. Durkin notified. Pt.
		asymptomatic. Peripheral
		pulses palpable; no edema
		noted. No murmurs,
		gallops or rubs. Denies
		chest pain/discomfort,
		SOB and palpitations. ——
		———— Diane Goldman, RN

- If cardiac monitoring will continue after the patient's discharge, document:
  - which caregivers can interpret dangerous rhythms and perform cardiopulmonary resuscitation
  - troubleshooting techniques to use if the monitor malfunctions
  - patient teaching and any referrals that were provided (such as to equipment suppliers).

Chest physiotherapy

Chest physiotherapy helps eliminate secretions, reexpand lung tissue, and promote efficient use of respiratory muscles. Whenever you perform chest physiotherapy, be sure to document:
- date and time of your interventions
- patient's positions for secretion drainage
- length of time the patient remains in each position
- chest segments percussed or vibrated

- characteristics of the secretion expelled (including color, amount, odor, viscosity, and the presence of blood)
- complications and subsequent interventions
- patient's tolerance of the treatment.

1/7/07	1415	Placed on ① side c̄ foot
		of bed elevated. Chest
		PT and postural drain-
		age performed for
		10 min. from lower to
		middle then upper
		lobes, as ordered. Pro-
		ductive cough and
		expelled large amt. of
		thick yellow sputum.
		Lungs clear p̄ chest PT.
		Procedure tolerated
		w/o difficulty. ————
		———— Jane Goddard, RN

Mechanical ventilation

Mechanical ventilation moves air in and out of the patient's lungs using ventilators that may use either positive or negative pressure. Whenever your patient is receiving mechanical ventilation, be sure to document:
- date and time that mechanical ventilation began
- type of ventilator
- ventilator settings
- patient's subjective and objective responses, including vital signs, breath sounds, use of accessory muscles, comfort level, and physical appearance
- complications and subsequent interventions
- pertinent laboratory data, including results of any arterial blood gas (ABG) analyses and oxygen saturation findings.

1/16/07	1015	Ventilator set at TV
		750; FIO₂, 45%; 5 cm
		PEEP; AC of 12. RR 20
		nonlabored. #8 ETT
		in ® corner of mouth,
		taped securely at
		22-cm mark. Suctioned
		via ETT for large amt.
		of thick white secre-
		tions. Pulse oximeter
		reading 98%. ① lung
		clear. ® lung with
		basilar crackles and
		expiratory wheezes. No
		SOB noted. ————
		— Janice Del Vecchio, RN

If the patient is receiving pressure support ventilation or using a T-piece or tracheostomy collar, be sure to document:
- duration of spontaneous breathing
- patient's ability to maintain the weaning schedule.

If the patient is receiving intermittent mandatory ventilation, with or without pressure-support ventilation, be sure to document:
- control breath rate
- time of each breath reduction
- rate of spontaneous respirations.

Throughout mechanical ventilation, follow these guidelines:
- Document any adjustments made in ventilator settings as a result of ABG levels, and document any adjustments of ventilator components.
- Document interventions implemented to promote mobility, to protect skin integrity, or to enhance ventilation. For example, document:

- when and how you perform active or passive range-of-motion exercises with the patient
- when you turn the patient or position him upright for lung expansion
- tracheal suctioning and the character of secretions.

● Document assessment findings related to peripheral circulation, urine output, decreased cardiac output, fluid volume excess, dehydration, and sleep and wake periods.

● Document patient teaching—which may involve the patient and his appropriate caregivers—that you carried out in preparation for the patient's discharge. Take special care to document teaching associated with:
- ventilator care and settings
- artificial airway care
- communication
- nutrition and exercise
- signs and symptoms of infection
- equipment functioning
- any referrals made to equipment vendors, home health agencies, and other community resources.

NG tube insertion and removal

An NG tube has many diagnostic and therapeutic uses but is usually inserted to decompress the patient's stomach and prevent vomiting after surgery. When you perform NG tube insertion, document:
● type and size of NG tube inserted
● date, time, and route of insertion
● reason for the insertion
● confirmation of proper placement
● type and amount of suction (if used)

● drainage characteristics, such as amount, color, consistency, and odor
● patient's tolerance of the insertion procedure
● when the NG tube was irrigated and the amount of solution used
● signs and symptoms signaling complications, such as nausea, vomiting, and abdominal distention
● subsequent irrigation procedures and continuing problems after irrigation.

1/15/07	1605	# 12 Fr. NG tube placed in Ⓛ nostril. Placement verified by grassy-green aspirate appearance and pH of 5.0. Attached to low intermittent suction as ordered. Drainage pale green; heme −. Irrigated with 30 ml NSS q 2 hr. Tolerated procedure. Hypoactive B.S. in all 4 quadrants. ———————— Vijay Rao, RN

For NG tube clamping or removal, be sure to document:
● date and time of the procedure
● patient's tolerance of the procedure
● unusual events accompanying the clamping or removal, such as nausea, vomiting, abdominal distention, and food intolerance.

Seizure management

When caring for a patient with seizure disorder, it's important to document in his medical record that he requires seizure precautions and what precau-

tions have been taken. Also be sure to document:

- date and time that a seizure began
- seizure's duration
- precipitating factors
- sensations that may be considered auras
- involuntary behavior occurring at onset, such as lip smacking, chewing movements, or hand and eye movements
- incontinence occurring during the seizure
- interventions performed, including medications that were administered
- complications
- assessment of the patient's postictal mental and physical status.

1/9/07	0830	At 1615 Pt. observed
		with generalized seizure
		activity lasting 2 1/2 min.
		Sleeping at time of
		onset. Urinary inconti-
		nence during seizure.
		Seizure pads in place
		on bed before seizure.
		Placed on ① side, air-
		way patent, no N/V.
		Dr. Gordon notified of
		seizure. Diazepam 10 mg
		given I.V. as ordered.
		VS taken q 15 min. and
		p.r.n. (see flow sheet).
		Currently obtunded
		(see neurologic flow
		sheet). No further
		seizure activity noted.
		—— Gale Hartman, RN

Tube feedings

In addition to frequently assessing and documenting the patient's tolerance of the procedure and the feeding formula, keep careful documentation of:

- tube placement verification
- kind of tube feeding the patient is receiving (for example, duodenal or jejunal feedings or continuous drip or bolus)
- amount, rate, route, and method of feeding
- dilution strength (for example, half- or three-quarters strength)
- time and the flushing solution (such as water or cranberry juice) to maintain patency
- intake amounts of feeding and flushing on intake and output records
- replacement of the feeding tube.

Also regularly assess and document:

- patient's gastric function
- prescribed medications or treatments to relieve constipation or diarrhea
- infusion rate when administering continuous feedings
- residual contents and amount when administering bolus feedings
- placement and patency of the tube prior to feeding when administering bolus feedings
- laboratory test findings, including the patient's urine and serum glucose, serum electrolyte, and blood urea nitrogen levels as well as serum osmolality
- feeding complications, such as hyperglycemia, glycosuria, and diarrhea.

If the patient will continue receiving tube feedings after discharge, be sure to document:

- instructions you give to the patient and his family
- referrals you make to suppliers or support agencies.

1/25/07	0700	Full-strength Pulmo-
		care infusing via Flexi-
		flow pump thru Dob-
		hoff tube in ® nostril
		at 50 ml/hr. Tube
		placement verified by
		grassy-green aspirate
		appearance and pH of
		5.0. Pt. maintained with
		HOB raised about 45°.
		5 ml residual obtained.
		Pt. denies any N/V.
		Normal active bowel
		sounds auscultated x 4
		quad. Diphenoxylate
		elixir 2.5 mg given via
		f.t. for continuous
		diarrhea. Tube flushed
		with 30 ml H₂O this
		shift as ordered. Pt.
		instructed to tell
		nurse of discomfort.
		—— Sandra Mann, RN

- length of time pressure was applied to the site to control bleeding
- type and amount of oxygen therapy that the patient was receiving, if appropriate.

1/12/07	1010	Blood drawn from ®
		radial artery p̄ + Allen's
		test c̄ brisk capillary
		refill. Pressure applied
		to site for 5 min. and
		pressure drsg. applied.
		No bleeding, hematoma,
		or swelling noted. Hand
		pink, warm c̄ 2-sec.
		capillary refill. Dr. Smith
		notified of ABG results.
		O₂ increased to 40%
		nonrebreather mask at
		0845. Pt. in no resp. dis-
		tress. — Pat Toricelli, RN

Withdrawal of arterial blood

ABG analysis evaluates lung ventilation by measuring arterial blood pH and partial pressure of arterial oxygen (PaO2) and carbon dioxide. When you must obtain blood for ABG analysis, keep careful documentation of:

- patient's vital signs and temperature
- arterial puncture site
- results of Allen's test
- indications of circulatory impairment, such as:
  – bleeding at the puncture site and swelling
  – discoloration
  – pain
  – numbness or tingling in the bandaged arm or leg.

When obtaining an ABG analysis, be sure to document:

- time that the blood sample was drawn

When filling out a laboratory request for ABG analysis, which is a computerized order in many facilities, be sure to include:

- patient's temperature and respiratory rate
- most recent hemoglobin level
- tidal volume and control rate, if he's on mechanical ventilation
- fraction of inspired oxygen.

ASSISTIVE PROCEDURES

When you assist a practitioner in such procedures as bone marrow aspiration, insertion or removal of arterial or central venous (CV) lines, lumbar puncture, paracentesis, or thoracentesis, your role also involves patient support, patient teaching, and evaluation of the patient's response. Careful documentation of these procedures is your responsibility. Make sure that you document:

- name of the practitioner performing the procedure
- equipment used
- patient's response to the procedure
- patient teaching provided
- other pertinent information.

Bone marrow aspiration

When assisting the physician with a bone marrow aspiration, document:
- time and date of the procedure
- name of the physician performing the procedure
- appearance of the specimen aspirated
- patient's response to the procedure
- appearance of the aspiration site
- patient's vital signs after the procedure
- signs of bleeding from the aspiration site
- pertinent information about the specimen sent to the laboratory.

1/3/07	1000	Assisted Dr. Shelbourne
		while he performed a
		bone marrow aspiration
		at 0915. The procedure
		was performed on the
		Ⓡ anterior iliac crest.
		Pt. tolerated the pro-
		cedure well with little
		discomfort. Specimens
		sent to lab, as ordered.
		No bleeding at site. VS:
		BP 142/82; P 88; RR 22.
		Pt. afebrile. Bed rest
		being maintained. ————
		——— Margaret Little, RN

Insertion and removal of an arterial line

When assisting with the insertion of an arterial line, document:
- time and date of the procedure

- name of the practitioner performing the procedure
- insertion site
- type, gauge, and length of the catheter
- whether the catheter is sutured in place.

When assisting with the removal of an arterial line, document:
- time and date of the procedure
- name of the practitioner performing the procedure
- length of the catheter
- length of time pressure was applied to the insertion site
- condition of the insertion site
- whether catheter specimens were obtained for culture.

1/5/07	0625	#20G arterial catheter
		placed in Ⓡ radial artery
		by anesthes. Dr. Mayer on
		2nd attempt after +
		Allen's test. Transducer
		leveled and zeroed.
		Readings accurate to
		cuff pressures. Site w/o
		redness or swelling. 4" x
		4" gauze pad c̄ povidone-
		iodine ointment applied.
		Ⓡ hand and wrist taped
		and secured to arm
		board. Line flushes easily.
		Good waveform on
		monitor. Hand pink and
		warm c̄ 2-sec. capillary
		refill. ——— Lisa Chang, RN

Insertion and removal of a CV line

Typically, when you assist the practitioner who's inserting a CV line, you'll need to document:
- time and date of the insertion
- name of the practitioner performing the procedure

- type, length, and location of the catheter
- solution infused
- patient's response to the procedure
- time of the X-ray performed to confirm the line's safe and correct placement
- X-ray results, along with your notification of the practitioner of the results.

After assisting with a CV line's removal, document:
- time and date of the removal
- name of the practitioner performing the procedure
- type of dressing applied
- length of the catheter
- condition of the insertion site
- collection of any catheter specimens for culture or other analysis.

1/3/07	1000	Procedure explained to
		pt. and consent obtained by Dr. Chavez.
		Placed in Trendelenburg position and
		triple-lumen catheter
		placed by Dr. Chavez on
		1st attempt in Ⓡ subclavian. Catheter sutured in place c̄ 3-0
		silk and sterile dressing
		applied per protocol.
		All lines flushed c̄ 100
		units heparin and
		portable chest X-ray
		obtained to confirm
		line placement. VSS. Pt.
		tolerated procedure
		well.— Louise Flynn, RN

Lumbar puncture

During lumbar puncture, observe the patient closely for such complications as a change in LOC, dizziness, and changes in vital signs. Report these observations to the physician, and document them carefully. Documentation should also include:
- date and the start and stop times of the procedure
- name of the physician performing the procedure
- number of test tube specimens of cerebrospinal fluid (CSF) obtained
- patient's tolerance of the procedure
- pertinent information about the specimens.

Make sure you also document your postprocedure interventions, which should include:
- monitoring the patient's condition
- assessing the patient for headache
- checking the puncture site for CSF leakage
- encouraging fluid intake
- keeping the patient in a flat supine position for 6 to 12 hours.

1/8/07	0900	Procedure explained to
		patient. Positioned, side
		lying for lumbar puncture.
		Procedure began at 0900
		and ended at 0935.
		Draped and prepped by
		Dr. Marshall. Specimen
		obtained on 1st attempt by
		Dr Marshall. Clear, straw-colored CSF noted. Tolerated procedure without
		difficulty. Vitals signs
		stable during procedure.
		Maintained in supine
		position as instructed. Due
		to flat positioning, and
		NPO status, NSS infusion
		started at 100 ml/hr.
		Puncture site dressed by
		Dr. Marshall. Site clean
		dry and intact. No leakage.
		Pt. without complaints of
		headache or dizziness. —
		— Jeanette Kane, RN

Paracentesis

When caring for a patient during and after paracentesis, be sure to document:
- date and time of the procedure
- name of the physician performing the procedure
- puncture site
- amount, color, viscosity, and odor of the initially aspirated fluid (both in your notes and in the intake and output record)
- total volume of fluid removed
- number of fluid specimens sent to the laboratory for analysis.

If you're responsible for ongoing patient care, be sure to document:
- a running record of the patient's vital signs
- nursing activities related to drainage and to dressing changes
- frequency of drainage checks (typically, every 15 minutes for the first hour, every 30 minutes for the next 2 hours, every hour for the next 4 hours, then every 4 hours for the next 24 hours)
- patient's response to the procedure
- drainage characteristics, including color, amount, odor, and viscosity
- daily patient weight
- abdominal girth measurements before and after the procedure.

If peritoneal fluid leakage occurs, notify the practitioner and document the time and date of your notification.

1/12/07	1100	After procedure ex-
		plained to pt. and con-
		sent obtained, Dr. Novello
		performed paracentesis
		in RLQ as per protocol.
		1,500 ml cloudy, pale-
		yellow fluid drained and
		sent to lab as ordered.
		Site sutured with one
		3-0 silk suture. Sterile
		4" x 4" gauze pad applied.
		No leakage noted at site.
		Abd. girth 44" prepro-
		cedure and $42^{3}/_{4}$" post-
		procedure. Pt. tolerated
		procedure w/o difficulty.
		VSS before and after
		procedure stable (see
		flow sheet). Emotional
		support given to pt. ———
		——— Carol Barsky, RN

Thoracentesis

When assisting with thoracentesis, assess the patient for any sudden or unusual pain, faintness, dizziness, or vital sign changes. Report these observations to the physician immediately, and document them as soon as possible. Also document:
- time and date of the procedure
- name of the physician performing the procedure
- amount and quality of fluid aspirated
- fluid specimens sent to the laboratory for analysis
- patient's response to the procedure.

If later symptoms of pneumothorax, hemothorax, subcutaneous emphysema, or infection occur, notify the practitioner immediately and document your observations and interventions on the chart.

1/10/07	1100	Procedure explained to
		patient and consent
		obtained by Dr. McCall.
		Positioned over secured
		bedside table. RLL thora-
		centesis performed by
		Dr. Garret without
		incident. Sterile 4" x 4"
		dressing applied to site.
		Site clean and dry, no
		redness or drainage
		present. 900 ml of
		blood-tinged serosan-
		guineous fluid aspirated.
		Specimen sent to lab
		as ordered. Vital signs
		stable. Denies SOB or
		dyspnea. Bilateral breath
		sounds auscultated. Chest
		X-ray results pending. —
		———— Ellen Pritchett, RN

INFECTION CONTROL

Meticulous record keeping is an important contributor to effective infection control. Various federal agencies require documentation of infections so that the data can be assessed and used to help prevent and control future infections. Typically, you must report to your facility's infection control department any culture result that shows a positive infection and any surgery, medication, elevated temperature, X-ray finding, or specific treatment related to infection. (See *Reportable diseases and infections,* page 34.)

If you suspect infection, document:
● to whom you reported the signs and symptoms of suspected infection
● instructions received
● treatments initiated
● that standard precautions were followed for direct contact with blood and body fluids—and that teaching was done with the patient and his family about these precautions
● dates and times of your interventions in the patient's chart and on the MAR
● any breach in an isolation technique, making sure you also file an incident report
● medications prescribed to treat the infection as well as the date and time initiated.

Be sure to communicate the results of any culture and sensitivity studies to the practitioner so that he can prescribe the appropriate medication to treat the infection. Also inform the infection control practitioner. Record the patient's response to this medication.

1/8/07	1300	Wound and skin pre-
		cautions maintained.
		Temperature remains
		elevated at 102.3° R.
		Amount of purulent
		drainage from the
		incision has increased
		since yesterday. Dr.
		Levick notified. Repeat
		C&S ordered. Specimen
		obtained and sent to
		the lab. ————
		———— Lynne Kasoff, RN

DIAGNOSTIC TESTS

Before receiving a diagnosis, most patients undergo testing, which can range from a simple blood test to a more complicated magnetic resonance imaging scan. When preparing a patient for diagnostic testing, follow these guidelines:

REPORTABLE DISEASES AND INFECTIONS

The Centers for Disease Control and Prevention (CDC), the Occupational Safety and Health Administration, the Joint Commission on Accreditation of Healthcare Organizations, and the American Hospital Association all require health care facilities to document and report certain diseases acquired in the community or in hospitals and other health care facilities.

Generally, the health care facility reports diseases to the appropriate local authorities. These authorities notify the state health department, which in turn reports the diseases to the appropriate federal agency or national organization.

The list of diseases that appears below is the CDC's list of nationally notifiable infectious diseases. Each state also keeps a list of reportable diseases appropriate to the region.

- Acquired immunodeficiency syndrome (AIDS)
- Anthrax
- Botulism (food-borne, infant, other [wound and unspecified])
- Brucellosis
- Chancroid
- *Chlamydia trachomatis*, genital infections
- Cholera
- Coccidioidomycosis
- Cryptosporidiosis
- Cyclosporiasis
- Diphtheria
- Ehrlichiosis (human granulocytic, human monocytic, human [other or unspecified agent])
- Encephalitis/meningitis: Arboviral California serogroup viral, eastern equine, Powassan, St. Louis, Western equine, West Nile
- Enterohemorrhagic *Escherichia coli* (O157:H7, shiga toxin positive [serogroup non-O157], shiga toxin positive [not sero-grouped])
- Giardiasis
- Gonorrhea
- *Haemophilus influenzae*, invasive disease
- Hansen disease (leprosy)
- *Hantavirus* pulmonary syndrome
- Hemolytic uremic syndrome, post-diarrheal
- Hepatitis, viral, acute (hepatitis A acute, hepatitis B acute, hepatitis B virus perinatal infection, hepatitis C acute)
- Hepatitis, viral, chronic (chronic hepatitis B, hepatitis C virus infection [past or present])
- Human immunodeficiency virus (adult [≥ 13 years], pediatric [< 13 years])
- Influenza-associated pediatric mortality
- *Legionella* infections (legionnaires' disease)
- Listeriosis

- Lyme disease
- Malaria
- Measles
- Meningococcal disease
- Mumps
- Pertussis
- Plague
- Poliomyelitis (paralytic)
- Psittacosis
- Q fever
- Rabies (animal, human)
- Rocky Mountain spotted fever
- Rubella (German measles) and congenital syndrome
- Salmonellosis
- Severe acute respiratory syndrome
- Shigellosis
- Smallpox
- Streptococcal disease, invasive, Group A
- Streptococcal toxic shock syndrome
- Streptococcus pneumoniae, drug resistant, invasive disease
- Streptococcus pneumoniae, invasive, in children < 5 years
- Syphilis (primary, secondary, latent, early latent, late latent, latent unknown duration, neurosyphilis, late non-neurologic)
- Syphilis, congenital (syphilitic stillbirth)
- Tetanus
- Toxic shock syndrome
- Trichinosis
- Tuberculosis
- Tularemia
- Typhoid fever
- Vancomycin intermediate *Staphylococcus aureus* (VISA)
- Vancomycin-resistant *Staphylococcus aureus* (VRSA)
- Varicella (morbidity)
- Varicella (deaths only)
- Yellow fever

- Begin your documentation by documenting any preliminary assessments you make of a patient's condition. (For example, if your patient is pregnant or has certain allergies, document this information because it might affect the test or the test result.)
- If the patient's age, illness, or disability requires special preparation for the test, document this information in his chart as well.
- Document patient compliance with other important factors that can affect diagnostic testing, such as follow-up care, the administration or withholding of medications and preparations, special diets, enemas, and specimen collection, as appropriate.

1/8/07	0700	24-hour urine test
		for creatinine clear-
		ance started. Pt. taught
		purpose of this test
		and how to collect
		urine. Sign placed on
		pt.'s door and in bath-
		room. Urine placed on
		ice in bathroom. ———
		——— Paul Steadman, RN

PAIN CONTROL

One of your main responsibilities to your patient is pain management. Determining pain's severity can be difficult, however, because pain is subjective. A number of tools can be used to assess pain; when you use them, always document the results. (See *Assessing and documenting pain,* page 36.)

When charting pain levels and characteristics, document:
- where the patient feels the pain
- whether it's internal, external, localized, or diffuse

- whether the pain interferes with the patient's sleep or other activities of daily living
- what the pain feels like in the patient's own words
- patient's pain rating using your facility's pain rating scale
- your observations of the patient's body language and behaviors, including whether the patient winces or grimaces, squirms in bed, and reacts to position changes or other measures (heat, cold massage, medications) that relieve or worsen the pain
- interventions you take to alleviate your patient's pain and the patient's response.

1/9/07	1600	Admitted to room 304
		with diagnosis of pan-
		creatic cancer. States
		he is having LLQ pain
		at 7 on a 0 to 10
		rating scale. Taking
		Percocet 2 tabs q 4 hr.
		at home without relief
		at present. Dr. Martin
		notified. Dilaudid 2 mg
		ordered and given I.V.
		@ 1600 VS stable. Rest-
		ing at present. ———
		——— K. Comerford, RN

Patient-controlled analgesia

Patient-controlled analgesia (PCA) allows patients to self-administer boluses of an opioid analgesic I.V. within limits prescribed by the practitioner, avoids overmedication with an adjustable lockout interval inhibiting delivery of additional boluses until the appropriate time has elapsed, increases the patient's sense of control and helps reduce anxiety, reduces medication use over the postoperative course, and gives enhanced pain con-

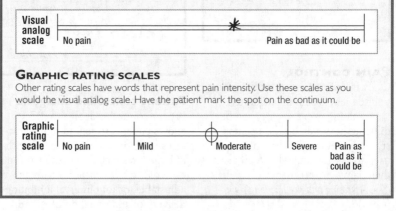

ASSESSING AND DOCUMENTING PAIN

Pain measurement tools, such as the pain flow sheet or the visual and graphic rating scales that appear below, provide a solid foundation for your nursing diagnoses and care plans. Whichever pain assessment tool you choose, remember to document its use and include the graphic record in your patient's chart.

PAIN FLOW SHEET

Possibly the most convenient tool for pain assessment, a flow sheet provides a standard for reevaluating the patient's pain at ongoing and regular intervals.

If possible, incorporate pain assessment into the flow sheet you're already using. Generally, the easier the flow sheet is to use, the more likely you and your patient will be to use it.

			Pain flow sheet		
Date and time	Pain rating (0 to 10)	Patient behaviors	Vital signs	Pain rating after intervention	Comments
1/16/07 0800	7	Wincing, holding head	186/88 98–22	5	Dilaudid 2 mg I.M. given in R glut.
1/16/07 1200	3	Relaxing, reading	160/80 84–18	2	Tylox ⊤ P.O. given

VISUAL ANALOG PAIN SCALE

In a visual analog pain scale, the patient marks a linear scale containing words or numbers that correspond to his perceived degree of pain. Draw a scale to represent a continuum of pain intensity. Verbal anchors describe the pain's intensity; for example, "no pain" begins the scale and "pain as bad as it could be" ends it. Ask the patient to mark the point on the continuum that best describes his pain.

Visual analog scale	No pain ⎯⎯⎯⎯⎯⎯⎯⎯⎯⎯⎯⎯⎯⎯⎯⎯⎯⎯⎯✳⎯⎯⎯ Pain as bad as it could be

GRAPHIC RATING SCALES

Other rating scales have words that represent pain intensity. Use these scales as you would the visual analog scale. Have the patient mark the spot on the continuum.

Graphic rating scale	No pain ⎯⎯⎯⎯ Mild ⎯⎯⎯⎯⊕ Moderate ⎯⎯⎯⎯ Severe ⎯⎯ Pain as bad as it could be

trol. When caring for a patient receiving PCA, use a PCA flow sheet to document:

- amount of medication used during your shift
- patient's response to the treatment
- patient teaching provided. (See *PCA flow sheet,* pages 38 and 39.)

CODES

If a code is called, American Heart Association guidelines direct you to

keep a written, chronological account of a patient's condition throughout resuscitative efforts. (See *Keeping a resuscitation record,* pages 40 and 41.) Two forms are particularly useful in accomplishing this:

● A *code record* is a form that incorporates detailed information about the code, including observations, interventions and any medications given to the patient.

● Some health care facilities use a *resuscitation critique form* to identify actual or potential problems with the resuscitation process. This form tracks personnel responses and response times as well as the availability of appropriate medications and functioning equipment.

1/4/07	2100	Summoned to the pt.'s room @ 2020 by a shout from roommate. Found pt. unresponsive without respirations or pulse. Roommate stated, "He was talking to me; then all of a sudden he started gasping and holding his chest." Code called. Initiated CPR with Ann Barrow, RN. Code team arrived @ 2023 and continued resuscitative efforts. (See code record.) Pt. groaned and opened eyes @ approx. 2030 (see neurologic flow sheet). Notified Dr. Cooper @ 2040 and explained situation— will be in immediately. Transferred to ICU @ 2035. Family notified of pt.'s condition and transfer. ——— Delia Landers, RN

CHANGE IN PATIENT'S CONDITION

One of your major documentation responsibilities is documenting any change in a patient's condition. Your documentation should include:
● patient's complaint
● your assessment
● interventions you performed
● name of personnel you notified
● what you reported
● what instructions you received.

Alert *When documenting your observations, avoid using vague words such as "appears." For example, instead of merely writing "stools appear bloody," describe the stool's characteristics, such as color, amount, frequency, and consistency.*

1/8/07	1500	Had moderate sized, soft, dark brown stools positive for blood c̄ a guaiac test. ——— Jackie Paterno, RN.

INTAKE AND OUTPUT MONITORING

Many patients require 24-hour intake and output monitoring, including surgical patients, patients on I.V. therapy, patients with fluid and electrolyte imbalances, and patients with burns, hemorrhage, and edema. When monitoring a patient's intake and output, follow these guidelines:

● If possible, keep intake and output sheets at the patient's bedside or by the bathroom door to remind you of this duty.

● Remember to include incontinent amounts; tube drainage; irrigation volumes, especially if not withdrawn; foods, such as gelatin and other liquids; I.V. piggyback infusions; med-

(Text continues on page 42.)

PCA FLOW SHEET

The form shown below is used to document the use of patient-controlled analgesia (PCA). PCA allows the patient to self-administer an opioid analgesic as needed yet within limits prescribed by the practitioner.

Date _____ 1/2/07 _____

Medication _____ Morphine 30 mg in 30 cc (1 mg/ml) _____

		0700 – 1500		
Time (enter in box)	1200	1400		
New cartridge inserted	JG			
PCA settings Lockout interval _7_ (minutes)		7		
Dose volume _1_ (ml/dose)				
Four-hour limit 30				
Continuous settings _1_ (mg/hr)				
Respiratory rate	18	20		
Blood pressure	150/70	130/62		
Sedation rating 1. Wide awake 2. Drowsy 3. Dozing, intermittent 4. Mostly sleeping 5. Only awakens when stimulated	1	2		
Analgesia rating (0–10) Minimal Pain – 0 Maximum Pain – 10	7	8		
Additional doses given (optional doses)	3 ml/JG			
Total ml delivered (total from ampule)	3	6		
ml remaining	27	24		

RN SIGNATURE	(0700–1500)	*Janet Green, RN*
RN SIGNATURE	(1500–2300)	*Karen Singleton, RN*
RN SIGNATURE	(2300–0700)	

	1500 – 2300				2300 – 0700			
1600								
7								
20								
128/70								
3								
6								
15								
15								

	Date	1/2/01	
	Date	1/2/07	
	Date		

KEEPING A RESUSCITATION RECORD

Here's an example of the completed resuscitation record for inclusion in the patient's chart.

CODE RECORD

Arrest Date: _1/9/07_
Arrest Time: _0630_
Rm/Location: _431-2_
Discovered by:
C. Brown
☑ RN ☐ MD
☐ Other

Methods of alert:
☑ Witnessed, monitored: rhythm
  V fib
☐ Witnessed, unmonitored
☐ Unwitnessed, unmonitored
☐ Unwitnessed, monitored; rhythm
  _____
Diagnosis: _Post anterior wall MI_

Condition when needed:
☑ Unresponsive
☐ Apneic
☐ Pulseless
☐ Hemorrhage
☐ Seizure

CPR PROGRESS NOTES

| | | | VITAL SIGNS | | | | I.V. PUSH | | | | |
Time	Pulse CPR	Resp. rate Spont; bag	Blood pressure	Rhythm	Defib (joules)	Atropine	Epinephrine	Lidocaine	NA bicarb		
0631	CPR	Bag	0	V fib	360						
0633	CPR	Bag	0	V fib	360		1 mg				
0634	40	Bag	60 palp	SB PVCs							
0645	60	Bag	80/40	SB PVCs							

| Time Spec Sent | ABGs & Lab Data | | | | | | |
	pH	PCO	Po$_2$	HCO$_3$	Sat%	Fio$_2$	Other
0633	7.1	76	43	14	80%		

Ventilation management:

Time: ___0635___

Method: ___oral ET tube___

Precordial thump:
___0631___

CPR initiated at:
___0631___

Previous airway:
- [ ] ET tube
- [ ] Trach
- [x] Natural

Addressograph

INFUSIONS				ACTIONS/PATIENT RESPONSE
Lidocaine	Procainamide	Isuprel	Dopamine	Responses to therapy, procedures, labs drawn/results
				ABGs drawn. ℞ fem pressure applied.
				Oral intubation by Dr. Hart
				ICU ready for patient

Resuscitation outcome

- [x] Successful [x] Transferred to ___CCU___ ___0648___
- [ ] Unsuccessful — Expired at _____ Pronounced by: _____ MD

Family notified by: ___S. Quinn, RN___ Time: ___0645___

Attending notified by: ___S. Quinn, RN___ Time ___0645___

Code Recorder ___S. Quinn, RN___

Code Team Nurse ___B. Mullen, RN___

Anesthesia Rep. ___J. Hanna, RN___

Other Personnel ___J. Hart, MD___
___B. Russo, RT___

ications given by I.V. push; PCA medication amounts; and fluids given to the patient orally or I.V. while he's in another unit.

- To simplify intake documentation:
  - document the volumes of specific containers
  - document amounts from infusion devices, such as enteral and I.V. intake, for accuracy
  - enlist the cooperation of the patient and his family members, who may bring him snacks and soft drinks or help him to eat.
- To simplify output documentation:
  - enlist the cooperation of staff members in other departments to report the patient's output while he's away from the unit
  - remind the patient to use a urinal or a commode if he's ambulatory
  - include drainage from suction devices and wound drains
  - document bleeding and other measurable sources of fluid loss
  - document vomitus amounts
  - count excessive or watery stools as output. (The amount of fluid lost through the GI tract is normally 100 ml or less daily. However, if the patient's stools become excessive or watery, they must be counted as output.) (See *Charting intake and output,* pages 44 and 45.)

SKIN AND WOUND CARE
The skin is the largest organ. Along with the hair, nails, and glands, it protects the body from microorganisms, ultraviolet light radiation, fluid loss, and the stress of mechanical forces. When serious wounds, such as pressure ulcers, fail to heal quickly and require long-term care and special

assessments, careful documentation is essential.

Pressure ulcers
The National Pressure Ulcer Advisory Panel defines a pressure ulcer as "any lesion caused by unrelieved pressure resulting in damage to underlying tissue." Because many patients are liable to develop pressure ulcers, always document findings related to the patient's skin condition. Follow these guidelines:

- Clearly document in the record whether the patient had the pressure ulcer upon admission or whether the ulcer developed in the health care facility. Failure to document an existing wound on admission can result in legal action.
- When a chronically ill or immobile patient enters your unit with a pressure ulcer, document the location, appearance, size, depth, color, and the appearance of exudate from that ulcer.

1/10/07	1400	Admitted by stretcher to room 418B. Lethargic, skin dry. Incontinent of urine. 1" wide black pressure ulcer noted on ℞ heel. Purulent, yellow drainage noted on ulcer's dressing. Dr. Kelly notified. Surgical consult ordered for debridement of ulcer. ℞ foot elevated on 2 pillows. Heel and elbow protectors applied. Skin lotion applied. Incontinent care given hourly. No other skin breakdown noted. Buttocks reddened but epidermis intact. ———— Rachel Moreau, RN

- Use flow sheets that have defined cues to make your documentation easier. However, even if you use a flow sheet, write a note in the medical record if and when you notify a practitioner about changes in the wound or surrounding tissue.
- Watch for and document the development of risk factors for pressure ulcers, such as obesity, poor nutritional status, decreased hemoglobin level, immobility, infection, incontinence, and fractures. If the patient's skin condition worsens during hospitalization, his stay may be extended, and you'll need a clear record of skin care and related factors.
- If your health care facility requires you to photograph pressure ulcers found at the time of admission, always date the photographs. You can then evaluate changes in a patient's skin condition by comparing his current skin integrity with previous photographs.

Wound care

Wound assessment and care has changed dramatically in the past several years and is continually evolving. However, one factor that hasn't changed is the need for good documentation. When documenting a wound assessment, be sure to include:
- wound size (including length, width, and depth in centimeters), shape, and stage
- wound site, drawn on a body plan to document the exact location
- characteristics of drainage, if any, including amount, color, and presence of odor
- characteristics of the wound bed, including description of tissue type, such as granulation tissue, slough, or epithelial tissue, and the percentage of each tissue type
- character of the surrounding tissue
- presence or absence of eschar, pain, or undermining or tunneling (in centimeters).

| 1/10/07 | 1400 | Admitted to unit for fem-pop bypass tomorrow. Has an open wound at tip of 2nd Ⓛ toe, approx. 0.5 cm X 1 cm X 0.5 cm deep. Wound is round with even edges. Wound bed is pale with little granulation tissue. No drainage, odor, eschar, or tunneling noted. Pt. reports pain at wound site, rates pain as 4/10, on 0-to-10 scale. Surrounding skin cool to touch, pale, and intact. Verbalizes understanding not to cross legs or wear tight garments. ——————— Mark Silver, RN |

Many facilities also have a special form or flow sheet on which to document wounds. (See *Wound care and skin assessment tool,* pages 46 and 47.)

PERSONAL PROPERTY

Encourage patients to send home their money, jewelry, and other valuable belongings. If a patient refuses to do so, make a list of his possessions and store them according to your facility's policy using the following guidelines:
- The list of the patient's valuables should include a description of each item and a signature from the patient or a responsible family member. (This

(Text continues on page 47.)

CHARTING INTAKE AND OUTPUT

As this sample shows, you can monitor your patient's fluid balance by using an intake and output record.

Name: _Josephine Klein_

Medical record #: _49731_

Admission date: _1/13/07_

INTAKE AND OUTPUT RECORD

	INTAKE					
	Oral	**Tube feeding**	**Instilled**	**I.V. and IVPB**	**TPN**	
Date _1/15/07_						
0700–1500	250	320	H_2O 50	1100		
1500–2300	200	320	H_2O 50	1100		
2300–0700	0	320	H_2O 50	1100		
24hr total	450	960	H_2O 150	3300		
Date						
24hr total						
Date						
24hr total						
Date						
24hr total						

Key: IVPB = I.V. piggyback   TPN = total parenteral nutrition   NG = nasogastric

Standard measures

Styrofoam cup	240 ml	Water (large)	600 ml
Juice	120 ml	Water pitcher	750 ml
Water (small)	120 ml	Milk (small)	120 ml

	OUTPUT				
Total	Urine	Emesis Tubes	NG	Other	Total
1720	1355			·	1355
1670	1200				1200
1470	1500				1500
4860	4055				4055

Milk (large)	600 ml		Ice cream, sherbet,	
Coffee	240 ml		or gelatin	120 ml
Soup	180 ml			

WOUND CARE AND
SKIN ASSESSMENT TOOL

When performing a thorough wound care and skin assessment, a pictorial demonstration is usually helpful to identify the wound site or sites. Using the wound care and skin assessment tool below, the nurse identified the left second toe as a partial-thickness wound, vascular ulcer, that's red in color using the classification of terms that follow.

PATIENT'S NAME (LAST, MIDDLE, FIRST)	ATTENDING PHYSICIAN	ROOM NUMBER	ID NUMBER
Brown, Ann	Dr. A. Dennis	123-2	01726

WOUND ASSESSMENT:

NUMBER	1	2	3	4	5
DATE	1/14/07				
TIME	1330				
LOCATION	Ⓛ second toe				
STAGE	II				
APPEARANCE	G				
SIZE-LENGTH	0.5 cm				
SIZE-WIDTH	1 cm				
COLOR/FLR.	RD				
DRAINAGE	O				
ODOR	O				
VOLUME	O				
INFLAMMATION	O				
SIZE INFLAM.					

KEY

Stage:
  I. Red or discolored
  II. Skin break/blister
  III. Sub 'Q' tissue
  IV. Muscle and/or bone

Appearance:
  D = Depth
  E = Eschar
  G = Granulation
  IN = Inflammation
  NEC = Necrotic
  PK = Pink
  SL = Slough
  TN = Tunneling
  UND = Undermining
  MX = Mixed (specify)

Color of Wound Floor:
  RD = Red
  Y = Yellow
  BLK = Black
  MX = Mixed (specify)

Drainage:
  0 = None
  SR = Serous
  SS = Serosanguinous
  BL = Blood
  PR = Purulent

Odor:
  0 = None
  MLD = Mild
  FL = Foul

Volume:
  0 = None
  SC = Scant
  MOD = Moderate
  LG = Large

Inflammation:
  0 = None
  PK = Pink
  RD = Red

WOUND ANATOMICAL LOCATION

(circle affected area)

Anterior Posterior Left lateral Right lateral

Left foot Right foot Left hand Right hand

Wound care protocol: *Clean wound with NSS.*

_____

_____

Signature: *Mark Silver, RN*   Date *1/14/05*

not only protects yourself and your employer, but also shows that you both understand which items you're responsible for.)

● Items to list include jewelry, money, dentures, eyeglasses or contact lenses, hearing aids, prostheses, and clothing.

● When documenting items, use objective language. Include the item's color, approximate size, style, type, serial number, and other distinguishing features in your description.

Alert *Don't assess the item's value or authenticity. For example, you might describe a diamond ring as a "clear,*

DOCUMENTING THE EVENTS OF YOUR SHIFT

Most health care facilities require the charge nurse to complete an end-of-shift report. The form below is an example of the information most facilities need to know.

Date: _1/6/07_ **Charge nurse:** _Donna Moriarty, RN_

Patient census: Start of shift _38_ End of shift: _37_

Number of admissions _2_ Number of transfers _2 in, 3 out_

Deaths _0_ Codes _0_

Comments

One patient transferred to SICU postop

Staff profile: Start of shift: _9_ End of shift: _7_

RNs _4_ Orientees _0_ LPNs _3_

Students _0_ Nursing assistants _2_

Agency _0_ Other _0_

Called in sick _Unit clerk — not replaced_

Late _0_ Floated _One aide, 1 LPN floated out halfway
through shift_

Unit workload during shift

Quiet _____ Busy but steady _____ Very busy _X_ Understaffed _X_

Equipment and supply problems

I.V. pumps not available. No sterile drsg. kits in supply cart. Not enough linen.

High-risk procedures performed

CVP line insertion, wound debridement, chest tube insertion

Assignment, personnel, or performance problems

_Staff floated out 4 hr. into shift to cover sick calls on another unit —
increased pt. ratio for rest of staff._

Patient or family problems

_Mr. Hale in room 516-B — his condition deteriorated rapidly — developed
acute abdomen and required emergency surgery. Family distraught — need
time and privacy to speak with doctor and clergy. Conference room is too
small to accommodate more than 10 people (18 family members present).
Because room doubles as staff lounge, privacy is difficult to maintain._

Number of incident reports filed: _None_

Number of problem logs completed: _None_

---

round stone set in a yellow metal band" or a ruby as "red stone."

1/18/07	1300	Admitted to room 318
		with one pair of brown
		glasses, upper and
		lower dentures, a
		yellow metal ring with
		a red stone, a pink
		bathrobe, and a black
		radio. — Paul Cullen, RN

SHIFT REPORTS

Your facility may require an end-of-shift report (sometimes called a unit report or a 24-hour report). Use these documents to:
- track conditions and activities on the unit
- provide a running record of the patient census
- list staff-to-patient ratio
- list bed utilization
- identify patient emergencies or acute changes
- make known patient or family problems
- list incidents
- log equipment and supply problems
- log high-risk procedures and other important data.

These reports are typically reviewed by nursing administrators charged with solving the day-to-day problems of a unit. (See *Documenting the events of your shift.*)

Challenging patient conditions

Some patient conditions, such as stroke and diabetic ketoacidosis, can be just as challenging to document as they are to provide care for. This section will help you to hone in on essential documentation for some challenging patient conditions.

ANAPHYLAXIS

A severe reaction to an allergen after reexposure to the substance, anaphylaxis is a potentially lethal response requiring emergency intervention. When anaphylaxis occurs, document:
- date and time the anaphylactic reaction started
- events leading up to the anaphylactic response
- patient's signs and symptoms, such as anxiety, agitation, flushing, palpitations, itching, chest tightness, light-headedness, throat tightness or swelling, throbbing in the ears, or abdominal cramping
- assessment findings, such as arrhythmias, skin rash, wheals or welts, wheezing, decreased LOC, unresponsiveness, angioedema, decreased blood pressure, weak or rapid pulse, and diaphoresis
- name of the practitioner notified and the time of notification
- emergency treatments and supportive care given
- patient's response.
Also follow these guidelines:
- If the allergen is identified, document the allergen on the medical record, MAR, nursing care plan, patient identification bracelet, practitioner's orders, and dietary and pharmacy profiles.
- Document that appropriate departments and individuals were notified, such as pharmacy, dietary, risk management, and the nursing coordinator.
- If required, fill out an incident report according to facility policy.

1/15/07	1600	Received Dilaudid 1 mg I.M. for abdominal incision pain at 1445. Rates pain 7 on a scale of 0 to 10. At 1520 pt. was SOB, diaphoretic, and c/o intense itching "every-where." Injection site on ⓁL buttock has 4-cm erythematous area. Skin is blotchy and upper anterior torso and face are covered with hives. BP 90/50, P 140, RR 44 in semi-Fowler's position. I.V. of D_5 ½ NSS infusing at 125 ml/hr in Ⓡ hand. O_2 sat. 94% via pulse oximetry on room air. O_2 at 2 L/min via NC started with no change in O_2 sat. Dr. Brown notified of pt.'s condition at 1525 and orders noted. Fluid challenge of 500 ml NSS over 60 min via Ⓛ antecubital began at 1535. O_2 changed to 50% humidified face mask with O_2 sat. increasing to 99%. After 15 min of fluid challenge, BP 110/70, P 104, RR 28. Benadryl 25 mg P.O. given for discomfort after fluid challenge absorbed. Allergy band placed on pt.'s Ⓛ hand for possible Dilaudid allergy. Chart, MAR, nursing care plan, and doctor's orders labeled with allergy information. Pharmacy, dietary, and nursing supervisor, Barbara Jones, RN, notified. Pt. told he had what appeared to be an allergic reaction to Dilaudid, that he shouldn't receive it in the future, and that he should notify all health care providers and pharmacies of this reaction. Recommended that pt. wear a Medic Alert ID noting his allergic reaction to Dilaudid. Medic Alert order form given to pt.'s wife. — Pat Sloan, RN

ARRHYTHMIAS

Arrhythmias occur when abnormal electrical conduction or automaticity changes heart rate or rhythm, or both. They vary in severity from mild, asymptomatic disturbances requiring no treatment to catastrophic ventricular fibrillation, which requires immediate resuscitation. In the event of an arrhythmia, document:

- date and time of the arrhythmia
- events prior to and at the time of the arrhythmia
- patient's symptoms and the findings of your cardiovascular assessment, such as pallor, cold and clammy skin, shortness of breath, palpitations, weakness, chest pain, dizziness, syncope, and decreased urine output
- patient's vital signs and heart rhythm (if the patient is on a cardiac monitor, place a rhythm strip in the chart)
- name of practitioner notified and the time of notification
- results of a 12-lead ECG, if ordered
- your interventions and the patient's response
- emotional support and patient teaching provided.

1/11/07	1700	While assisting pt. with ambulation in the hallway at 1640, pt. c/o feeling weak and dizzy. Pt. said he was "feeling my heart hammering in my chest." Pt. stated he never felt like this before. Apical rate 170, BP 90/50, RR 24, peripheral pulses weak, skin cool, clammy, and diaphoretic. Denies chest pain or SOB. — Cathy Doll, RN

1/11/07	1700	Breath sounds clear
		bilaterally. Placed in
		wheelchair and assisted
		back to bed without
		incident. Dr. Brown
		notified at 1645 and
		orders noted. Lab
		called to draw stat
		serum electrolyte and
		digoxin levels. O_2 via
		NC started at 2 L/min.
		Stat ECG revealed
		PSVT at a rate of 180.
		I.V. infusion of D_5W
		started in ® hand at
		KVO rate with 18G
		cannula. Placed on con-
		tinuous cardiac moni-
		toring. At 1650 apical
		rate 180, BP 92/52,
		and pulses weakened
		all 4 extremities, lungs
		clear, skin cool and
		clammy. Still c/o weak-
		ness and dizziness.
		Transferred to telem-
		etry unit. Report given
		to Nancy Powell, RN.
		Nursing supervisor,
		Carol Jones, RN, noti-
		fied. — Cathy Doll, RN

BRAIN DEATH

In 1981, the American Medical Association, the American Bar Association, and the President's commission for the Study of Ethical Problems in Medicine and Behavioral Research derived a working definition of brain death. The Uniform Determination of Death Act (UDODA) was then developed, which defines brain death as the cessation of all measurable functions or activity in every area of the brain, including the brain stem. This definition excludes comatose patients as well as those in a persistent vegetative state.

It's important to know your state's laws regarding the definition of death. Exact criteria may also vary for determining brain death, depending on the facility. (See *Know your state's laws concerning brain death,* page 52.) Your documentation for a patient undergoing testing for brain death should include:

- date and time of each test
- name of the test
- name of the person performing the test and their required documentation
- response of the patient to the test, if any
- actions taken in response to the patient, such as your course of action if the patient had gone into ventricular fibrillation
- time and names of people notified of the results
- support given to family members if they're present.

1/9/07	0800	ABG specimen obtained by
		Michael Burke, R.T., at
		0730. Results pH 7.40,
		PO_2 100, PCO_2 40. Pt.
		taken off ventilator by
		respiratory therapist and
		placed on 100% flowby.
		Dr. Brown in attendance.
		Cardiac monitor showing
		NSR at a rate of 70, O_2
		sat. via continuous pulse
		oximetry 99%. Within 1
		min of testing, heart rate
		150 with PVCs, and O_2
		sat. dropped to 95%. Pt.
		without spontaneous
		respirations. O_2 sat
		continued to decrease.
		Pt. placed back on venti-
		lator. — Dawn Silfies, RN

KNOW YOUR STATE'S LAWS CONCERNING BRAIN DEATH

In states without laws defining death or without judicial precedents, the common law definition of death (cessation of circulation and respiration) is still used. In these states, physicians are understandably reluctant to discontinue artificial life support for brain-dead patients. If you're likely to be involved with patients on life-support equipment, protect yourself by finding out how your state defines death.

CHEST PAIN

When your patient complains of chest pain, you'll need to act quickly to determine its cause. When caring for a patient with chest pain, be sure to document:

- date and time of pain onset
- what the patient was doing when the pain started
- how long the pain lasted, whether it had ever occurred before, and whether the onset was sudden or gradual
- whether the pain radiates
- factors that improve or aggravate the pain
- exact location of the pain, which can be derived by asking the patient to point to the pain
- pain's severity, which can be derived by asking the patient to rank the pain on a 0-to-10 scale, with 0 indicating no pain and 10 indicating the worst pain imaginable
- results of your patient assessment, including vital signs
- time and name of people notified, such as the practitioner, nursing supervisor, and the admission's department (if the patient is transferred)
- patient education and emotional support given.

| 1/9/07 | 0410 | Pt. c/o sudden onset of a sharp chest pain while sleeping. Points to center of chest, over sternum. States, "It feels like an elephant is sitting on my chest." Pain radiates to the neck and shoulders. Rates pain as 7 on a scale of 0 to 10. P 112, BP 90/62, RR 26. Lungs have fine rales in the bases on auscultation. Dr. Romano notified and orders received. Morphine 2 mg I.V. given. O₂ at 4 L/min started by NC. Continuous pulse oximetry started with O₂ sat. 94%. 12-lead ECG and MI profile obtained. — Martha Wolcott, RN |
| 1/9/07 | 0415 | Dr. Romano here to see patient. Pt. states pain is now a 5 on a scale of 0 to 10. Morphine 2 mg I.V. repeated. ECG interpreted by Dr. Romano to show acute ischemia. Pt. prepared for transport to CCU. — Martha Wolcott, RN |

DIABETIC KETOACIDOSIS

Characterized by severe hyperglycemia, diabetic ketoacidosis (DKA) is a potentially life-threatening condition that most commonly occurs in people with type 1 diabetes. When caring for a patient with DKA, follow these guidelines:

- Perform frequent documentation of specific parameters—such as blood and urine glucose levels, intake and output, mental status, ketone levels, and vital signs—on a frequent assessment flow sheet.
- Document the clinical manifestations of DKA assessed, such as:
  - changes in LOC
  - fruity breath odor
  - hypotension
  - Kussmaul's respirations
  - polydipsia
  - polyphagia
  - polyuria
  - poor skin turgor
  - warm, dry skin and mucous membranes.
- Document all interventions, such as fluid and electrolyte replacement and insulin therapy, and document the patient's response.
- Document any procedures performed, which may include ABG analysis, blood samples sent to the laboratory, cardiac monitoring, and insertion of an indwelling urinary catheter.
- Document results, the name of persons notified, and the time of notification.
- Document emotional support and patient teaching provided.

1/11/07	0810	Admitted at 0730 with serum blood glucose level of 500 with c/o nausea, vomiting, and excessive urination. Urine positive for ketones. P 112, BP 94/58, RR 28 deep and rapid, oral T 96.8° F. Skin warm, dry, with poor skin turgor. Mucous membranes dry. Resting with eyes closed. Confused to time and date. —— Louise May, RN

1/11/07 continued	0810	States, "I didn't take my insulin for 2 days because I ran out." Dr. Bernhart notified and came to see pt. Blood sample sent to lab for ABG, electrolytes, BUN, creatinine, serum glucose, CBC. Urine obtained and sent for UA. O₂ 2L via NC started with O₂ sat. 94% by pulse oximetry. 1000 ml of NSS being infused over 1 hr through I.V. line in ℝ forearm. 100 units I.V. bolus of regular insulin infused through I.V. line in ℝ antecubital followed by an infusion of 100 units regular insulin in 100 ml NSS at 5 units/hr. Monitoring blood glucose with hourly fingersticks. Next due at 0900. See frequent parameter flow sheet for I/O, VS, and blood glucose results. Notified diabetes educator, Teresa Mooney, RN, about pt.'s admission —— —— Louise May, RN

HYPERTENSIVE CRISIS

Hypertensive crisis is a medical emergency in which the patient's diastolic blood pressure suddenly rises above 120 mm Hg. When caring for a patient with hypertensive crisis, be sure to document:
- patient's blood pressure and vital signs
- findings of your assessment of the patient's cardiopulmonary, neurologic, and renal systems, such as headache, nausea, vomiting, seizures, blurred vision, transient blindness, confusion, drowsiness, heart failure, pulmonary edema, chest pain, and oliguria
- measures you've taken to ensure a patent airway

- name of the practitioner notified and the time of the notification
- patient's response to interventions, such as I.V. fluids and medication given
- intake and output
- emotional support and patient teaching provided.

1/15/07	1100	Arrived in ED with c/o head-
		ache, blurred vision, and
		vomiting. BP 220/120, P 104
		bounding, RR 16 unlabored, oral
		T 97.4° F. Pt. states, "I
		stopped taking my blood
		pressure pills 2 days ago when
		I ran out." Drowsy, but
		oriented to place and person,
		knew year but not day of week
		or time of day. No c/o chest
		pain, neck veins not distended,
		lungs clear. Cardiac monitor –
		sinus tachycardia, no arrhyth-
		mias noted. Dr. Kelly notified
		and in to see pt. at 1045,
		orders written. O₂ at 4 L/min.
		administered via NC. Dr. Kelly
		explained need for arterial
		line for BP monitoring. Pt.
		understands procedure and
		signed consent. Assisted Dr.
		Kelly with insertion of arterial
		line in ® radial artery using
		20G 2½" arterial catheter,
		after a positive Allen's test.
		Catheter secured with 1 suture.
		4" X 4" gauze pad with
		povidone-iodine ointment
		applied. ® hand and wrist
		secured to arm board. Trans-
		ducer leveled and zeroed.
		Initial readings 238/124 mean
		arterial pressure 162 mm Hg.
		Readings accurate to cuff
		pressures. Line flushes easily.
		Pt. tolerated procedure well.
		I.V. line inserted in ® fore-
		arm with 18G catheter. Nitro-
		prusside sodium 50 mg in
		250 ml D₅W started at 0.30
		mcg/kg/min. See frequent vital
		sign flow sheet for frequent
		vital signs. — Alan Walker, RN

1/15/07	1100	Blood sent to lab for stat CBC,
continued		ABG, electrolytes, BUN, creati-
		nine, blood glucose level. Stat
		ECG and portable CXR done,
		results pending. Foley catheter
		inserted, urine sent for UA.
		Side rails padded, bed in low
		position, airway taped to head-
		board of bed, suction equip-
		ment placed in room. All pro-
		cedures explained to pt. and
		wife. —— Alan Walker, RN

HYPOTENSION

Defined as blood pressure below 90/60 mm Hg or 30 mm Hg below baseline, hypotension reduces perfusion to the tissues and organs of the body. Severe hypotension is a medical emergency that may progress to shock and death. When caring for a patient with hypotension, be sure to document:

- patient's blood pressure and other vital signs
- assessment findings, such as bradycardia; tachycardia; weak pulses; cool, clammy skin; oliguria; reduced bowel sounds; dizziness; syncope; reduced LOC; and myocardial ischemia
- name of the practitioner notified and the time of notification
- orders given, such as continuous blood pressure and cardiac monitoring, obtaining a 12-lead ECG, administering supplemental oxygen, and inserting an I.V. line for fluids and vasopressor medications
- interventions, such as lowering the head of the bed, inserting an indwelling urinary catheter, and assisting with insertion of hemodynamic monitoring lines, and the patient's response
- emotional support and patient teaching provided.

HYPOXEMIA

Defined as a low concentration of oxygen in arterial blood, hypoxemia occurs when the PaO_2 falls below 60 mm Hg. Hypoxemia causes poor tissue perfusion and may lead to respiratory failure. When caring for a patient with hypoxemia, be sure to document:

- vital signs and laboratory findings including PaO_2 level
- cardiopulmonary assessment findings, such as change in LOC, tachycardia, increased blood pressure, tachypnea, dyspnea, mottled skin, cyanosis and, in patients with severe hypoxemia, bradycardia and hypotension
- name of the practitioner notified, the time of notification, and any orders given
- interventions—such as measuring oxygen saturation by pulse oximetry, obtaining ABG values, providing supplemental oxygen, positioning the patient in high Fowler's position, assisting with endotracheal intubation, monitoring mechanical ventilation, and providing continuous cardiac monitoring—and the patient's response
- emotional support and patient teaching provided.

1/19/07	1400	Restless and confused,
		SOB, skin mottled. P
		116, BP 148/78, RR 32
		labored, rectal T 97.4°
		F. Dr. Bouchard noti-
		fied and came to see
		pt. ABGs drawn by
		doctor and sent to lab.
		Pulse oximetry 86% on
		O_2 3 L/min by NC.
		Placed on O_2 100% via
		nonrebreather mask
		with pulse oximetry
		92%. Positioned in high
		Fowler's position. Con-
		tinuous cardiac moni-
		toring shows sinus
		tachycardia at 116, no
		arrhythmias noted.
		Radiology called for
		stat portable CXR.
		Doctor notified wife
		of change in husband's
		status. ————————
		—— Donna Damico, RN

INTRACEREBRAL HEMORRHAGE

Intracerebral hemorrhage is the result of the rupture of a cerebral vessel that causes bleeding into the brain tissue. This type of hemorrhage may cause extensive loss of function and may have a very slow recovery and poor prognosis. When caring for a patient with intracerebral hemorrhage, be sure to document:

● evaluation of the patient's airway, breathing, and circulation
● neurologic assessment, such as reduced LOC, confused, restless, agitated, lethargic, comatose, pupillary changes (including unequal size, sluggish or absent response to light), headache, seizures, focal neurologic signs, increased blood pressure, widened pulse pressure, bradycardia, decorticate or decerebrate posturing, and vomiting

● name of the practitioner notified and the time of notification
● interventions—such as medication and fluid administration, assisting with intracranial pressure monitoring insertion, administering oxygen, assisting with intubation, and maintaining mechanical ventilation—and the patient's response
● emotional support and patient teaching provided.

Also follow these guidelines:
● Assess your patient frequently, and document the specific time and results of your assessments.
● Use the appropriate flow sheets to record intake and output, I.V. fluids, medications, and frequent hemodynamic measurements and vital signs. A critical care flow sheet may also be used to document frequent assessments; a neurologic flow sheet, such as the Glasgow Coma Scale or the National Institutes of Health (NIH) Stroke Scale, may be used to document your frequent neurologic assessments.

1/1/07	0810	Found in bed at 0735
		unresponsive to verbal
		stimuli but grimaces
		and opens eyes with
		painful stimuli. PERRL.
		Moving ® side of body
		but not Ⓛ. Airway is
		patent, with unlabored
		breathing. BP 100/60,
		P 72 reg, RR 16. Breath
		sounds clear, normal
		heart sounds. Skin cool,
		dry. Peripheral pulses
		palpable. Dr. Martinez
		notified at 0740 and
		orders given. Adminis-
		tering O_2 at 2 L/min
		by NC. ————————
		—— Juanita Perez, RN

1/1/07	0810	I.V. infusion started
continued		in ® forearm with 18G
		catheter. NSS infusing
		at KVO rate. Foley
		catheter inserted. Dr.
		Martinez in to see pt.
		at 0750. Dr. called
		family to notify them
		of change in condition.
		Glasgow score of 7.
		See Glasgow Coma
		Scale, I.V., I/O, and VS
		flow sheets for fre-
		quent assessments. —
		— Juanita Perez, RN

MYOCARDIAL INFARCTION, ACUTE

A myocardial infarction (MI) is an occlusion of a coronary artery that leads to oxygen deprivation, myocardial ischemia and, eventually, necrosis. Mortality is high when treatment for MI is delayed; however, prognosis improves if vigorous treatment begins immediately. Whenever caring for a patient with an acute MI, be sure to document:

- date and time of your entry
- patient's chest pain and other symptoms of MI, using his own words whenever possible
- your assessment findings, such as feelings of impending doom, anxiety, restlessness, fatigue, nausea, vomiting, dyspnea, tachypnea, cool extremities, weak peripheral pulses, diaphoresis, third or fourth heart sounds, a new murmur, pericardial friction rub, low-grade fever, hypotension or hypertension, bradycardia or tachycardia, and crackles on lung auscultation
- name of the practitioner notified, the time of notification, and the orders given, such as transfer to the coronary care unit, continuous cardiac monitoring, supplemental oxygen,

12-lead ECG, I.V. therapy, cardiac enzymes (including troponin and myoglobin), nitroglycerin (sublingual or via an I.V. line), thrombolytic therapy, aspirin, morphine, bed rest, antiarrhythmics, beta-adrenergic blockers, angiotensin-converting enzyme inhibitors, and heparin

- interventions and the patient's response
- emotional support and patient teaching provided.

1/10/07	2310	C/o severe crushing
		midsternal chest pain
		with radiation to Ⓛ
		arm at 2240. Pt.
		pointed to center of
		chest and stated, "I
		feel like I have an
		elephant on my chest."
		Rates pain at 9 on a
		0 to 10 scale w/ 10
		being worst pain imag-
		inable. Restless in bed
		and diaphoretic, c/o
		nausea. P 84 and reg-
		ular, BP 128/82, RR 24,
		oral T 98.8° F. Extrem-
		ities cool, pedal pulses
		weak, normal heart
		sounds, breath sounds
		clear. Dr. Boone noti-
		fied of pt.'s chest pain
		and physical findings at
		2245 and came to see
		pt. and orders given.
		O₂ started at 2 L by
		NC. 12-lead ECG ob-
		tained; showed ST-
		segment elevation in
		anterior leads. Placed
		on portable cardiac
		monitor. I.V. line
		started in Ⓛ forearm
		with 18 G catheter with
		NSS at KVO rate. Lab
		called for stat cardiac
		enzymes, troponin,
		myoglobin, and electro-
		lytes. — Patricia Silver, RN

1/10/07	2310	Nitroglycerin 1/150 gr
continued		given SL, 5 minutes
		apart X 3 with no
		relief. Explaining
		all procedures to pt.
		Assuring him that he's
		being monitored closely
		and will be trans-
		ferred to CCU for
		closer monitoring and
		treatment. Dr. Boone
		called wife and noti-
		fied her of husband's
		chest pain and trans-
		fer. Report called to
		CCU at 2255 and given
		to Laurie Feldman, RN.
		— Patricia Silver, RN

PULMONARY EDEMA

Pulmonary edema is a diffuse extravascular accumulation of fluid in the tissues and airspaces of the lungs due to increased pressure in the pulmonary capillaries. When caring for a patient with pulmonary edema, be sure to document:

- assessment findings of pulmonary edema, such as dyspnea, orthopnea, use of accessory muscles, pink frothy sputum, diaphoresis, cyanosis, tachypnea, tachycardia, adventitious breath sounds (such as crackles, wheezing, or rhonchi), and jugular vein distention
- name of the practitioner notified, the time of notification, and orders given, such as oxygen and medication administration
- interventions—such as patient positioning, inserting I.V. lines, administering oxygen and medications, assisting with the insertion of hemodynamic monitoring lines, and suctioning, and the patient's response
- frequent assessments, vital signs, hemodynamic measurements, intake and output, I.V. therapy, and laboratory and ABG values using the appropriate flow sheets
- emotional support and patient teaching provided.

1/12/07	0310	Discovered lying flat
		in bed at 0230 trying
		to sit up and stating,
		"I can't breathe."
		Coughing and bringing
		up small amount of
		pink frothy sputum.
		Skin pale, lips cyanotic,
		sluggish capillary re-
		fill, +1 ankle edema.
		Lungs with crackles $^1/_2$
		way up bilaterally, S₃
		heard on auscultation.
		P 120 and irregular,
		BP 140/90, RR 30
		and shallow, tympanic
		T 98.8° F. Restless,
		alert, and oriented
		to time, place, and
		person. Dr. Green
		notified of assessment
		findings at 0235 and
		came to see pt. at
		0245. Placed in sitting
		position with legs
		dangling. O_2 via NC at
		2 L/min changed to
		nonrebreather mask at
		12 L/min. Explained to
		pt. that mask would
		give her more O_2 and
		help her breathing. O_2
		sat. by pulse oximetry
		88%. Stat portable CXR
		done. 12-lead ECG
		sinus tachycardia with
		occasional PVCs. CBC
		and electrolytes drawn
		and sent to lab stat.
		— Rachel Moreau, RN

1/12/07	0310	Morphine, furose-
continued		mide, and digoxin I.V.
		ordered and given
		through saline lock in
		Ⓛ forearm. See MAR.
		Indwelling urinary
		catheter inserted to
		straight drainage,
		drained 100 ml on
		insertion. Explained all
		procedures and drugs
		to pt. See flow sheets
		for documentation of
		frequent VS, I/O, and
		lab values. ————
		——— Rachel Moreau, RN

STROKE

Stroke is a sudden impairment of cerebral circulation in one or more of the blood vessels supplying the brain that can be caused by thrombosis, embolus, or intracerebral hemorrhage. When caring for a patient who has suffered a suspected stroke, be sure to document:

- events leading up to the suspected stroke and date and time of the event
- patient's symptoms in his own words, if he can talk
- assessment findings, including evaluation of the patient's airway, breathing, and circulation; neurologic assessment; and vital signs
- name of the practitioner notified and time of the notification
- interventions performed and the patient's response
- times and results of your frequent assessments, using a frequent vital sign assessment sheet to document vital signs and a neurologic flow sheet such as the NIH Stroke Scale to record your frequent neurologic assessments. (See *Using the NIH Stroke Scale,* pages 60 and 61.)

1/10/07	2030	When giving pt. her medi-
		cation at 2015, noted
		drooping of Ⓛ eyelid and
		Ⓛ side of mouth. Pt. was
		in bed breathing comfort-
		ably with RR 24, P 112, BP
		142/72, axillary T 97.2° F.
		PERRL, awake and aware
		of her surroundings,
		answering yes and no by
		shake of head, speech
		slurred with some words
		inappropriate. Follows
		simple commands. Ⓛ hand
		grasp weaker than Ⓡ hand
		grasp. Ⓛ foot slightly
		dropped and weaker than
		Ⓡ. Glasgow score of 13.
		See Glasgow Coma Scale
		flow sheet for frequent
		assessments. Skin cool, dry.
		Peripheral pulses palpable.
		Brisk capillary refill. Called
		Dr. Lee at 2020. Stat CT
		scan ordered. Adminis-
		tered O_2 at 2 L/min by
		NC. I.V. infusion of NSS
		at KVO rate started in Ⓡ
		forearm with 18G catheter.
		Continuous pulse oximetry
		started with O_2 sat. of
		96% on 2 L O_2. Dr. Lee in
		to see pt. at 2025. Pre-
		pared for transfer to
		ICU. Dr. Lee will notify
		family of transfer. ———
		——— Luke Newell, RN

(Text continues on page 62.)

USING THE NIH STROKE SCALE

CATEGORY	DESCRIPTION	SCORE	BASELINE DATE/TIME	DATE/ TIME
1a. Level of conscious- ness (LOC)	Alert	0	1/15/07	
	Drowsy	1	1100	
	Stuporous	2	1	
	Coma	3		
1b. LOC questions (Month, age)	Answers both correctly	0		
	Answers one correctly	1	0	
	Incorrect	2		
1c. LOC commands (Open/close eyes, make fist, let go)	Obeys both correctly	0		
	Obeys one correctly	1	1	
	Incorrect	2		
2. Best gaze (Eyes open — patient follows examiner's finger or face.)	Normal	0		
	Partial gaze palsy	1	0	
	Forced deviation	2		
3. Visual (Introduce visual stimu- lus/threat to patient's visual field quadrants.)	No visual loss	0		
	Partial hemianopia	1	1	
	Complete hemianopia	2		
	Bilateral hemianopia	3		
4. Facial palsy (Show teeth, raise eyebrows, and squeeze eyes shut.)	Normal	0		
	Minor	1	2	
	Partial	2		
	Complete	3		
5a. Motor arm — left (Elevate extremity to 90 degrees and score drift/movement.)	No drift	0		
	Drift	1		
	Can't resist gravity	2		
	No effort against gravity	3	4	
	No movement	4		
	Amputation, joint fusion (explain)	9		
5b. Motor arm — right (Elevate extremity to 90 degrees and score drift/movement.)	No drift	0		
	Drift	1		
	Can't resist gravity	2		
	No effort against gravity	3	0	
	No movement	4		
	Amputation, joint fusion (explain)	9		

CATEGORY	DESCRIPTION	SCORE	BASELINE DATE/TIME	DATE/TIME
6a. Motor leg — left (Elevate extremity to 30 degrees and score drift/movement.)	No drift Drift Can't resist gravity No effort against gravity No movement Amputation, joint fusion (explain)	0 1 2 3 4 9	4	
6b. Motor leg — right (Elevate extremity to 30 degrees and score drift/movement.)	No drift Drift Can't resist gravity No effort against gravity No movement Amputation, joint fusion (explain)	0 1 2 3 4 9	0	
7. Limb ataxia (Finger-nose, heel down shin)	Absent Present in one limb Present in two limbs	0 1 2	0	
8. Sensory (Pinprick to face, arm, trunk, and leg — compare side to side.)	Normal Partial loss Severe loss	0 1 2	R L 0 2	R L
9. Best language (Name items; describe a picture and read sentences.)	No aphasia Mild to moderate aphasia Severe aphasia Mute	0 1 2 3	1	
10. Dysarthria (Evaluate speech clarity by patient repeating listed words.)	Normal articulation Mild to moderate dysarthria Near to unintelligible or worse Intubated or other physical barrier	0 1 2 9	1	
11. Extinction and inattention (Use information from prior testing to identify neglect or double simultaneous stimuli testing.)	No neglect Partial neglect Complete neglect	0 1 2	0	
		Total	17	
Individual Administering Scale:	*Helen Hareson, RN*			

Common charting flaws

Ideally, every chart you receive from the nurses on the previous shift will be complete and accurate. Unfortunately, this isn't always the case. Although you can't necessarily affect what other nurses do, you can try to make your own charting flawless, so it doesn't mislead other caregivers.

BLANK SPACES IN CHART OR FLOW SHEET

A blank space may imply that you failed to give complete care or assess the patient fully. In order to ensure that your documentation is complete, follow your facility's policy regarding blank spaces, which may require you to:

● fill in only those fields or prompts that apply to your patient
● draw a line through empty spaces or write "N/A" (not applicable) in empty spaces, which leaves no doubt that you addressed every part of the record and prevents others from inserting information that could change the meaning of your original documentation.

1/9/07	1500	20 y/o male admitted
		to room 418B by wheel-
		chair. #20 angiocath in-
		serted in ① antecubital
		vein with I.V. of 1,000
		ml D$_5$¹/₂ NSS infusing at
		125 ml/hr. O$_2$ at 2 L/
		min. via NC. Dilaudid
		1 mg given I.M. for ab-
		dominal pain. Rates pain
		8 on a scale of 0 to 10.
		Relief reported. ————
		———— David Dunn, RN

CARE GIVEN BY SOMEONE ELSE

Unless you document otherwise, anyone reading your notes assumes that they're a firsthand account of care provided. In some settings, nursing assistants and technicians aren't allowed to make formal charting entries. If this is the case in your facility, be sure to document:

● that the appropriate care was provided
● your assessment of the patient
● your assessment of the task performed (such as a dressing change)
● full names and titles of unlicensed personnel who provided care—not just their initials.

1/13/07	0600	Morning care provided
		by Kevin Lawson, NA,
		who stated that patient
		moaned and opened
		eyes when being turned.
		———— Camille Dunn, RN

If your facility's policy requires you to countersign the notes of unlicensed personnel, follow these guidelines:

● If unlicensed personnel must provide care in your presence, don't countersign for care unless you actually witnessed the action detailed in the note.
● If unlicensed personnel are allowed to provide care without supervision, verify that the documentation describes care that the other person had the authority and competence to perform and that the care was performed.
● If necessary, specifically document that you reviewed the documentation

and consulted with the technician or assistant on certain aspects of care.

- Document any follow-up care you provide. (For more information on countersigning, see chapter 4, Legally perilous documentation.)

LATE AND ALTERED ENTRIES

Late and altered entries can arouse suspicions and be a significant problem in the event of a malpractice lawsuit. It's best to avoid them, if you can. (See *Avoiding late additions*.) However, they're appropriate in several situations:

- if the chart was unavailable when you needed it—for example, when the patient was away from the unit
- if you need to add important information after completing your notes
- if you forgot to write notes on a particular chart.

1/14/07	0900	(Chart not available 2/13/07 @ 1500.) On 2/13 @ 1300, stated she felt faint when getting OOB on 2/13 @ 1200 and fell to the floor. States she did not hurt herself and did not think she had to tell anyone about this until her husband encouraged her to report it. No bruises or lacerations noted. Denies pain. Dr. Muir examined pt. at 1320 on 2/13. ———— Elaine Kasmer, RN

If you must make a late entry or alter an earlier entry, follow these guidelines:

- Find out if your health care facility has a protocol for making late or altered entries. If so, follow it. If there isn't a protocol, the best approach is to add the entry to the first available line and label it "late entry" to indicate that it's out of sequence.

In court

AVOIDING LATE ADDITIONS

If the court uncovers alterations in a patient's chart during the course of a trial, suspicions may be aroused and the court may logically infer that additional alterations were made. In such situations, the value of the entire medical record may be brought into question.

That's what happened to the nurse involved in one case. She failed to chart her observations of a postoperative patient for 7 hours, during which time the patient died. The patient's family later sued the hospital, charging the nurse with malpractice. The nurse insisted that she had observed the patient, but because her particular unit was understaffed and overpopulated, she wasn't able to record her observations. She explained that the assistant director of nursing later instructed her about the hospital's policy on charting late additions. The nurse subsequently added her observations to the patient's medical record.

However, the court wasn't convinced that the nurse had indeed observed the patient during the postoperative period. Suspicious of the altered record, it ruled that the nurse's failure to chart her observations at the proper time supported the plaintiff's claim that she had made no such observations.

● Record the time and date of the entry and, in the body of the entry, record the time and date it should have been made.

CORRECTIONS

As with late and altered entries, corrected entries can also arouse suspicions. If a chart with corrected entries ends up in court, the plaintiff's attorney will try to exploit the corrections to cast doubt on the chart's accuracy. If you must make a correction, follow these guidelines:

● When you make a mistake on a chart, correct it promptly.

● Make your corrections as neat and legible as possible. If appropriate, explain why the correction needed to be made. (See *Correcting a charting error.*)

● Never erase, cover, completely scratch out, or otherwise obscure an erroneous entry because this may imply a cover-up. Erasures or the use of correction fluid or heavy black ink to obliterate an error are red flags.

Patient noncompliance

Patients commonly refuse to comply with or unintentionally violate such common instructions as "Follow your diet," "Don't get out of bed without assistance," "Take your medicine as directed," or "Keep your practitioner's appointment for a checkup." Beyond reexplaining the importance of following such instructions after an incident occurs, there's little you can do. However, by documenting the noncompliance, you're creating an important record should the patient's care be questioned later. In the chart, be sure to document:

● any patient behavior that goes against your instructions

● that you reported the problem to the appropriate person

In court

CORRECTING A CHARTING ERROR

When you make a mistake documenting on the medical record, correct it by drawing a single line through it and writing the words "mistaken entry" below or beside it. Follow these words with your initials and the date. If appropriate, briefly explain the necessity for the correction.

Make sure that the mistaken entry is still readable. This indicates that you're only trying to correct a mistake, not cover it up.

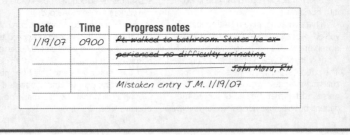

Date	Time	Progress notes
1/19/07	0900	~~Pt. walked to bathroom. States he ex-~~
		~~perienced no difficulty urinating.~~
		~~John Mora, RN~~
		Mistaken entry J.M. 1/19/07

- that you attempted to encourage the patient's compliance, even if unsuccessful.

DIETARY RESTRICTIONS

If your patient is on dietary restrictions, and you discover unauthorized food or beverages at his bedside, be sure to document:
- patient's noncompliance
- your patient teaching reemphasizing the importance of the need to follow the prescribed dietary plan
- other patient teaching you provide
- your notification of the patient's practitioner and the time of the notification.

1/17/07	1400	Milkshake and cookies found at bedside. Discussed with pt. his need to maintain 1800-calorie diet. States, "I'll eat what I want." Dr. Mayer notified that pt. is not complying with prescribed diabetic diet. Dietitian called to meet with pt. and wife. ——— Claire Bowen, RN

OUT OF BED AGAINST ADVICE

Even after you've told a patient that he must not get out of bed without assistance, he may attempt to do so—which puts him at risk for a fall and you at risk for a lawsuit. To safeguard yourself, be sure to:
- clearly document your instructions and anything that the patient does in spite of them
- include in your documentation any devices being used to ensure patient safety such as bed alarms.

1/10/07	0300	Assisted to bathroom. Weak, unsteady on feet. States she gets dizzy when she stands. Instructed pt. to call for assistance to get OOB. Side rails up. Call button within reach. ——— Joseph Romano, RN
1/10/07	0430	Found pt. walking to bathroom. Stated she got OOB by herself. Reminded her to call for assistance. Said she understood. ——— ——— Joseph Romano, RN

MEDICATION ABUSE OR REFUSAL

If the patient refuses or abuses prescribed medication, document the event in his chart. Follow these guidelines:
- If you find medications not ordered by the practitioner at the patient's bedside, document the type of medication (pills or powders), the amount, and its appearance (color and shape).
- If you find a supply of his prescribed medications in his bedside table, indicating that he's hoarding his medication instead of swallowing each dose, document the type of medication that you found and the amount.
- If you give the patient prescribed medications and he refuses, document his refusal, the reason for the refusal, and the medications refused. Taking these steps will ensure that the patient's refusal isn't misinterpreted as an omission or a medication error on your part.

- If you observe that the patient's behavior suddenly changes after he has visitors, and you suspect the visitors of providing him with contraband (opioids or other medications, for example), document how the patient appeared before and after the visitors came to see him.

1/2/07	1100	Alert, oriented. Visitor present at bedside. I.V. D$_5$1/2 NSS infusing at 125 ml/hr. ———— Eileen Sullivan, RN
1/2/07	1125	Upon entering room, found lethargic, pupils were constricted, speech was slurred. Stated, "My friend gave me something to help with the pain." Dr. Ettingoff notified and told of lethargy, slurred speech, and pinpoint pupils. ———— Eileen Sullivan, RN
1/2/07	1130	Dr. Ettingoff in to see pt. Narcan administered as ordered. ———— Eileen Sullivan, RN

DISCHARGE INSTRUCTIONS

At discharge, review the discharge instructions and discuss the date on which the patient will have a follow-up evaluation.

Patient safety *According to JCAHO's National Patient Safety Goals, the patient must be given a complete list of discharge medications.*

Make sure that your documentation includes:

- date on which the patient is expected to return for a follow-up visit and the date on which you discussed the appointment with him

- related patient teaching that you provided
- written instructions and medicaton lists that you provided.

1/12/07	1300	Instructed to return to see Dr. Bonn on 1/26/07 at 0900. Discussed this with pt. and his wife. Wrtten list of discharge medications provided. ———— ———— Laura E. Cray, RN

REFUSING TREATMENT

The courts recognize a competent adult's right to refuse medical treatment, even when that refusal will clearly result in his death. In most cases, the health care personnel who are responsible for the patient's care can remain free from legal jeopardy as long as they fully inform the patient about his medical condition and the likely consequences of refusing treatment. When your patient refuses treatment, be sure to document:

- that you informed him of the risks involved in making such a decision, in writing if possible
- that you notified the practitioner and the time of the notification
- patient's exact words in the chart.

To help protect yourself legally:

- Document that you didn't provide the prescribed treatment because the patient refused it.
- Ask the patient to sign a refusal-of-treatment release form; if he refuses to sign the release form, document this refusal in the progress notes.
- Ask the patient's spouse or closest relative to sign another refusal-of-treatment release form, if facility policy. Document whether the spouse or

another relative does this. (See chapter 3, Legal and ethical implications.)

1/8/07	2000	Refusing to have I.V.
		inserted, stating that
		he's "sick and tired of
		being stuck." Explained
		to pt. the need for
		I.V. fluids and anti-
		biotics and likely result
		of refusing treatment.
		Dr. Eisenberg notified.
		Dr. Eisenberg spent
		time with pt. Pt. still
		refusing I.V. Orders
		written to force
		fluids, repeat electro-
		lytes in morning, and
		give amoxicillin orally.
		—— Barbara Tyson, RN

Interdisciplinary communication

Because health care involves teamwork, all interdepartmental and interdisciplinary communication about the patient must be documented, including:

● calls from the laboratory informing you of a patient's test results
● calls you make to the practitioner about the patient's condition
● calls from patients requesting advice
● giving a patient's family bad news over the telephone.

INFORMATION FROM OTHER DEPARTMENTS

When a department, such as the laboratory or radiology, notifies your unit of a patient's test results, follow these guidelines:

● Notify the practitioner of abnormal results and then document your notification, including the practitioner's name, the time he was notified, and orders received.
● Document patient interventions and the patient's response.

1/4/07	1400	Laboratory technician
		Donald Boyle called floor
		to report random blood
		glucose level of 486. Dr.
		Somers notified. Stat
		blood glucose ordered.
		Pt. being monitored
		until results available.
		—— Peggy Irwin, RN

REPORTS TO PHYSICIANS

You've just phoned the physician to tell him about his patient's deteriorating condition. He listens as you give laboratory test results and the patient's signs and symptoms, thanks you for the information, and hangs up—without giving you an order. What do you do?

● Document what exactly you told the physician and the physician's response, or lack thereof. Be specific. Don't simply write, "Notified physician of patient's condition." This statement is too vague. In the event of a malpractice suit, it allows the plaintiff's lawyer (and the physician) to imply that you didn't communicate the essential data. (See *Ensuring clear communication,* page 68.)
● If you think a physician's failure to order an intervention puts your patient's health at risk, follow your facility's chain of command, notify your supervisor, and document your actions.

1/15/07	2215	Called Dr. Spencer
		regarding increased
		serous drainage from Ⓛ
		chest tube. Dr. Spencer's
		order was to observe
		the drainage for 1 more
		hr and then call him.
		— Danielle Bergeron, RN

TELEPHONE ADVICE TO PATIENTS

Nurses, especially those working in hospital emergency departments (ED), commonly get requests to give advice to patients by telephone. A hospital has no legal duty to provide a telephone-advice service, and you've no legal duty to give advice to anyone who calls. (See *Accepting responsibility.*) The best response is to tell the caller to come to the hospital because you can't assess his condition or treat him over the phone. As with all rules, however, this one has its exceptions—for example, a life-threatening situation when someone needs immediate care, treatment, or referral.

When dispensing advice over the phone, follow these guidelines:

• Document the call in the telephone log, if available. In your notes, be sure to include the date and time of the call, name of the caller, address of the caller, caller's request or chief complaint, disposition of the call, and name of the person who made that disposition. (See *Benefits of the telephone log.*)

• Document your interventions. For example, you may give the caller a poison-control number or suggest that he come to the ED for evaluation. Document whatever information you give.

1/6/07	1615	Louis Chapman phoned
		asking how big a cut
		has to be to require
		stitches. He was asked
		to describe the injury.
		He described a 4" gash
		in his Ⓛ leg from a
		fall. Instructed to
		apply pressure to the
		cut and come into the
		ED to be assessed. —
		—— Claire Bowen, RN

ENSURING CLEAR COMMUNICATION

To ensure clear communication when discussing a patient's care with a physician on the phone, remember to keep the following points in mind:

■ If you don't know the physician, ask him to state and spell his full name.

■ Include the exact time you contacted the physician. To establish proof, you could have another nurse listen in and then cosign the time of notification. If you don't note the time you called, allegations may later be made that you failed to obtain timely medical treatment for the patient.

■ Always note in the chart the specific change, problem, or result you reported to the physician, along with the physician's orders or response. Use his own words, if possible.

■ If you're reporting a critical laboratory test result (for example, a low serum potassium level of 3.2 mEq/L) but don't receive an order for intervention (such as potassium replacement therapy), be sure to verify with the physician that he doesn't want to give an order. Then document this fact in the progress notes. For example, you would write: "Dr. P. Jones informed of potassium of 3.2 mEq/L. No orders received."

BENEFITS OF THE TELEPHONE LOG

In court, the telephone log can provide evidence and refresh your recollection of an event. For example, the plaintiff may claim that you told him to take two acetaminophen tablets to reduce his fever of 105° F (40.6° C) when, in fact, you told him to come to the emergency department. Even if you can't recall the conversation, if you've filled out the telephone log properly, the notes in the log will aid in your defense. When you log such information, the law presumes that it's true because you wrote it in the course of ordinary business.

ACCEPTING RESPONSIBILITY

If you dispense advice over the phone, keep in mind that a legal duty arises the minute you say, "Okay, let me tell you what to do." You now have a nurse-patient relationship, and you're responsible for any advice you give. You can't decide midway through that you're in over your head and simply hang up; that could be considered abandonment. You must give appropriate advice or a referral—for example, "After listening to you, I strongly suggest that you come to the emergency department or call your practitioner."

If the patient has specific questions, direct them to the practitioner, especially if the patient's symptoms have changed.

Physician's orders

Most patient treatments require physician's orders; therefore, careful and accurate documentation of these orders is crucial.

WRITTEN ORDERS

No matter who transcribes a physician's orders—a registered nurse, licensed practical nurse, or unit secretary—a second person needs to double-check the transcription for accuracy. Your unit should have a method of checking for errors in written orders, such as performing 8-hour or 24-hour chart checks and verifying preprinted order forms. Night-shift nurses usually do the 24-hour check by:

● placing a line across the order sheet to indicate that all orders above the line have been checked

● signing and dating the sheet to verify that they have done the 24-hour medication check.

The nurse caring for the patient will perform the 8-hour check, which includes:

● making sure that the orders were written for the intended patient

● asking the physician to clarify unclear orders

● asking a physician who is known to have poor handwriting to read his orders to you before he leaves the unit.

If your facility uses preprinted order forms, don't automatically assume that it's a flawless document. You may still need to clarify its meaning with the physician who filled it out. (See *Avoiding pitfalls of preprinted order forms,* page 70.)

AVOIDING PITFALLS OF PREPRINTED ORDER FORMS

When documenting the execution of a practitioner's preprinted order, make sure that you've interpreted and carried out the order correctly. Even though these forms aim to prevent problems (caused by illegible handwriting, for example), they may still be misread. Here are some considerations for using preprinted forms.

INSIST ON APPROVED FORMS

Use only preprinted order forms that have your health care facility's approval and seal of approval by the medical records committee. Most facilities stamp or print an identification number or code on the form. When in doubt, call the medical records department—the practitioner may be using a form he developed or one provided by a drug manufacturer.

REQUIRE COMPLIANCE WITH POLICIES

To enhance communication and continuity, a preprinted order form needs to comply with facility policies and other regulations. For example, a postoperative preprinted order form shouldn't say, "Renew all previous orders" if facility policy requires specific orders. Alert your nurse-manager if any order form requires you to perform duties that are outside your scope of practice.

MAKE SURE THAT THE FORM IS COMPLETED CORRECTLY

Many preprinted order forms list more orders than the practitioner wants you to follow, so he'll need to indicate which specific interventions he's ordering. For example, he may check the appropriate orders, put his initials next to them, or cross out the ones he doesn't want.

ASK FOR CLARITY AND PRECISION

Make sure that the practitioner orders drug doses in the unit of measure in which they're dispensed. For example, make sure that the form uses the metric system instead of the error-prone apothecary system. Report any errors to your nurse-manager.

PROMOTE PROPER NOMENCLATURE

Ask practitioners to use generic drug names, especially when more than one brand of a generic drug is available (for example, "acetaminophen" instead of "Tylenol"). If only one brand of a drug is available, its name can be included in parentheses after the generic name—for example, "dobutamine (Dobutrex)."

TAKE STEPS TO AVOID MISINTERPRETATION

Unapproved, potentially dangerous abbreviations and symbols—such as q.d., U, and q.o.d.—don't belong on preprinted order forms. Improper spacing between a drug name and its dosage can also contribute to medication errors. For example, a 20-mg dose of Inderal written as, "Inderal20 mg" could be misinterpreted as 120 mg.

ENSURE THAT THE COPY IS READABLE

If your facility uses a no-carbon-required form, make sure that the bottom copy contains an identical set of preprinted orders; this is the copy that goes to the pharmacy. All lines on the bottom copy should also appear on the top copy—extra lines on the pharmacy copy can hide decimal points (making 1.5 look like 15, for example) and the tops of numbers (making 7 look like 1 and 5 look like 3).

VERBAL ORDERS

Errors made in the interpretation or documentation of verbal orders can lead to mistakes in patient care and liability problems for you. Clearly, they can be a necessity—especially if you're providing home health care. However, in a health care facility, try to take verbal orders only in an emergency when the physician can't immediately attend to the patient and follow these guidelines:

● Carefully follow your facility's policy for documenting a verbal order, and use a special form if one exists.

● If possible, write the order out while the physician is still present.

Patient safety *JCAHO's Patient Safety Goals require that for verbal or telephone orders, the complete order should be verified by having the person receiving the information read back the complete order and document that the order was read back and verified.*

● Read the order back for verification and note it in the chart.

● Document the order on the physician's order sheet, and read it back to him. Note the date and time.

● On the following line, write "VO" for verbal order. Then write the physician's name and the name of the nurse who read the order back to the physician.

● Sign your name and draw a line for the physician to sign.

● Draw lines through any spaces between the order and your verification of the order.

● Document the type of medication, the dosage, the time you administered it, and any other information your facility's policy requires.

● Make sure that the physician countersigns the order within the time limits set by your facility's policy.

1/17/07	1500	V.O. by Dr. Blackstone
		taken for digoxin
		0.125 mg P.O. now and
		daily in a.m. Furose-
		mide 40 mg P.O. now
		and daily starting in
		a.m. Order read back
		and confirmed. ———
		— Judith Schilling, RN
		———— Carla Roy, RN
		MD sig.: _____

TELEPHONE ORDERS

Normally, you should accept only written orders from a physician. However, in emergency situations in which the patient needs immediate treatment, and the physician isn't available to write an order, and when new information is available that doesn't require a physical examination, telephone orders are acceptable. Carefully follow your facility's policy for documenting a telephone order. Generally, you'll follow this procedure:

● Document the order on the physician's order sheet, and read the order back to the physician before he hangs up.

● Document the date and time, then write the order verbatim. On the next line, write "T.O." for telephone order. (Don't use "P.O." for phone order; that abbreviation could be misinterpreted to mean "by mouth.")

● Write the physician's name, and sign your name.

ADVANTAGES OF FAXING ORDERS

Most hospital units now have a facsimile, or fax, machine at their disposal. Faxing has two main advantages: It speeds the transmittal of practitioner's orders and test results to different departments, and it reduces the likelihood of errors.

SPEEDS COMMUNICATION

Faxing allows practitioners to back up phone orders in writing for the patient's chart. Orders can be faxed to you on the unit and also to the pharmacy, radiology department, and other relevant departments. The results: no more time wasted calling the department and waiting to get through and no more time spent waiting for orders to be picked up.

In return, the receiving department gets a copy of the original order (needed for filling the order and for department files). If an order can't be filled, the receiving department can contact the practitioner for clarification or for a new order, again reducing delays in filling orders and wasting your time as a go-between. An additional advantage comes from the fax machine itself, which prints the date and time the order was sent and the department it came from.

Faxing also allows staff members to transmit exact copies of X-rays, laboratory test results, and electrocardiogram strips in as little as 15 seconds.

REDUCES ERRORS

Using a fax network helps you and other staff members prevent errors by checking one another's work and consulting the practitioner directly about unresolved problems. In addition, faxing provides printed accounts, promoting accurate documentation.

HIPAA COMPLIANCE

The goal of the Health Insurance Portability and Accountability Act (HIPAA) is to provide safeguards against the inappropriate use and release of personal medical information, including all medical records and identifiable health information in any form (electronic, paper, or oral). When faxing patient information, remember to protect patient confidentially by verifying that you're sending the information to the correct fax number, properly disposing of unneeded information, and not leaving faxes and other computer printouts unattended.

• If another nurse listened to the order with you, have her sign the order too.

1/4/07	1100	Codeine 30 mg orally now and every 12 hr for pain. Bisacodyl suppos. ī rectally now. May repeat x 1 if no results. Order read back to Dr. Kaufman who confirmed it. ——————— T.O. Dr. Kaufman/ Jane Goddard, RN. ———— Carol Barsky, RN

Also follow these guidelines:
• Draw lines through any blank spaces in the order.
• Make sure that the physician countersigns the order within the set time limits.
• To save time and avoid errors, consider asking the physician to send a copy of the order by fax. (See *Advantages of faxing orders*.)

CLARIFYING PHYSICIAN'S ORDERS

Although unit secretaries may transcribe orders, the nurse is ultimately

WHEN IN DOUBT, QUESTION ORDERS

Always question a physician's order if it seems strange or "not right."

In *Poor Sisters of Saint Francis Seraph of the Perpetual Adoration, et al. v. Catron* (1982), a hospital was held liable for negligence because a nurse failed to question a physician's order about an endotracheal tube.

The physician ordered that the tube be left in the patient's trachea for an excessively long period: 5 days instead of the standard 2 to 3 days. The nurse knew that 5 days was exceptionally long, but instead of clarifying the physician's order and documenting her actions, she followed the order. As a result, the patient's voice box was irreparably damaged, and the court ruled the hospital negligent.

responsible for the accuracy of the transcription. Only you have the authority and knowledge to question the validity of orders and to spot errors. When clarifying orders, follow these guidelines:

● Follow your facility's policy for clarifying orders that are vague or possibly erroneous. If you don't have a policy to cover a particular situation, contact the prescribing physician.

● Always document your actions, including your efforts to clarify the order and whether the order was carried out.

● If you believe a physician's order is in error, you must not carry it out until you receive clarification. Document your refusal together with the reasons and an account of all communication with the physician. (See *When in doubt, question orders.*)

Do-not-resuscitate orders

When a patient is terminally ill, and his death is expected, his physician and family (and the patient if appropriate) may agree that a do-not-resuscitate (DNR), or no-code, order is appropriate. The physician writes the order, and the staff carries it out when the patient goes into cardiac or respiratory arrest.

1/19/07	1900	DO NOT RESUSCITATE THIS PATIENT ——— Deepak Patel, MD

Every patient with a DNR order should have a written order on file. If a terminally ill patient without a DNR order tells you verbally that he doesn't want to be resuscitated in a crisis, be sure to document:

● his statement

● his degree of awareness and orientation

● notification of the patient's physician and your nurse-manager and the times of these notifications

● requests for assistance from administration or risk management.

Advance directives

Health care facilities must provide written information to all patients concerning their rights under state law to make decisions regarding their care, including the right to refuse medical treatment and the right to

DOCUMENTING
ADVANCE DIRECTIVES

Spurred by patients' requests and the passage of self-determination laws in many states, many health care facilities are requiring documentation of advance directives or lack of the same.

An advance directive is a legal document by which a person tells his medical caregivers how he prefers to be treated in an illness from which he can't reasonably expect to recover. Advance directives also include living wills (which instruct the practitioner to administer no life-sustaining treatment) and durable powers of attorney (which name another person to act in the patient's behalf for medical decisions in the event that the patient can't act for himself).

Because these laws vary from state to state, be sure to find out how your state's law applies to your practice and to the medical record.

PREVIOUSLY EXECUTED DIRECTIVE

If a patient has previously executed an advance directive, request a copy of it for his chart, and make sure that his practitioner is aware of it. Some health care facilities routinely make this request a part of admission or preadmission procedures.

Also, be sure to document the name, address, and phone number of the person entrusted with decision-making power.

PRESENTLY EXECUTED DIRECTIVE

If a patient wants to execute an advance directive during his stay in your facility, he can do so as long as he's a competent adult. In such a case, the record should include documented proof of competence (usually the responsibility of the medical, legal, social services, or risk management department) along with the signed and witnessed, newly executed advance directive.

DIRECTIVES ABOUT NUTRITION AND HYDRATION

If you practice in an area with laws related to artificial nutrition and hydration (nourishment provided by invasive tubes and I.V. lines), record the patient's wishes if these issues aren't addressed in his advance directive.

REVOCATION OF THE DIRECTIVE

Legally, the patient can revoke an advance directive at any time either orally or in writing. In such a case, include a copy of the written revocation in the record, or sign and date a statement in the patient's medical record explaining that the patient made the request orally. Consult your facility's policy and state laws pertaining to living wills and advance directives; revocation statements may need to be countersigned.

---

formulate an advance directive. (See *Documenting advance directives*.)

Incidents

A patient injury—typically referred to as an incident—is a serious situation. It may be the result of patient action, staff action, or equipment failure, but no matter the reason, an incident requires the filing of an incident report. (See *Functions of the incident report*.)

When filing an incident report, follow these guidelines:
● Only a person with firsthand knowledge of an incident should file a report, and only the person making the report should sign it.

- Never sign a report describing circumstances or events that you didn't witness.
- Each person with firsthand knowledge should fill out and sign a *separate* report. Your report should:
  - identify the person involved in the incident
  - document accurately and objectively unusual occurrences that you witnessed
  - include details of what happened and the consequences for the persons involved, with enough sufficient information so that administrators can decide whether the matter requires further investigation
  - avoid opinions, judgments, conclusions, or assumptions about who or what caused the incident
  - avoid making suggestions about how to prevent the incident from happening again.
- Don't include detailed statements from witnesses and descriptions of remedial action in the incident report itself. They're normally part of an investigative follow-up.
- Treat the patient's chart and the incident report separately.
  - Don't note in the chart that you filed an incident report, but do include the clinical details of the incident in the chart.
  - Make sure that the descriptions in the incident report are consistent with those in the chart; after it's filed, it may be reviewed by the nursing supervisor, the practitioner called to examine the patient, appropriate department heads and administrators, the health care facility's attorney, and the insurance company. (See *What happens to an incident report,* page 76.)

FUNCTIONS OF THE INCIDENT REPORT

An incident report serves two functions:
- It informs the administration of the incident, allowing the risk management team to consider changes that might prevent similar incidents in the future.
- It alerts the administration and the health care facility's insurance company to a potential claim and the need for further investigation.

Incidence reports should be filed in compliance with your health care facility's procedures. Chart all patient injuries caused by falls, restraints, burns, or other factors. Also file an incident report whenever a patient insists on being discharged against medical advice.

FALLS

Current research shows that falls—involving patients, visitors, and staff—constitute most of the incidents reported on clinical units. Among the events qualifying as falls are slips, slides, knees giving way, faints, or tripping over equipment. Consequences of falls include prolonged hospitalization, increased hospital costs, and liability problems. Because they raise so many problems, your health care facility may require an all-out risk assessment and prevention effort. (See *Determining a patient's risk for falling,* page 78.)

If a patient falls despite precautions, be sure to document the event and file an incident report, follow these documentation guidelines:
- Document bruises, lacerations, or abrasions.
- Document pain or deformity in the extremities, particularly the hip, arm, leg, or lumbar spine.

WHAT HAPPENS TO AN INCIDENT REPORT

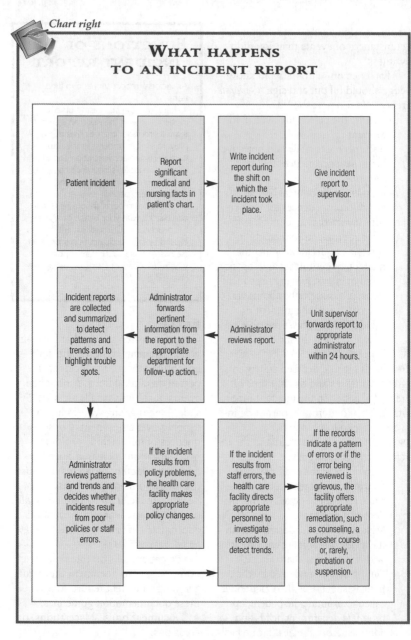

Patient incident → Report significant medical and nursing facts in patient's chart. → Write incident report during the shift on which the incident took place. → Give incident report to supervisor.

Incident reports are collected and summarized to detect patterns and trends and to highlight trouble spots. ← Administrator forwards pertinent information from the report to the appropriate department for follow-up action. ← Administrator reviews report. ← Unit supervisor forwards report to appropriate administrator within 24 hours.

Administrator reviews patterns and trends and decides whether incidents result from poor policies or staff errors. → If the incident results from policy problems, the health care facility makes appropriate policy changes.

If the incident results from staff errors, the health care facility directs appropriate personnel to investigate records to detect trends.

If the records indicate a pattern of errors or if the error being reviewed is grievous, the facility offers appropriate remediation, such as counseling, a refresher course or, rarely, probation or suspension.

- Document the patient's vital signs.
- Document that you performed a neurologic assessment and any abnormalities you find, including slurred speech, weakness in the extremities, or a change in mental status.
- Document that you notified the patient's practitioner and the time of the notification.

1/6/07	1400	Pt. found lying on
		floor beside her bed
		and chair. C/o pain in
		her Ⓡ hip area and
		difficulty moving Ⓡ leg.
		No abrasions or lacera-
		tions noted. BP ele-
		vated at 158/94; P 94;
		RR 22. States she fell
		trying to get to her
		chair. Mental status
		unchanged. Dr. Dayoub
		notified. Returned to
		bed. Hip X-ray reveals
		fractured Ⓡ hip. Pt.
		medicated for hip pain.
		Family notified by Dr.
		Dayoub. Assessed hourly.
		Discussed the need for
		side rails with pt. In-
		structed her in use of
		call button. Side rails
		up at present. ————
		—— Beverly Kotsur, RN

RESTRAINTS

Restraints are defined as any method of physically restricting a person's freedom of movement, physical activity, or normal access to his body. They can cause numerous problems, such as limited mobility, skin breakdown, impaired circulation, incontinence, and strangulation. Because of these complications, restraints are "prescriptive devices"—you can't use them unless you have a practitioner's order. In most facilities, the practitioner must renew the order every 24 hours. (See *Physical restraint order,* page 79.)

The medical record of all restrained patients must show evidence of:

- written orders for restraint or seclusion
- name of the licensed independent practitioner who ordered the restraint
- reason for the restraint
- type of restraint

- attempted alternatives to restraints, if any
- reassessment by a licensed independent practitioner for a continuation of the original order
- monitoring and reassessment of the patient in restraints. (See *Performance improvement outcome monitor for soft restraints,* page 80.)

BURNS

Burns are another common cause of injury to patients. Patients are burned by spilled hot food or liquids, hot baths, and electrical equipment. Always assess the risk of burns and take appropriate precautions. Document that you:

- cautioned patients with hand tremors not to handle hot foods or liquids by themselves
- taught patients with decreased sensation in their feet or hands to test bathwater with an unaffected extremity
- explained to patients taking medications that cause drowsiness that they may be more prone to burns and need to be cautious.

If a patient in your care does burn himself, always document the injury in his chart.

1/8/07	1100	Dropped hot cup of
		tea on Ⓡ thigh. Area
		slightly pink, sensitive
		to touch, with no
		edema. Dr. Adler noti-
		fied. Cold compresses
		ordered and applied.
		Pt. tolerates cold com-
		press well. Tylenol
		Extra-Strength 500 mg
		X 1 given with relief.
		—— Colleen Cameron, RN

DETERMINING A PATIENT'S RISK FOR FALLING

The Morse Fall Scale is one method of rapidly assessing a patient's likelihood of falling. It's widely used in hospital and long-term-care inpatient settings.

To use the scale, score each item and total the number of points. A score between 0 and 24 indicates no risk, 25 to 50 indicates low risk, and a score greater than 50 indicates a high risk for falling.

ITEM	SCALE		SCORING
History of falling; immediate or within 3 months	No Yes	0 25	*0*
Secondary diagnosis	No Yes	0 15	*0*
Ambulatory aid ■ Bed rest/nurse assist ■ Crutches/cane/walker ■ Furniture		0 15 30	*15*
I.V./Heparin Lock	No Yes	0 20	*20*
Gait/Transferring ■ Normal/bedrest/immobile ■ Weak ■ Impaired		0 10 20	*20*
Mental status ■ Oriented to own ability ■ Forgets limitations		0 15	*0*
TOTAL			55

Adapted with permission from Morse, J.M. *Preventing Patient Falls.* Thousand Oaks, Calif.: Sage Pubs., 1997.

DISCHARGE AMA

Although a patient can choose to leave a health care facility against medical advice (AMA) at any time, the law requires clear evidence that he's mentally competent to make that choice. In most facilities, an AMA form serves as a legal document to protect you, the practitioners, and the facility should any problems arise from a patient's unapproved discharge. The AMA form should clearly document:

● that the patient knows he's leaving against medical advice

PHYSICAL RESTRAINT ORDER

A form such as the one shown here must be in the patient's chart before physical restraints are applied. If a competent patient makes an informed decision to refuse restraints, the facility may require the patient to sign a release that would absolve the facility of liability should injury result from the patient's refusal to be restrained.

Date: _1/12/07_   **Time:** _0315_

Reason for restraint use (circle all that apply):

To prevent:

    1. High risk for self-harm

    2. High risk for harm to others

    ③ High potential for removing tubes, equipment, or invasive lines
         ℞ subclavian CV line

    4. High risk for causing significant disruption in the treatment environment

Duration of restraint: (Not to exceed 24 hr) _24 hr_

Type of restraint (circle all that apply):

    Vest

    Left mitt   Right mitt

    (Left wrist)   (Right wrist)

    Left ankle   Right ankle

    Other _____

Physician's signature _Colette Hendler, MD_

- that he has been advised of the risks of leaving and understands them
- that he knows he can come back.

If a patient refuses to sign the AMA form:

- document this refusal on the form
- document his refusal in his chart, using his own words to describe the refusal.

Include the following information on the AMA form:

- patient's reason for leaving AMA
- names of relatives or others notified of the patient's decision and the dates and times of the notifications
- an explanation of the risks and consequences of the AMA discharge, as told to the patient, including the name of the person who provided the explanation
- instructions regarding alternative sources of follow-up care given to the patient
- list of those accompanying the patient at discharge and the instructions given to them
- patient's destination after discharge.

Also follow these guidelines:

- Document statements and actions reflecting the patient's mental state at the time he chose to leave the facility. This will help protect you, the practitioners, and the facility against a charge of negligence. The patient may later claim that his discharge occurred while he was mentally incompetent

PERFORMANCE IMPROVEMENT OUTCOME MONITOR FOR SOFT RESTRAINTS

This form lists criteria for the use of soft restraints and for ensuring that interventions are properly documented.

Date: _1/3/07_   **Department:** _Nursing_

Room No.: _325_   **Staff signature:** _Pamela Petrakis, RN_

Criteria: Soft restraint: Any use of soft restraints (padded mitts, cloth wrist or ankle restraints, cloth vests)	Satisfactory	Unsatisfactory
1. Is there documentation of clinical justification for restraint?	✓	
2. Does the documentation show that less restrictive measures were attempted prior to restraints?	✓	
3. Is a clinical assessment documented prior to the use of restraint by an RN?	✓	
4. Is there a physician's order for each incident of restraint documented within 8 hours of restraints? Signed within 24 hours?	✓	
5. Is the time of going into restraint specified in the physician's order?	✓	
6. Is the physician's order time limited? Use "Not to exceed 24 hours" instead of "up to."	✓	
7. Is there an RN progress note written describing this incident? (Prior to and after discontinuation of restraint)	✓	
8. Does the restraint documentation reflect that the patient's needs were not neglected? (Review flow sheet.)	✓	
9. Does documentation reflect interventions of staff with patient after restraint?	✓	
10. Is the restraint record complete?	✓	
11. Does the documentation reflect the physical status of the patient prior to use of restraint and after removal of restraint?	✓	
12. Is the order renewed every 24 hours?	✓	

Comments:

and that he was improperly supervised while he was in that state.

● Check your facility's policy regarding incident reports. If the patient leaves without anyone's knowledge or if he refuses to sign the AMA form, you'll probably be required to complete an incident report.

In the patient's chart, be sure to document:

● time that you discovered the patient missing
● your attempts to find him
● people notified
● other pertinent information.

1/4/07	1500	Pt. found in room packing his clothes. When asked why he was dressed and packing, he stated, "I'm tired of all these tests. They keep doing tests, but they still don't know what's wrong with me. I can't take any more. I'm going home." Dr. Giordano notified and came to speak with pt. Wife notified and she came to the hospital. She was unable to persuade husband to stay. Pt. willing to sign AMA form. AMA form signed. Advised of possible risks of his leaving the hospital with headaches and hypertension. Pt. agrees to see Dr. Giordano in his office in 2 days. Discussed appointment with pt. and wife. Pt. going home after discharge. Accompanied patient in wheelchair to main lobby, with wife. Left at 1445. ———— Lynn Nakashima, RN

Missing patient

If you discover that a patient is missing, try to find him in the building and attempt to contact his home. Notify your nurse-manager, the patient's practitioner, and the police if there's a possibility of the patient hurting himself or others—especially if he has left the facility with any medical devices.

2

DOCUMENTING FROM ADMISSION TO DISCHARGE

Documentation must reflect the nursing process, which is based on theories of nursing and other disciplines and follows the scientific method. This problem-solving process:

● systematically organizes nursing activities to ensure the highest quality of care

● allows you to determine which problems you can help alleviate and which potential problems you can help prevent

● helps you to identify what kind and how much assistance a patient requires

● helps you to identify the person who can best provide assistance to the patient and the desired and actual treatment outcomes.

To get a complete picture of the patient's situation, you'll need to systematically follow and document the six steps of the nursing process—assessment, nursing diagnosis, outcome identification, planning, implementa-

---

SIX-STEP NURSING PROCESS

This flowchart shows the six steps of the nursing process and lists the forms you should use to document them.

Step 1
Assessment
Gather data from the patient's health history, physical examination, medical record, and diagnostic test results.
Documentation tools
Initial assessment form, flow sheets

Step 2
Nursing diagnosis
Make judgments based on assessment data.
Documentation tools
Nursing care plan, patient care guidelines, clinical pathway, progress notes, problem list

Step 3
Outcome identification
Set realistic, measurable goals with outcome criteria and target dates.
Documentation tools
Nursing care plan, clinical pathway, progress notes

tion, and evaluation. (See *Six-step nursing process*.)

Fundamentals of nursing documentation

To ensure clear communication and complete, accurate documentation of nursing care, you must keep in mind the fundamentals of documentation.

WRITE NEATLY AND LEGIBLY

Documentation allows you to communicate with other members of the health care team. Clean, legible documentation eases the communication process. Sloppy or illegible handwriting:
● confuses other members of the health care team and wastes time
● causes a patient potential injury if other caregivers can't understand crucial information.

If you don't have room to document something legibly:
● leave that section blank, put a bracket around it, and write, "see progress notes"
● document the information fully and legibly in the progress notes
● indicate the date and time when cross-referencing a progress note.

WRITE IN INK

Complete documentation in ink, not in pencil, which is susceptible to erasure and tampering. Also follow these guidelines:
● Use black or blue ink because other colors may not photocopy well.
● Don't use felt-tipped or gel ink pens on charts containing carbon paper; the pens may not produce sufficient pressure for copies.

USE CORRECT SPELLING AND GRAMMAR

Documentation filled with misspelled words and incorrect grammar creates the same negative impression as illegible handwriting. To avoid spelling and grammatical errors:

Step 4	Step 5	Step 6
Planning	**Implementation**	**Evaluation**
Establish care priorities, select interventions to accomplish expected outcomes, and describe interventions.	Carry out planned interventions.	Use objective data to assess outcome.
Documentation tools	**Documentation tools**	**Documentation tools**
Nursing care plan, patient care guidelines, clinical pathway	Progress notes, flow sheets	Progress notes

- keep a general and medical dictionary in documentation areas
- post a list of commonly misspelled words, especially terms and medications regularly used on the unit.

USE STANDARD ABBREVIATIONS

✦ *Patient safety* *Joint Commission on Accreditation of Healthcare Organizations (JCAHO) standards and many state regulations require health care facilities to use an approved abbreviation list to prevent confusion. To make sure that your documentation meets applicable standards:*
- *Know and use your facility's approved abbreviations.*
- *Place a list of approved abbreviations in documentation areas.*
- *Avoid using unapproved abbreviations because they may result in ambiguity, which may endanger the patient's health. (See* Abbreviations to avoid.*)*

WRITE CLEAR, CONCISE SENTENCES

- Avoid using a long word when a short word will do.
- Clearly identify the subject of the sentence.
- Use "I," as in "I contacted the patient's family at 1300 hours, and I explained the change in his condition." Doing so differentiates your actions from those of the patient, physician, or another staff member.

SAY WHAT YOU MEAN

- Be precise. Don't use inexact qualifiers such as "appears" or "apparently" because other caregivers reading the patient's chart may conclude that you weren't sure what you were describing or doing.
- State clearly and succinctly what you see, hear, and do.
- Don't sound tentative.

DOCUMENT PROMPTLY

- Document observations and nursing actions as soon as possible. If you put off documentation until the end of your shift, you may forget important details.
- Use bedside flow sheets to facilitate documentation throughout the shift. Keep these flow sheets in a secure place, such as a locked fold-down desk outside the patient's room, so confidentiality can't be breached.
- Use bedside computers to document promptly.
- Document on a worksheet or pad that you keep in your pocket when time is an issue. Jot down key phrases and times; then transcribe the information into the chart as soon as possible.

DOCUMENT THE TIME

- Be specific about times in the chart. Particularly document the exact time of:
  – sudden changes in the patient's condition
  – significant events
  – nursing actions.
- Avoid block documentation such as "0700 to 1500." This sounds vague and implies inattention to the patient.

DOCUMENT IN CHRONOLOGICAL ORDER

- Document observations, assessments, and interventions as you make them to keep them in chronological order and establish the pattern of care.

DOCUMENT ACCURATELY AND COMPLETELY

- Document facts, not opinions or assumptions.

ABBREVIATIONS TO AVOID

To reduce the risk of medical errors, the Joint Commission on Accreditation of Healthcare Organizations (JCAHO) has created an official "Do Not Use" list of abbreviations. In addition, JCAHO offers suggestions for other abbreviations and symbols to avoid.

OFFICIAL "DO NOT USE" LIST[1]

DO NOT USE	POTENTIAL PROBLEM	USE INSTEAD
U (unit)	Mistaken for "0" (zero), the number "4" (four) or "cc"	Write "unit"
IU (International Unit)	Mistaken for IV (intravenous) or the number 10 (ten)	Write "International Unit"
Q.D., QD, q.d., qd (daily) Q.O.D., QOD, q.o.d., qod (every other day)	Mistaken for each other Period after the Q mistaken for "I" and the "O" mistaken for "I"	Write "daily" Write "every other day"
Trailing zero (X.0 mg)* Lack of leading zero (.X mg)	Decimal point is missed	Write X mg Write 0.X mg
MS	Can mean morphine sulfate or magnesium sulfate	Write "morphine sulfate"
MSO_4 and $MgSO_4$	Confused for one another	Write "magnesium sulfate"

1 Applies to all orders and all medication-related documentation that is handwritten (including free-text computer entry) or on pre-printed forms.
* Exception: A "trailing zero" may be used only where required to demonstrate the level of precision of the value being reported, such as for laboratory results, imaging studies that report size of lesions, or catheter/tube sizes. It may not be used in medication orders or other medication-related documentation.

ADDITIONAL ABBREVIATIONS, ACRONYMS, AND SYMBOLS
(For possible future inclusion in the Official "Do Not Use" List)

DO NOT USE	POTENTIAL PROBLEM	USE INSTEAD
> (greater than) < (less than)	Misinterpreted as the number "7" (seven) or the letter "L" Confused for one another	Write "greater than" Write "less than"
Abbreviations for drug names	Misinterpreted due to similar abbreviations for multiple drugs	Write drug names in full
Apothecary units	Unfamiliar to many practitioners Confused with metric units	Use metric units
@	Mistaken for the number "2" (two)	Write "at"
cc	Mistaken for U (units) when poorly written	Write "ml" or "milliliters"
µg	Mistaken for mg (milligrams) resulting in one thousand-fold overdose	Write "mcg" or "micrograms"

© Joint Commission on Accreditation of Healthcare Organizations, 2006. Reprinted with permission.

Alert

WATCH YOUR
DOCUMENTATION LANGUAGE

At times, some of us may speak and write in a vague or judgmental manner without being aware of it. However, when you're documenting, you should conscientiously avoid including ambiguous statements and subjective judgments.

AMBIGUOUS TIME PERIODS

"Mrs. Brown asks for pain medication every so often." How would you interpret "every so often"—once an hour, once per shift, or once per day? Although you can't time each and every interaction or occurrence precisely, you should document time relationships when appropriate. In this case, for example, you might document, "Mrs. Brown asked for pain medication at 0800 and again at 1300."

AMBIGUOUS QUANTITIES

"A large amount of bloody drainage drained from the nasogastric tube." "A large amount" could mean 75 ml of fluid to you and 150 ml to another nurse. Document a specific measurement.

SUBJECTIVE JUDGMENTS

"Mr. Russo has a good attitude." How do you know? Support your judgment with an objective rationale—for example, "Mr. Russo states that he intends to learn insulin injection techniques before discharge."

Don't be afraid to give your impressions of the patient; just make sure that you support your observations—for example, "Leslie was frustrated, voicing dismay at being unable to walk around the room without help." Avoid using words such as "seems" or "appears"—they make you sound unsure of your observations.

- Document all relevant information relating to patient care and to the nursing process.
- Don't document routine tasks such as changing bed linens.

DOCUMENT OBJECTIVELY

- Document exactly what you see, hear, and do. (See *Watch your documentation language*.)
- When you document a patient's statement, use his exact words and quotation marks.
- Avoid making subjective statements such as "Patient's level of cooperation has deteriorated since yesterday." Instead, include the facts that led you to this conclusion. If you must document a conclusion, make sure to document the objective assessment data that supports it.
- Document data you have witnessed or data witnessed by a reliable source—such as the patient or another nurse. When you include information reported by someone else, cite your source.

SIGN EACH ENTRY

- Sign each entry you make in your progress notes with your first name or initial, full last name, and professional licensure, such as RN or LPN.
- If you find the last entry unsigned, immediately contact the nurse who made the entry and have her sign her name. If you can't locate her, notify the supervisor, who will follow up on the unsigned entry, and simply write and sign your progress notes. The different times and handwriting on the chart should dispel confusion as to the author. (See *Signing nurses' notes*.)

SIGNING NURSES' NOTES

To discourage others from adding information to the nurses' notes, draw a line through any blank spaces and sign your name at the far right of the column.

1/5/07	1200	Will continue plan and request enterostomal
		therapist to assess patient's knowledge and
		acceptance of colostomy on the 2nd postop
		day. ———————— Nora Martin, RN

If you don't have enough room to sign your name after the last word of your entry, draw a line from the last word to the end of the line. Then go to the next line and draw a line from the left margin toward the right margin, leaving room to sign your name on the far right side.

1/5/07	0900	Pt.'s respiratory status markedly improved after
		diuretic and O_2 therapy. Continue to monitor
		ABGs, urine output, weight, and breath sounds.
		Continue diuretic therapy as prescribed. ———
		————————— Nora Martin, RN

If you want to document a lot of information but think you'll run out of room on the page, leave space at the bottom of the page to write your signature. Start the next page with the date, time and the word "continued," then finish your notes and sign the second page as usual.

| 1/5/07 | 1500 | Morphine sulfate effective. Patient drowsy |
| | | and relaxed ——————— Nora Martin, RN |

| 1/5/07 | 1500 | Patient verbalized that pain is now 2 on a |
| (continued) | | scale of 0 to 10. ——————— Nora Martin, RN |

Assessment

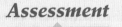

Assessment of a patient begins with the first encounter and continues throughout the patient's hospitalization as you obtain more information about his changing condition. The initial step of the nursing process, assessment includes collecting relevant information from various sources and analyzing it to form a complete picture of your patient. Accurate assessments:

● help guide you through the rest of the nursing process
● help you formulate nursing diagnoses, create patient problem lists, and write nursing care plans
● serve as a vital communication tool for other health care team members
● form a baseline from which to evaluate a patient's progress
● help you meet the requirements of JCAHO and other regulatory agencies
● provide a means of indicating that quality care has been given (Peer re-

view organizations and other quality assurance reviewers commonly look to the nursing assessment data as proof of quality care.)
- serve as evidence in court.

INITIAL ASSESSMENT

Perform an initial assessment when first meeting a patient. Before getting started, consider two questions:
- Which information will be most relevant for this patient?
- How much time do I have to gather the information?

Collecting relevant information

In your initial patient assessment, make sure to document:
- signs and symptoms
- chief complaint or medical diagnosis

- type of care received in another unit, such as the intensive care unit or the emergency department, if appropriate
- time the assessment was performed. (See *Complying with the time frame.*)

Also consider these questions:
- Why has the patient sought health care?
- What are his immediate problems and are they life-threatening?
- Does a potential for injury exist?
- What other influences—such as advanced age, fear, cultural differences, or lack of understanding—might affect treatment outcomes?
- What medications does he take?

● Does he have allergies to latex, medications, or foods? (See *Handling latex allergy.*)

Categorizing assessment data

Subjective information represents the patient's perception of his problem. A patient's complaint of chest pain, for example, is subjective information. Objective information is something you can observe and verify without interpretation—such as a patient's blood pressure reading. (See *Documenting subjective and objective information.*)

Sources of data

Information gathered directly from the patient (primary source data) is the most valuable because it reflects his situation most accurately. However, additional data about a patient can be obtained from secondary sources, including:

● family members
● friends
● other members of the health care team
● written records, such as past clinical records, transfer summaries, and personal documents such as a living will.

Gather as much information from secondary sources as possible. You'll find that it's helpful because:

● it gives you alternative viewpoints from the patient's
● the information you find may be essential to establish a complete profile because of a patient's condition or age
● family members and friends give important indications of family dy-

MAKING GENERAL OBSERVATIONS

Your general observations of the patient's appearance, mobility, communication ability, and cognitive function form an important part of your initial assessment. To save time, here are some specific characteristics to look for and document.

APPEARANCE
AGE
- Appears to be stated age
- Appears older or younger than stated age

PHYSICAL CONDITION
- Physically fit, strong, and appropriate weight for height
- Deconditioned, weak, and either underweight or overweight
- Apparent limitations, such as an amputation or paralysis
- Obvious scars or rash

DRESS
- Dressed appropriately or inappropriately for season
- Clean and wellkept clothes
- Soiled or torn clothes; smell of alcohol, urine, or feces

PERSONAL HYGIENE
- Clean and wellgroomed
- Unkempt; unshaved; dirty skin, hair, and nails
- Body odor or unusual breath odor

SKIN COLOR
- Appropriate for race
- Pale, ruddy, cyanotic, jaundiced, or tanned

MOBILITY
AMBULATION
- Walks independently; steady gait
- Uses a cane, crutches, or walker
- Unsteady, slow, hesitant, or shuffling gait; leans to one side; can't support own weight
- Transfers from chair to bed independently
- Needs assistance (from one, two, or three people) to transfer from chair to bed

MOVEMENT
- Moves all extremities
- Has right or leftsided weakness; paralysis
- Can't turn in bed independently
- Has jerky or spastic movements of body parts (specify)

COMMUNICATION
SPEECH
- Speaks clearly in English or other language
- Speaks only with one-word responses; doesn't respond to verbal stimuli
- Speech is slurred, hoarse, loud, soft, incoherent, hesitant, slow, fast, or nonsensical
- Has difficulty completing sentences because of shortness of breath or pain

HEARING
- Hears well enough to respond to questions
- Hard of hearing; wears hearing aid; must speak loudly into left or right ear
- Deaf; reads lips or uses sign language

VISION
- Sees well enough to read instructions in English or other language
- Wears corrective lenses to see or read
- Can't read
- Blind

COGNITIVE FUNCTIONS
AWARENESS
- Oriented; aware of surroundings
- Disoriented; unaware of time, place, and person

MOOD
- Responds appropriately; talkative
- Answers in one-word responses; offers information only in response to direct questions

■ Hesitates in answering questions; looks to family member before answering
■ Angry; states "Leave me alone" (or similar response); speaks loudly and abruptly to family members
■ Maintains or avoids eye contact

THOUGHT PROCESSES
■ Maintains a conversation; makes relevant statements; follows commands appropriately
■ Mind wanders; makes irrelevant statements; follows commands inappropriately

namics, educational needs, and available support systems
● including people close to the patient helps alleviate their feelings of helplessness during the hospitalization.

PERFORMING THE INITIAL ASSESSMENT
An initial assessment consists of your general observations, the patient's health history, and the physical examination. Remember to document the assessment as you perform it.

General observations
Observations can begin as soon as you meet the patient. By looking critically at him, you can collect valuable information about his:
● emotional state
● immediate comfort level
● mobility status
● general physical condition. (See *Making general observations.*)
　　When making observations, follow these guidelines:
● Document general observations made during the interview and physical examination as well as throughout the patient's hospitalization.
● Keep your observations objective, and don't draw conclusions.
● Document the facts.

Health history
The health history organizes pertinent physiologic, psychological, cultural, and psychosocial information. (See *Conducting the patient interview,* pages 92 and 93.) When documenting your patient's health history, include:
● subjective data about the patient's current health status that provide clues that point to actual or potential health problems
● the patient's ability to comply with health care interventions and his expectations for treatment outcomes
● details about the patient's lifestyle, family relationships, and cultural influences—all of which may affect his health care needs
● patient problems that your nursing interventions can help resolve.

Physical examination
Perform the physical examination by using the assessment techniques of inspection, palpation, percussion, and auscultation. When you document the physical examination, include:
● the scope of the physical examination
● objective data that may confirm or rule out suspicions raised during the health history interview
● findings that will enable you to plan care and start teaching the patient about his condition
● abnormal findings that require a more in-depth assessment.

CONDUCTING THE PATIENT INTERVIEW

When conducting a patient interview, show empathy, compassion, self-awareness, and objectivity to promote a trusting relationship with your patient.

TECHNIQUES TO USE

■ *Use general leads.* Broad opening questions allow the patient to relate information that he deems essential. Asking such questions as "What brought you to the hospital?" or "What concerns do you have?" encourages the patient to discuss what's most important to him.

■ *Restate information.* To help clarify the patient's meaning, restate or summarize the essence of his comments. For instance, suppose a patient says, "I have pain after I eat," and you respond, "So, you have pain about three times per day." This might prompt the patient to reply, "Oh no, I eat only breakfast, and then the pain is so severe that I don't eat for the rest of the day."

■ *Use reflection.* Asking a question in a different way offers the patient an opportunity to reconsider his response. A patient might say, "I've told you everything about my home life." Using reflection, you might respond, "Do you have other concerns about your situation after you leave the hospital?"

■ *State the implied meaning.* A patient may hint at difficulties or problems. By stating what he has left unspoken, you give him an opportunity to clarify his thoughts and accurately interpret the meaning of his statements. For example, a patient who remarks, "I'm sure my wife is glad that I'm in the hospital," may be implying several things. To clarify this statement, you might respond, "By saying your wife is glad, do you mean she has been concerned about your condition, or do you feel that you've been a burden to her at home?"

■ *Focus the discussion.* The patient may stray from the topic at hand to relate other information he feels you should know. You need to get the conversation back on track without insulting the patient or making him feel that the information isn't important. To help him refocus the conversation, you might say, "That's very interesting, but first

I'd like to get back to our discussion about your last hospitalization."

■ *Ask open-ended questions.* Questions that encourage the patient to express himself elicit more information than questions that call for a one-word response. If you ask, "Do you take your medications?" the patient may respond with a simple "Yes." But if you ask, "How do you take your medications?" you might discover that the patient takes his antihypertensive pills sporadically because they make him feel dizzy.

TIMESAVING MEASURES

■ Before the interview, fill in as much of the health history information as you can from secondary sources, such as admission forms, transfer summaries, and the medical history. This avoids duplication of effort and reduces interview time. If some of this information needs clarification, you can ask the patient to give you a fuller explanation.

■ Check your facility's policy regarding who can gather assessment data. You may be able to have a nursing assistant collect routine information, such as allergies and past hospitalizations. Remember, however, that you must review the information and verify it, as necessary.

■ Begin by asking about the patient's chief complaint and the reason for his hospitalization. Then, if the interview is interrupted, you'll have some initial information on which to base a care plan.

■ Use your facility's nursing assessment documentation form as a guide to organize information.

■ Take only brief notes during the interview to avoid interrupting the flow of conversation.

■ Document your findings using concise, specific phrases and approved abbreviations.

TECHNIQUES TO AVOID

■ *Don't ask judgmental or threatening questions.* A patient shouldn't have to justify his feelings or actions. Questions such as "Why did you do that?" or demanding statements such as "Explain your behavior" may be

perceived as a threat or challenge. When a patient doesn't have a specific answer to this type of question, he may invent an appropriate response merely to satisfy you.

■ *Don't ask probing and persistent questions.* This style of questioning can make the patient feel manipulated and defensive, so only make one or two attempts to obtain information about a particular subject. If the patient seems to be avoiding the topic or is reluctant to answer, reevaluate the relevance of the information.

■ *Don't use inappropriate language or technical terms or jargon.* Questions such as "Do you take that med q.i.d. or p.r.n.?" can intimidate or alienate the patient and his family. It can also make the patient feel that you're unwilling to share information about his condition or to converse on his level.

■ *Don't give advice.* Giving advice implies that you know what's best for the patient. Instead, you should encourage the patient and his family to participate in health care decisions. If the patient asks for advice, inform him about available options and then help him explore his own opinions about them.

■ *Don't provide false reassurance.* Statements such as "You'll be all right" or "Everything will work out fine" tend to devalue a person's feelings. By recognizing those feelings, you can open communication channels. Saying something such as, "You seem worried or frightened" encourages the patient to speak candidly. Always try to be honest and sensitive. Even when a patient asks, "Am I going to die?" you can honestly state, "I don't know. Tell me what makes you ask that."

A routine review for an adult patient on a medical-surgical unit includes a general survey of his height, weight, vital signs, and pulse oximetry as well as a review of the following body systems.

Respiratory system

After examining the respiratory system, document that you:
● assessed rate and rhythm of respirations and auscultated the lung fields
● inspected the lips, mucous membranes, and nail beds
● inspected any sputum for color, consistency, and other characteristics.

Cardiovascular system

After examining the cardiovascular system, document that you:
● auscultated for heart sounds
● assessed heart rate and rhythm
● assessed the color and temperature of the extremities
● assessed the peripheral pulses
● checked for edema
● inspected the neck veins.

Neurologic system

After examining the neurologic system, document that you:
● inspected the patient's head for evidence of trauma
● assessed the patient's level of consciousness, including his orientation to time, place, and person and his ability to follow commands
● assessed the patient's pupillary reactions and cranial nerve function
● assessed the patient's extremities for movement and sensation.

Eyes, ears, nose, and throat

After examining the eyes, ears, nose, and throat, document that you:
● assessed the patient's ability to see objects with or without corrective lenses as appropriate
● assessed the patient's ability to hear spoken words clearly
● inspected the patient's eyes and ears for discharge; the nasal mucous membranes for dryness, irritation, and the presence of blood; and teeth for cleanliness

- assessed how well the patient's dentures fit, if appropriate
- assessed the condition of the oral mucous membranes
- palpated the lymph nodes in the neck.

Gastrointestinal system

After examining the GI system, document that you:
- auscultated for bowel sounds in all quadrants
- assessed for abdominal distention or ascites
- palpated the abdomen to assess for tenderness.

Musculoskeletal system

After examining the musculoskeletal system, document that you:
- assessed the range of motion of major joints
- assessed for swelling at the joints as well as for contractures, muscular atrophy, or obvious deformity.

Genitourinary system

After examining the genitourinary system, document that you:
- assessed for bladder distention or incontinence
- inspected the genitalia for rashes, edema, or deformity, if indicated. (Inspection of the genitalia may be waived at the patient's request or if no dysfunction was reported during the interview.)

Reproductive system

After examining the reproductive system, document that you:
- inspected the genitalia for sexual maturity and abnormal discharge, if indicated
- performed a breast examination, if permitted, and whether you found abnormalities.

Integumentary system

After examining the integumentary system, document that you:

- inspected the patient for sores, lesions, scars, pressure ulcers, rashes, bruises, or petechiae
- assessed the patient's skin turgor.

MEETING JCAHO REQUIREMENTS

JCAHO requires health care professionals in accredited facilities to meet certain standards for performing patient assessments, determines whether these standards have been met by reviewing the documentation of patient assessments, and requires you to obtain assessment information from the patient's family or friends when appropriate. Make sure that you document the nature of the relationship and the time the person has known the patient.

Patient safety *Current JCAHO standards mandate that each patient's initial assessment include three key categories: physical, psychological and social, and environmental factors. To make sure that your assessment meets these standards, follow these guidelines:*

- *Document your findings from your review of the patient's major body systems.*
- *Document the patient's expectations, fears, anxieties, and other concerns related to his hospitalization as well as his support system. In your documentation, include information on the patient's family structure and role and roles within that structure, work status, income level, and socioeconomic concerns.*
- *Document where the patient lives (whether it's a house or an apartment) and whether he has adequate heat, ventilation, hot water, and bathroom facilities. Also document how many flights of stairs he has to climb, whether the layout of his home poses hazards, whether his home is convenient to stores and physicians' offices, and whether he uses equipment that isn't available in*

the hospital when he performs activities of daily living (ADLs) at home.

- *Document the patient's food and fluid intake and his elimination patterns. Also document recent weight gain or loss. A registered dietitian should be consulted as warranted by the patient's needs or condition.*
- *Document how the patient's ability to perform ADLs affects his compliance with his treatment regimen before and after discharge. Assess his ability to eat, wash, dress, use the bathroom, turn in bed, get out of bed, and get around. (Some health care facilities use a checklist to indicate if a patient can perform these tasks independently or if he needs partial or total assistance.) Document the use of assistive devices.*
- *Document your patient's knowledge of the disease process, self-care, diet, medications, lifestyle changes, treatment measures, and limitations resulting from the disease or its treatment. If he has factors that may hinder his learning—such as the nature of his illness or injury, health and religious beliefs, cultural practices, educational level, sensory deficits, language barriers, stress level, age, and pain or discomfort—document these as well.*
- *Document the patient's discharge planning needs as soon as possible. Document where he'll go after discharge and whether follow-up care will be accessible. Also document whether community resources, such as visiting nurse services and Meals On Wheels, are available where the patient lives.*

DOCUMENTING THE INITIAL ASSESSMENT

Initial assessment information can be referred to by any of several names, including the "nursing admission assessment" and the "nursing database." Some facilities have adopted initial assessment forms that include information gathered from different members of the health care team. These forms may be called "integrated," "interdisciplinary," or "multidisciplinary" care team assessment forms. (See *Integrated admission database form,* pages 96 to 104.)

Documentation styles

Initial assessment findings are documented in one of three basic styles:
- narrative notes
- standardized open-ended style
- standardized closed-ended style.

Many assessment forms use a combination of all three styles.

Narrative notes

Narrative notes consist of handwritten accounts in paragraph form that summarize information obtained by general observation, interview, and physical examination.

Advantages
- Allow findings to be listed in order of importance
- Are most practical for independent practitioners

Disadvantages
- Mimic the medical model by focusing on a review of body systems
- Are time-consuming to write and read
- Require the nurse to remember and document all significant information in a detailed, logical sequence—typically an unrealistic goal
- Can contain illegible handwriting that can easily lead to misinterpretation of findings
- Can waste time and jeopardize quality monitoring if used exclusively

Standardized open-ended style

The standardized open-ended style of documentation is the typical "fill-in-the-blanks" assessment form that comes with preprinted headings and

(Text continues on page 105.)

INTEGRATED
ADMISSION DATABASE FORM

Most health care facilities use a multidisciplinary admission form. The sample form here has spaces that can be filled in by the nurse, physician, and other health care providers.

Name _Beatrice Perry_   Admission Date _1/26/07_

Address _2 Clayton Street_   Time _1345_

    Dallas, Texas

Admitted per: _____ Ambulatory ✔ Stretcher _____ Wheelchair

T _97_   P _92_   R _24_   BP _98/52_   Ht. _5'2"_   Wt. _225 lb_

                   (estimated/actual)

ORIENTATION TO ROOM/UNIT POLICIES EXPLAINED

✔ Call light   _____ Living will on chart

✔ Bed operation   _____ Valuables form completed

✔ Phone   ✔ Elec.

✔ Television   ✔ Smoking

✔ Meals   _____ Side rails

_____ Advance directive explained   ✔ ID bracelet on

_____ Living will   _____ Visiting hours

SECTION COMPLETED BY: _P. Lippman, CST_   **TIME:** _1350_

Name and phone numbers of two people to call if necessary:

Name	Relationship	Phone#
Mary Ryan	daughter	665-2190
Thomas Perry	son	630-4785

REASON FOR HOSPITALIZATION (patient quote:) _I go numb in my rt. arm and leg_

ANTICIPATED DATE OF DISCHARGE: _1/28/07_

PREVIOUS HOSPITALIZATIONS: SURGERY/ILLNESS	DATE
TIA	12/15/06

Name _Beatrice Perry_   Date _1/26/07_

HEALTH PROBLEM

HEALTH PROBLEM	Yes	No	?
Arthritis		✔	
Blood problem (anemia, sickle cell, clotting, bleeding)		✔	
Cancer		✔	
Diabetes	✔		
Eye problems (cataracts, glaucoma)		✔	
Heart problem		✔	
Liver problem		✔	
Hiatal hernia		✔	
High blood pressure	✔		
HIV/AIDS		✔	
Kidney problem		✔	
Lung problem (emphysema, asthma, bronchitis, TB, pneumonia, shortness of breath)	✔		
Stroke		✔	
Ulcers		✔	
Thyroid problem		✔	
Psychological disorder		✔	
Alcohol abuse		✔	
Drug abuse			
Drug(s) _____		✔	
_____			
Smoking	✔		
Other _____			

Comments: _____

_____

ALLERGIES: ☐ no known allergies ☐ TAPE ☐ IODINE ☐ LATEX
☐ FOOD: _____
☑ DRUG: _Penicillin_
☐ BLOOD REACTION: _____
☐ OTHER: _____

MEDICATIONS: _____

HERBAL PREPARATIONS: _____

Information received from:
☑ Patient ☐ Relative _____ ☐ Friend _____ ☐ Other _____

Section completed by:
Jill O'Brien, RN   Date _1/26/07_   Time _1405_

(continued)

Name _Beatrice Perry_   Date _1/26/07_

All assessment sections are to be completed by a professional nurse.

✔ _____ Clean   _____ Disheveled

SKIN INTEGRITY: Indicate the location of any of the following on the chart below using the designated letter: a = rashes, b = lesions, c = significant bruises/abrasions, d = burns, e = pressure sores, f = recent scars, g = presence of tubes/appliances, h = other _b: ischemic ℞ leg ulcer (2 cm – healing)_

Comments: _____

GENERAL PHYSICAL APPEARANCE

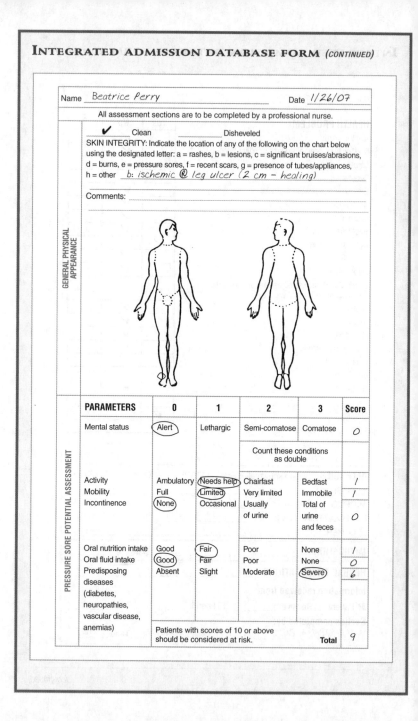

PRESSURE SORE POTENTIAL ASSESSMENT

PARAMETERS	0	1	2	3	Score
Mental status	(Alert)	Lethargic	Semi-comatose	Comatose	0
			Count these conditions as double		
Activity	Ambulatory	(Needs help)	Chairfast	Bedfast	1
Mobility	Full	(Limited)	Very limited	Immobile	1
Incontinence	(None)	Occasional	Usually of urine	Total of urine and feces	0
Oral nutrition intake	Good	(Fair)	Poor	None	1
Oral fluid intake	(Good)	Fair	Poor	None	0
Predisposing diseases (diabetes, neuropathies, vascular disease, anemias)	Absent	Slight	Moderate	(Severe)	6
	Patients with scores of 10 or above should be considered at risk.			**Total**	9

Name _Beatrice Perry_   Date _1/26/07_

FALL-RISK

Impaired: ____ Sensory function   ____ Mental status
         ____ Urinary/GI function   ____ General debility/weakness
         ____ Mobility function
         ✔ History of recent falls/dizziness/blackouts
            (automatically designates patient as prone-to-fall)
         ✔ Prone-to-fall risk (indicated on nursing Kardex ___✔___)

NEUROLOGICAL ASSESSMENT

____ Dizziness ____ Syncope ____ Headache ____ Blurred vision
____ Recent seizure ✔ Numbness/tingling location: _Rt. arm and leg_
LOC: ✔ Alert ____ Lethargic ____ Semi-comatose ____ Comatose
Mental Status: ✔ Oriented ____ Confused ____ Disoriented
Speech: ✔ Clear ____ Slurred ____ Garbled ____ Aphasic

Neurological Checklist

Right Arm / Left Arm	Right Leg / Left Leg	R. Pupil / L. Pupil	Pupil Reaction	Eyes Open	Best Verbal Response	Best Motor Response	Total
				Coma Scale			
+2/+4	+2/+4	5/6	+	4	5	6	15

+1: cannot move   +3: move against gravity
+2: cannot move against gravity   +4: move strongly against gravity

Pupil Reaction
+ Reactive   > Greater than
− Nonreactive   < Less than
D Dilated   = Equal
C Constricted   S Sluggish

CODE
Pupils (mm):
● ● ● ● ● ● ⬤ ⬤
1 2 3 4 5 6 7 8

COMA SCALE CODE	Response	1	2	3	4	5	6
	EYES OPEN	Never	To Pain	To Sound	Spontaneously		
	VERBAL	None	Incomprehensible Sounds	Inappropriate Words	Confused Conversation	Oriented	
	MOTOR	None	Extension	Flexion Abnormal	Flexion Withdrawal	Localizes Pain	

Comments: _numbness transient_

Signature _T. Jones, MD_

(continued)

Name *Beatrice Perry*   Date *1/26/07*

BEHAVIORAL

Behavior: ✔ Cooperative   ___ Depressed
           ___ Combative   ___ Unresponsive
           ___ Uncooperative ___ Restless
           ✔ Anxious   ___ Other _____
Religious/Spiritual beliefs: *Lutheran*
P. request to contact minister/priest/rabbi? ✔ Y   ___ N
Name *Rev. William Lacy*
Phone # *(555)726-8039*
Comments: _____

PAIN

Pt. having pain at present? ___ Y ✔ N
Pt. had pain in last several months? ___ Y ✔ N
Rate pain on a scale of 0 to 10 (0 = no pain, 10 = severe pain) _____
Pain location _____ Quality _____
Radiation ___ Y ___ N Duration _____
What aggravates pain? _____
What alleviates pain? _____
Effects on ADLs _____
Pt. pain goals _____

CARDIOVASCULAR

Skin color: ___ Normal ___ Flushed ___ Pale ✔ Cyanotic
Apical pulse: ___ Regular ✔ Irregular
Pacemaker: Type _____ Rate _____
Peripheral pulses: ✔ Present ___ Equal ✔ Weak ___ Absent
Comments: *bilat. weak lower extremities*
Specify: R ___ radial ___ pedal L ___ radial ___ pedal
Comments: _____
Edema: ___ No ✔ Yes *+1 bilat. pretibial*
Numbness: ___ No ✔ Yes Site: *Rt. arm and leg*
Chest pain: ✔ No ___ Yes ____
Family cardiac history: ___ No ✔ Yes
Telemetry Monitor: ___ No ✔ Yes Rhythm *normal sinus*
Comments: _____

PULMONARY

Respirations: ✔ Regular ___ Irregular
              ___ Shortness of breath ___ Dyspnea on exertion
O_2 use at home? ___ Yes ✔ No
Chest expansion: ✔ Symmetrical
                 ___ Asymmetrical (explain: _____)
Breath sounds: ___ Clear ___ Crackles ___ Rhonchi ✔ Wheezing
               ___ Location *bilat upper lobe, inspiratory*
Cough: None ✔ Nonproductive ___ Productive ___ Describe ____
Comments: *pulse oximetry 98% on 2 L; sleeps with 2 pillows*

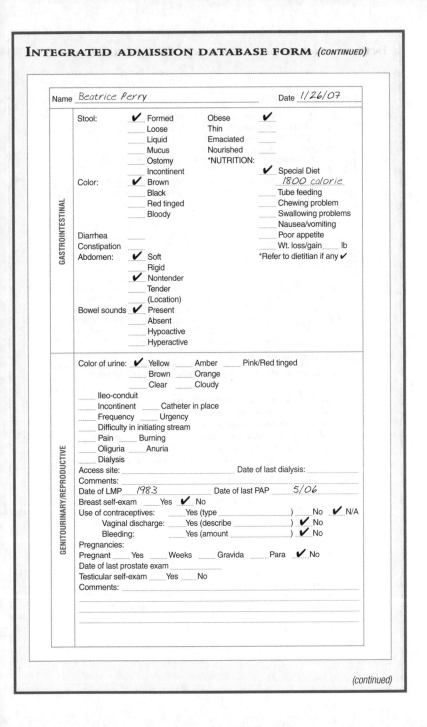

Name *Beatrice Perry*   Date *1/26/07*

GASTROINTESTINAL

Stool:
- ✔ Formed
- ___ Loose
- ___ Liquid
- ___ Mucus
- ___ Ostomy
- ___ Incontinent

- ___ Obese ✔
- ___ Thin
- ___ Emaciated
- ___ Nourished
- *NUTRITION:

Color:
- ✔ Brown
- ___ Black
- ___ Red tinged
- ___ Bloody

- ✔ Special Diet
  1800 calorie
- ___ Tube feeding
- ___ Chewing problem
- ___ Swallowing problems
- ___ Nausea/vomiting
- ___ Poor appetite
- ___ Wt. loss/gain ___ lb

Diarrhea ___
Constipation ___
Abdomen:
- ✔ Soft
- ___ Rigid
- ✔ Nontender
- ___ Tender
- ___ (Location)

*Refer to dietitian if any ✔

Bowel sounds ✔ Present
- ___ Absent
- ___ Hypoactive
- ___ Hyperactive

GENITOURINARY/REPRODUCTIVE

Color of urine: ✔ Yellow ___ Amber ___ Pink/Red tinged
___ Brown ___ Orange
___ Clear ___ Cloudy
___ Ileo-conduit
___ Incontinent ___ Catheter in place
___ Frequency ___ Urgency
___ Difficulty in initiating stream
___ Pain ___ Burning
___ Oliguria ___ Anuria
___ Dialysis
Access site: _____ Date of last dialysis: _____
Comments: _____
Date of LMP ___ *1983* ___ Date of last PAP ___ *5/06*
Breast self-exam ___ Yes ✔ No
Use of contraceptives: ___ Yes (type _____) ___ No ✔ N/A
Vaginal discharge: ___ Yes (describe _____) ✔ No
Bleeding: ___ Yes (amount _____) ✔ No
Pregnancies:
Pregnant ___ Yes ___ Weeks ___ Gravida ___ Para ✔ No
Date of last prostate exam _____
Testicular self-exam ___ Yes ___ No
Comments: _____

(continued)

Name _Beatrice Perry_   Date _1/26/07_

ACTIVITY/MOBILITY PATTERNS

____ Ambulates independently ____ Full ROM
____ Limited ROM (explain: _____)
✔ Ambulates with assistance (explain: _____)
✔ cane ____ walker ____ crutches
____ Gait steady/unsteady ____ Mobility in bed (ability to turn self) ____
Musculoskeletal
____ Pain ____ Weakness ____ Contractures ____ Joint swelling
____ Paralysis ____ Deformity ____ Joint stiffness ____ Cast
____ Amputation
Describe: _____
Comments: _____

REST/SLEEP PATTERNS

____ Use of sleeping aids _____ Sleeps _6_ hr/day
Comments: _____

Additional assessment comment: _On arrival, diaphoretic and ⊕ hand tremors. Vital signs stable. glucose 56 mg/dl. Orange juice and lunch given to patient. 2 hr postprandial glucose 204. Symptoms subsided with juice. Nutrition and diabetes educator consulted._ _____ _Jill O'Brien, RN_
MRI shows no cerebral lesions. Carotid doppler ultrasound pending. _____ _B. Mayer MD_

EDUCATION/DISCHARGE SECTION
Instructions: Assessment sections must be completed within 8 hours of admission. Discharge planning and summary must be completed by day of discharge.

Yes	No	
✔		Patient understands current diagnosis
✔		Family/significant other understands diagnosis
✔		Patient able to read English
✔		Patient able to write English
✔		Patient able to communicate
	✔	Patient/family understands pre-hospital medication/treatment regimen

Yes	No	**Emotional factors:**
✔		Patient appears to be coping
✔		Family appears to be coping
	✔	Any suspicion of family violence
	✔	Any suspicion of family abuse
	✔	Any suspicion of family neglect

Comments: _diabetic teaching_ _____

Language spoken, written, and read (other than English): _____
Interpreter services needed: ✔ No ____ Yes
Are there any barriers to learning (e.g., emotional, physical, cognitive)? _No_
Religious or cultural practices that may alter care or teaching needs?
____ Yes ✔ No Describe: _____
Is pt/family motivated to learn? ✔ Yes ____ No Describe: _____

INTEGRATED ADMISSION DATABASE FORM *(CONTINUED)*

Name _Beatrice Perry_   Date _1/26/07_

DISCHARGE ASSESSMENT

Living arrangements/caregiver (relationship): _____ lives alone _____

Type of dwelling:

___Apartment ✔House ___Nursing home

___More than 1 floor? ✔Yes___No Describe: _____

___Boarding home ___Other _____

Physical barriers in home:

✔No ___Yes (explain: _____)

Access to follow-up medical care:

✔Yes ___No (explain: _____)

Ability to carry out ADLs: ___Self-care ✔Partial assistance ___Total assistance

Needs help with:

✔Bathing ___Feeding ___Ambulation ___Other _____

Anticipated discharge destination:

✔Home ___Rehab. ___Nursing home ___SNF ___Boarding home

___Other _____

Currently receiving services from a community agency? ___Yes ✔No

If yes, check which one ___Visiting nurses ___Meals on Wheels

Concerned about returning home?

___Being alone ___Financial problems ___Homemaking ___Meal prep.

✔Managing ADLs ___Other _____

Assessment completed by:

J. OBrien, RN   Date _1/26/07_ Time _1430_

Assessment completed by:

B. Mayer, MD   Date _1/26/01_ Time _1445_

DISCHARGE PLANNING

Resources notified	Name	Date	Time	Signature
Social worker				
Home care coordinator	M. Murphy, RN	1/28/07	0900	J. OBrien, RN
Other_____				

Equipment/supplies needed: _stair chair_ _____

Arranged for by:

M. Murphy, RN   Date _1/28/07_ Time _0930_

Comments: _Daughter to stay with pt at home_ _____

(continued)

Name _Beatrice Perry_   Date _1/26/07_

DISCHARGE SUMMARY

Alterations in patterns (If yes, explain.)	Yes	No	Explanation
Nutrition	✔		adherence to diet regimen
Elimination		✔	
Self-care		✔	
Skin integrity		✔	
Mobility	✔		needs help with stairs
Comfort pain		✔	
Mental status/behavior		✔	
Vision/hearing/speech		✔	

Discharge instructions given (specify): _standard hosp. discharge instruction sheet_

Effects of illness on employment/lifestyle: _____

Central venous line removed: _N/A_ By whom: _____

Belongings sent with patient:

✔ clothes ✔ dentures ✔ eyeglasses

___ hearing aid ___ prosthesis ___ valuables

✔ prescriptions ✔ other _cane_

Follow-up medical supervision to be provided by: _Dr. Schneider_

✔ Patient/family instructed to call for follow-up appointment

Discharge destination: _pt's home with daughter_

Section completed by:

C. Rafferty, RN   Date _1/28/07_   Time _1130_

DOCUMENTING ASSESSMENT ON AN OPEN-ENDED FORM

At some health care facilities, you may use a standardized open-ended form to document initial assessment information. Below, you'll find a portion of such a form.

Reason for hospitalization *"My blood sugar is high."*
Expected outcomes *By discharge, the patient and his family will understand the disease process of diabetes mellitus, demonstrate correct insulin administration techniques, and identify signs and symptoms of hyperglycemia and hypoglycemia.*

Last hospitalization
Date *1/05/07*   Reason *high blood pressure*

Medical history   *hypertension, diabetes mellitus*

Medications and allergies

Drug	Dose	Time of last dose	Patient's statement of drug's purpose
Humulin N	30 units	0730	for sugar
Humulin R	5 units	0730	for sugar
furosemide	20 mg	1000	water pill
atenolol	50 mg	0800	for BP

Allergy	Reaction
shellfish	hives

---

questions. (See *Documenting assessment on an open-ended form.*)

Advantages
● Allows information to be categorized under specific headings and questions
● Can be completed using partial phrases and approved abbreviations

Disadvantages
● Doesn't always provide enough space or instructions to encourage thorough descriptions
● Can contain nonspecific responses that can lead to misinterpretation

Standardized closed-ended style
Standardized closed-ended assessment forms provide preprinted headings, checklists, and questions with specific responses. You simply check

DOCUMENTING ASSESSMENT ON A CLOSED-ENDED FORM

At some health care facilities, you may use a standardized closed-ended form to document initial assessment information. Below you'll find a portion of such a form.

SELF-CARE ABILITY

Activity	1	2	3	4	5	6
Bathing		✔				
Cleaning		✔				
Climbing stairs			✔			
Cooking	✔					
Dressing and grooming		✔				
Eating and drinking	✔					
Moving in bed	✔					
Shopping					✔	
Toileting			✔			
Transferring			✔			
Walking		✔				
Other home functions			✔			

Key
1 = Independent
2 = Requires assistive device
3 = Requires personal assistance
4 = Requires personal assistance and assistive device
5 = Dependent
6 = Experienced change in last week

Assistive devices
- ☑ Bedside commode
- ☐ Brace or splint
- ☐ Cane
- ☐ Crutches
- ☐ Feeding device
- ☐ Trapeze
- ☑ Walker
- ☐ Wheelchair
- ☐ Other
- ☐ None

Activity tolerance
- ☐ Normal
- ☑ Weakness
- ☐ Dizziness
- ☑ Exertional dyspnea
- ☐ Dyspnea at rest
- ☐ Angina
- ☐ Pain at rest
- ☐ Oxygen needed
- ☐ Intermittent claudication
- ☐ Unsteady gait
- ☐ Other

Rest pattern
Sleep habits
- ☑ Less than 8 hours
- ☐ 8 hours
- ☐ More than 8 hours
- ☐ Morning nap
- ☑ Afternoon nap

Sleep difficulties
- ☐ Insomnia
- ☑ Early awakening
- ☐ Unrefreshing sleep
- ☐ Nightmares
- ☐ None

off the appropriate response. (See *Documenting assessment on a closed-ended form*.)

Advantages
- Saves time
- Eliminates the problem of illegible handwriting and makes checking documented information easy
- Can be easily incorporated into most computerized systems
- Clearly establishes the type and amount of information required by the health care facility
- Uses guidelines that clearly define responses, even though closed-ended forms usually use nonspecific terminology, such as "within normal limits" or "no alteration"

Disadvantages
- May not provide a place to document relevant information that doesn't fit the preprinted choices
- Can be lengthy, especially when a facility's policy calls for documenting in-depth physical assessment data

Documentation formats
Historically, nursing assessment has followed a medical format emphasizing the patient's initial symptoms and a comprehensive review of body systems. However, some facilities have adopted formats that more readily reflect the nursing process. Other documentation formats are modeled on specific conceptual frameworks based on published nursing theories and include the following systems.
- *Human response patterns*. NANDA-International (NANDA-I) has developed a classification system for nursing diagnoses based on human response patterns that relate directly to actual or potential health problems, as indicated by assessment data. Using an assessment form organized by these patterns allows you to easily es-

tablish appropriate diagnoses while you document assessment data—especially if a listing of diagnoses is included with the form.
- *Functional health care patterns*. Developed by Marjory Gordon, this system classifies nursing data according to the patient's ability to function independently. Many nurses consider this system easier to understand and remember than human response patterns.
- *Conceptual frameworks*. These assessment forms, which are based on nursing philosophies, reflect the individual theory's approach to nursing care. Some examples include:
  - Dorothea Orem's self-care model
  - Imogene King's theory of goal attainment
  - Sister Callista Roy's adaptation model.

Documenting learning needs
Most initial assessment forms have a separate section for documenting a patient's learning needs. When you reassess your patient's learning needs, document your findings in:
- the progress notes
- an open-ended patient education flow sheet
- a structured patient education flow sheet designed for a specific problem such as diabetes mellitus.

Documenting discharge planning needs
Effective discharge planning begins when you identify and document the patient's needs during the initial assessment. (See *Documenting discharge planning needs*, pages 108 and 109.) Document the patient's discharge needs on:
- the initial assessment form (in a designated section)

DOCUMENTING
DISCHARGE PLANNING NEEDS

How and where you document your discharge planning will depend on the policy at the health care facility where you work. Here's one of the more common ways of documenting this information.

DISCHARGE PLANNING NEEDS

Occupation _Retired college professor_

Language spoken _English_

Patient lives with _Wife_

Self-care capabilities _Needs extensive assistance_

Assistance available

☐ Cooking

☐ Cleaning

☑ Shopping

☑ Dressing changes/treatments   _Irrigate Ⓛ lower leg wound b.i.d._
with ½ strength H_2O_2, followed by rinse with normal saline so-
lution. Pack with ½" iodoform gauze. Apply dry sterile dressing.

Medication administration routes

☑ P.O.	☐ S.C.
☐ I.V.	☐ Other: _____
☐ I.M.	_____

Dwelling

☐ Apartment	☑ Kitchen
☑ Private home	(gas stove)
☐ Single room	electric stove
☐ Institution	wood stove
☐ Elevator	☐ Other: _____
☑ Outside steps	☑ Bathrooms (number) _2_
(number) _6_	(location) _one upstairs, one_
☑ Inside steps	_downstairs_
(number) _12_	☑ Telephones (number) _1_
	(location) _kitchen_

Transportation
- ☐ Drives own car
- ☐ Takes public transportation
- ☑ Relies on family member or friend

After discharge, patient will be:
- ☐ Home alone
- ☑ Home with family
- ☐ Other: _____

Patient has had help from:
- ☑ Visiting nurse
- ☑ Housekeeper
- ☑ Other: *social worker* _____

Anticipated needs *Nurse for dressing changes, transportation*
for groceries, etc.
Social service requests *VNA*
Date contacted *1/16/07* **Reason** *Contacted VNA for*
dressing changes and transportation needs. —Susan Reed, RN

- a specially designed discharge planning form
- a separate section on the patient care card file
- the progress notes
- a discharge planning flow sheet.

Documenting incomplete initial data

You may not always be able to obtain a complete health history during the initial assessment. When this occurs, base your initial assessment on your observations and physical examination of the patient. When documenting your findings, follow these guidelines:

- Be sure to write something such as, "Unable to obtain complete data at this time." Otherwise, it might appear that you failed to perform a complete assessment.
- Obtain missing information as soon as possible, either when the patient's condition improves or when family members or other secondary sources are available.
- Document how and when you obtained the missing data.
- When adding information to complete an initial assessment, be sure to revise your nursing care plan accordingly. Depending on your facility's policy:

JCAHO REASSESSMENT GUIDELINES

The following reassessment guidelines are suggested by the Joint Commission on Accreditation of Healthcare Organizations (JCAHO).
- Reassessment occurs at regular intervals in the course of care.
- Reassessment determines a patient's response to care.
- Significant change in a patient's condition results in reassessment.
- Significant change in a patient's diagnosis results in reassessment.

– *Document the information on the progress notes.* This method aids in the day-to-day communication with others who read the notes, but makes it difficult to retrieve the data later.

– *Return to the initial assessment form and add the new information along with the date and your signature.* This method makes it easy to retrieve data when needed—either during the patient's hospitalization or after discharge for quality assurance.

ONGOING ASSESSMENT

Assessment of a patient is a continuous process; how often you reassess a patient depends primarily on his condition, JCAHO requirements, and your facility's policy. (See *JCAHO reassessment guidelines.*)

Reassessment and effective documentation of your findings:
- allow you to evaluate the effectiveness of nursing interventions and determine your patient's progress toward the desired outcomes
- facilitate communication with other health care practitioners
- allow you to plan the most appropriate patient care.

USING FLOW SHEETS

You'll usually document ongoing assessment data on flow sheets or in narrative notes on the patient's progress report. Ideally, though, you should use flow sheets to document all routine assessment data and routine interventions. They:
- allow you to shorten the narrative notes to include only information regarding the patient's progress toward achieving desired outcomes as well as any unplanned assessments.
- are a quick and consistent way to highlight trends in the patient's condition, when used to document routine assessment data.

Because flow sheets are legally accepted components of the patient's medical record, they must be documented correctly. Follow these guidelines:
- Give yourself enough time to evaluate each piece of information on the flow sheet.
- Make sure that your documentation accurately reflects the patient's current clinical status.
- When documenting only the information requested on a flow sheet isn't sufficient to give a complete picture of the patient's status, document additional information in the space provided on the flow sheet. If your

flow sheet doesn't have additional space, and you need to document more information, use the progress notes.

• If additional information isn't necessary, draw a line through the space. Doing so indicates that, in your judgment, further information isn't required.

Nursing diagnosis and care plan

Identify nursing diagnoses carefully. Then write a plan that not only fits your nursing diagnoses but also fits your patient. The plan should consider the patient's needs, age, developmental level, culture, strengths and weaknesses, and willingness and ability to take part in his care.

FORMULATING NURSING DIAGNOSES

Unlike a medical diagnosis, which focuses on the patient's pathophysiology or illness, a nursing diagnosis focuses on the patient's responses to illness. (See *Nursing diagnoses: Avoiding the pitfalls.*)

Types of nursing diagnoses
Depending on the policy of your health care facility, you'll either use standardized diagnoses or formulate your own diagnoses.

NURSING DIAGNOSES: AVOIDING THE PITFALLS

To avoid making common mistakes when formulating your nursing diagnoses, follow these guidelines.

USE NURSING DIAGNOSES
Don't use medical diagnoses or interventions. Terms such as *angioplasty* and *coronary artery disease* belong in a medical diagnosis—not in a nursing diagnosis.

USE ALL RELEVANT ASSESSMENT DATA
If you focus only on the physical assessment, for instance, you might miss psychosocial or cultural information relevant to your diagnoses.

TAKE YOUR TIME
Take enough time to analyze the assessment data. If you rush, you might easily miss something important.

INTERPRET THE ASSESSMENT DATA ACCURATELY
Make sure that you follow established norms, professional standards, and interdisciplinary expectations in interpreting the assessment data. In addition, don't permit your biases to interfere with your interpretation of information.

For instance, don't assume your patient is exaggerating if he states that he feels pain during what you would consider a painless procedure. If possible, have the patient verify your interpretation.

KEEP DATA UP-TO-DATE
Don't stop assessing and updating your diagnoses after the initial examination. As the patient's condition changes, your evaluation should be updated.

To formulate your nursing diagnoses, you must evaluate the essential assessment information. These questions will help you quickly zero in on the appropriate data.
- Which signs and symptoms does the patient have?
- Which assessment findings are abnormal for this patient?
- How do particular behaviors affect the patient's wellbeing?
- What strengths or weaknesses does the patient have that affect his health status?
- Does he understand his illness and treatment?
- How does the patient's environment affect his health?
- Does he want to change his state of health?
- Do I need to gather more information for my diagnoses?

Benefits of using standardized diagnoses

- By using nationally standardized diagnoses, such as NANDA-I's Taxonomy II, health care facilities make communication easier and diagnoses more precise.
- Diagnoses can be categorized according to nursing models, but other ways of categorizing diagnoses—for instance, according to Orem's self-care model—may also be used.
- Health care facilities or units can establish their own list of nursing diagnoses, categorizing them according to medical diagnoses and surgical procedures.

Benefits of formulating your own nursing diagnoses

- Developing your own diagnoses prevents the usage of standardized diagnoses that may be incomplete or that use overly formal or abstract language.
- Developing your own diagnoses can help you characterize a problem that standardized diagnoses don't readily address.

Deciding on a diagnosis

Evaluate relevant assessment data by looking at a standardized assessment form that groups related information into categories. Looking at the data in these groupings lets you determine which patient needs require nursing intervention and associate relevant nursing diagnoses with specific assessment findings. (See *Evaluating assessment data.* Also see *Relating assessment data to nursing diagnoses.*)

Components of the diagnosis

- *The human response or problem.* The first part of the diagnosis, the human response, identifies an actual or a potential problem that can be affected by nursing care.
- *Related factors.* The second part of the nursing diagnosis identifies related factors, which may precede, contribute to, or simply be associated with the human response. They make your diagnosis more closely fit the particular patient and help you choose the most effective interventions.

RELATING ASSESSMENT DATA TO NURSING DIAGNOSES

Some assessment forms group assessment information and relevant nursing diagnoses together so that you can immediately relate one to the other. This saves you from looking back through the form for assessment data when determining the nursing diagnosis. Here's a section of this type of form.

Patient *Michael Ramsey*   **Age** *72*
Medical diagnosis: *Heart failure*

ASSESSMENT FINDINGS	NURSING DIAGNOSES

Cardiopulmonary

Breath sounds
crackles, bilateral bases

Breathing pattern
☑ cough   *dry*   ☐ smoker

Dyspnea
☐ on exertion   ☐ nocturnal

Sputum
color _____

consistency _____

Heart sounds
S₃ and S₄ present

Peripheral pulses
all peripheral pulses +1

Edema
☑ Extremities *ankles*
☐ Other _____

Cyanosis
☑ Extremities *nail beds*
☑ Other *lips*

☑ Impaired gas exchange
☐ Ineffective airway clearance
☐ Impaired spontaneous ventilation
☑ Ineffective breathing pattern
☑ Decreased cardiac output
☐ Ineffective tissue perfusion (peripheral)
☐ Ineffective tissue perfusion (cardiopulmonary)

(continued)

Patient *Michael Ramsey*   Age *72*
Medical diagnosis: *Heart failure*

ASSESSMENT FINDINGS	NURSING DIAGNOSES
Nutrition	
Diet __2G Na, low cholesterol__	☑ Imbalanced nutrition: Less than body requirements
Appetite	☐ Imbalanced nutrition: More than body requirements
☐ normal	☐ Risk for imbalanced nutrition: More than body requirements
☐ increased	
☑ decreased	
☐ vomiting	
☐ nausea	

• *Signs and symptoms.* A complete nursing diagnosis includes the signs and symptoms that lead you to the diagnosis—what NANDA calls the "defining characteristics."

Outcome identification

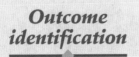

After you've determined your nursing diagnoses, rank them based on which problems require immediate attention. Maslow's hierarchy of needs is generally accepted as the basis for setting priorities. (See *Maslow's hierarchy of needs.*) When ranking diagnoses, follow these guidelines:

• Typically, the first nursing diagnosis will stem from the primary medical diagnosis or from the patient's chief complaint. This nursing diagnosis points out a threat to the patient's physical well-being.

• Rank related nursing diagnoses, which pose less immediate threats to the patient's well-being, next.

• In most cases, list nursing diagnoses that pertain to the patient's psychosocial, emotional, or spiritual needs last.

• Keep in mind that although a nursing diagnosis may have a lower priority, you shouldn't wait to intervene until you've resolved all the higher-priority problems. Meeting a lower-priority goal may help resolve a higher-priority problem.

• Whenever possible, include the patient in this process.

Maslow's hierarchy of needs

Abraham Maslow's hierarchy of needs, shown below, is a system for classifying human needs that may prove useful when establishing priorities for your patient's care, especially if he has several nursing diagnoses. According to Maslow, a person's lower-level physiologic needs must be met before higher-level needs—those less crucial to survival—can be addressed. In fact, higher-level needs may not become apparent until lower-level needs are at least partially met.

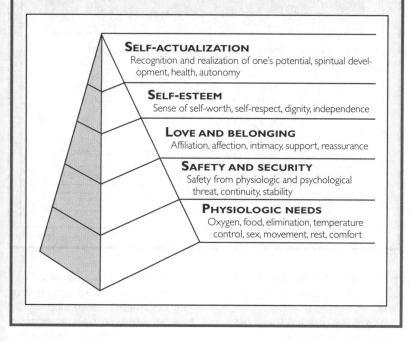

SELF-ACTUALIZATION
Recognition and realization of one's potential, spiritual development, health, autonomy

SELF-ESTEEM
Sense of self-worth, self-respect, dignity, independence

LOVE AND BELONGING
Affiliation, affection, intimacy, support, reassurance

SAFETY AND SECURITY
Safety from physiologic and psychological threat, continuity, stability

PHYSIOLOGIC NEEDS
Oxygen, food, elimination, temperature control, sex, movement, rest, comfort

DEVELOPING EXPECTED OUTCOMES

Based on the nursing diagnoses, expected outcomes are measurable goals that the patient should reach as a result of planned nursing interventions and may specify an improvement in the patient's ability to function. When developing expected outcomes, remember that:

● one nursing diagnosis may require more than one expected outcome.

● each outcome should call for the maximum realistic improvement for a particular patient.

Writing outcome statements

An outcome statement should include four components:
● specific behavior that will demonstrate the patient has reached his goal
● criteria for measuring the behavior
● conditions under which the behavior should occur

WRITING AN OUTCOME STATEMENT

An outcome statement should consist of four components:

B	M	C	T

BEHAVIOR
A desired behavior for the patient. This behavior must be observable.

MEASURE
Criteria for measuring the behavior. The criteria should specify how much, how long, how far, and so on.

CONDITION
The conditions under which the behavior should occur.

TIME
The time by which the behavior should occur.

As indicated, the two outcome statements below have these four components.

Limit sodium intake	2 g/day	using hospital menu	by 1/21/07
Eat	50% of all meals	unassisted	by 1/21/07

● time by which the behavior should occur. (See *Writing an outcome statement.*)

When you're writing outcome statements, follow these guidelines:
● *Make your statements specific.* Use action verbs, such as *walks, demonstrates, consumes,* and *expresses.* Clearly state which behaviors you expect the patient to exhibit and when.
● *Focus on the patient.* The outcome statement should reflect the patient's behavior—not your intervention.
● *Let the patient help you.* A patient who takes part in developing outcome statements is more motivated to achieve his goals. His input—and the input of family members—can help you set realistic goals.

● *Take medical orders into account.* Don't write outcome statements that ignore or contradict medical orders.
● *Adapt the outcome to the circumstances.* Consider the patient's coping ability, age, educational level, cultural influences, support systems, living conditions, and socioeconomic status. Consider his anticipated length of stay when you're deciding on time limits for achieving goals, and consider the health care setting itself.
● *Change your statements as necessary.* Sometimes you may need to revise even the most carefully written outcome statements. If the patient has trouble reaching his goal, choose a later target date or change the goal to one the patient can reach more easily.

- *Use shortcuts.* Save documenting time by including only the essentials in your outcome statements. Omit the words "Patient will" from your outcomes because "patient" is understood. Rather than writing "Patient will demonstrate insulin self-administration by 1/18/07," simply write "Demonstrate insulin self-administration by 1/18/07." Many facilities use abbreviations for target dates, such as "HD2" for "hospital day 2" and "POD3" for "postoperative day 3."

Planning

Planning interventions is a nursing action that you and your patient agree will help him reach the expected outcomes. Their proper selection is important. When selecting interventions, follow these guidelines:

- Base interventions on the second part of your nursing diagnosis, the related factors.
- Write at least one intervention for each outcome statement.
- Start by considering interventions that you or your patient have previously used successfully.
- Select interventions from standardized care plans.
- Talk and brainstorm with your colleagues about interventions they have used successfully, and check nursing journals that discuss interventions for standardized nursing diagnoses.

WRITING INTERVENTION STATEMENTS

Intervention statements must communicate your ideas clearly to other staff members. When writing your interventions, follow these guidelines:

- *List assessment as an intervention.* One of the first interventions in your care plan must include an assessment intervention to allow for reevaluation of the problem in the nursing diagnosis.
- *Clearly state the necessary action.* Include as much specific detail as possible in your interventions to allow continuity of care. Note how and when to perform the intervention as well as any special instructions.
- *Tailor the intervention to the patient.* Keep in mind the patient's age, condition, developmental level, environment, and value system when writing your interventions.
- *Keep the patient's safety in mind.* Take into account the patient's physical and mental limitations so that your interventions don't worsen existing problems or create new ones.
- *Follow the rules of your health care facility.* If your facility has a rule that only nurses may administer medications, don't write an intervention calling for the patient to "administer hemorrhoidal suppositories as needed."
- *Take other health care activities into account.* Necessary activities may interfere with interventions you want to use. Adjust your interventions accordingly.
- *Include available resources.* Make use of the facility's resources as well as available outside sources.

WRITING YOUR CARE PLAN

A good care plan is the blueprint for concise, meaningful documentation. If you write a good care plan, your nurses' notes will practically write themselves. A good plan consists of:

- prioritized patient problems identified during the admission interview and hospitalization
- realistic, measurable expected outcomes and target dates
- specific nursing interventions that will help the patient or his family achieve these outcomes
- an evaluation of the patient's responses to intervention and progress toward outcome achievement
- patient teaching and discharge plans.

Types of nursing care plans

Two basic types of care plans exist: traditional and standardized. No matter which you choose, your plan should cover all nursing care from admission to discharge and should be a permanent part of the patient's medical record.

Traditional care plan

Also called the *individually developed care plan,* the traditional care plan is written from scratch for each patient. The basic form and what you must include can vary, depending on the health care facility or department. When writing one of these plans, keep these points in mind:
- Most forms have four main columns: one for nursing diagnoses, another for expected outcomes, a third for interventions, and a fourth for outcome evaluation. Other columns allow you to enter the date you initiated the care plan, the target dates for expected outcomes, and the dates for review, revisions, and resolution.

- Most forms also have a place to sign or initial when you make an entry or a revision.
- Most facilities require you to write only short-term outcomes that the patient should reach before discharge. However, some facilities—particularly long-term care facilities—want to include long-term outcomes that reflect the maximum functional level the patient can reach. (See *Using a traditional care plan,* pages 120 and 121.)

Standardized care plan

Developed to save documentation time and improve the quality of care, standardized care plans provide a series of standard innovations for patients with similar diagnoses. (See *Using a standardized care plan,* pages 122 and 123.)

When writing one of these plans, customize it to fit your patient's specific needs. To do this, fill in:
- related factors and signs and symptoms for a nursing diagnosis
- time limits for the outcomes
- frequency of interventions
- specific instructions for interventions.

Practice guidelines

Also referred to as protocols, practice guidelines give specific sequential instructions for treating patients with a particular problem. They're used to manage patients with specific nursing diagnoses. (See *Practice guidelines for acute pulmonary edema,* pages 124 and 125. Also see *Managing ineffective breathing pattern,* page 126.)

Advantages of practice guidelines

- Because they spell out the steps to follow for a patient with a particular

nursing diagnosis, practice guidelines help you provide thorough care and ensure that the patient receives consistent care from all caregivers.

- They specify what to teach the patient and what to document, and include a reference section that lets you quickly determine how up-to-date they are.
- They spell out the role of other health care professionals, helping all team members coordinate their efforts.
- They supply comprehensive instruction and help teach inexperienced staff members.
- They save documentation time.

Using practice guidelines

- Choose the guidelines that best fit your patient. You'll probably use some practice guidelines, such as the generic one for pain, and rarely use other guidelines.
- Note in the interventions section that you'll follow the guideline.
- List the practice guidelines you plan to use on a flow sheet.
- Document any modifications you'll need to make.
- After your interventions, document in your progress notes that you followed the practice guidelines, or check off the practice guidelines box on your flow sheet and initial it.
- If you find that a practice guideline doesn't exist for a patient problem, help develop a new one. Tailor it to fit your patient's needs, and document any modifications you made on the patient's care plan.
- Keep the guidelines at the nurses' station.

Patient-teaching plan

Patient-teaching plans help all the patient's educators coordinate their teaching, serve as legal proof that the patient received appropriate instruction, and satisfy the requirements of regulatory agencies such as JCAHO. When creating a patient-teaching plan, follow these guidelines:

- Include the patient-teaching plan on your main plan, or write a separate plan, according to your facility's guidelines.
- Be sure to document what the patient needs to learn, how he'll be taught, and what criteria will be used for evaluating his learning.
- Work closely with other health care team members as well as with the patient and his family to make the plan's content realistic and attainable.
- Include provisions for follow-up teaching at home.
- Keep your patient-teaching plan flexible. Take into account such variables as the patient being unreceptive because of a poor night's sleep as well as your own daily time limits.

Components of the plan

Although the scope of each teaching plan differs, all should contain the same elements:

- *Patient-learning needs,* which you identify, help you decide which outcomes you should establish for your patient. When identifying these needs, consider what you, the physician, and other health care team members want the patient to learn as well as what the patient wants to learn.

(Text continues on page 123.)

USING A TRADITIONAL CARE PLAN

Here's an example of a traditional care plan. It shows how these forms are typically organized. Remember that a traditional plan is written from scratch for each patient.

DATE	NURSING DIAGNOSIS	EXPECTED OUTCOMES	
1/8/07	Decreased cardiac output R/T reduced stroke volume secondary to fluid volume overload	Lungs clear on auscultation by 1/10/07. BP will return to baseline by 1/10/07.	

REVIEW DATES

Date	Signature
1/8/07	Karen Kramer, RN

INTERVENTIONS	OUTCOME EVALUATION (INITIALS AND DATE)
Monitor for signs and symptoms of hypoxemia, such as dyspnea, confusion, arrhythmias, restlessness, and cyanosis. Ensure adequate oxygenation by placing patient in semi-Fowler's position and administering supplemental O_2 as ordered. Monitor breath sounds q 4 hr. Administer cardiac medications as ordered and document pt's response, drugs' effectiveness, and any adverse reactions. Monitor and document heart rate and rhythm, heart sounds, and BP. Note the presence or absence of peripheral pulses. —————— KK	

Initials
KK

USING A STANDARDIZED CARE PLAN

The standardized care plan below is for a patient with a nursing diagnosis of *Impaired tissue integrity*. To customize it to your patient, complete the diagnosis—including signs and symptoms—and fill in the expected outcomes. Also modify, add, or delete interventions as necessary.

Date
1/15/01

Nursing diagnosis
Impaired tissue integrity related to arterial insufficiency

Target date
1/11/01

Expected outcomes
Attains relief from immediate symptoms: *pain, ulcers, edema*

Voices intent to change aggravating behavior:
will stop smoking immediately

Maintains collateral circulation: *palpable peripheral pulses, extremities warm and pink with good capillary refill*

Voices intent to follow specific management routines after discharge: *foot care guidelines, exercise regimen as specified by physical therapy department*

Date
1/15/01

Interventions
- Provide foot care. Administer and monitor treatments according to facility protocols.
- Encourage adherence to an exercise regimen as tolerated.
- Educate the patient about risk factors and prevention of injury. Refer the patient to a stop-smoking program.
- Maintain adequate hydration. Monitor I/O *every 8 hours*
- To increase arterial blood supply to the extremities, elevate head of bed *6" to 8"*

- Additional interventions: *inspect skin integrity every 8 hours*

Date	Outcomes evaluation
_____	Attained relief of immediate symptoms: _____
	Voiced intent to change aggravating behavior: _____
	Maintained collateral circulation: _____
	Voiced intent to follow specific management routines after discharge: _____

● *Expected learning outcomes* should focus on the patient and be readily measurable. (See *Writing clear learning outcomes,* page 127.) They should also fall into one of three categories:
  – cognitive, relating to understanding
  – psychomotor, covering manual skills
  – affective, dealing with attitudes.
● *Teaching content,* organized from the simplest concept to the most complex, includes what the patient needs to be taught to achieve the expected outcomes. Include family members and other caregivers into the plan so that they can serve as a source of information in case the patient forgets some aspect of his care.
● *Teaching methods* include one-on-one teaching, demonstration, practice, return demonstration, role playing, and self-monitoring.
● *Teaching tools*—ranging from printed pamphlets to closed-circuit television programs—can familiarize the patient with a specific topic. When choosing your tools, focus on what will work best for the particular patient, and keep your patient's abilities and limitations in mind.
● *Barriers to learning and the patient's readiness to learn* can comprise physical conditions that may impede the learning process and the patient's unwillingness or inability to learn because he's overwhelmed by illness, frightened, in denial, or all three.

Documenting the patient-teaching plan
Several forms are available for documenting patient-teaching plans—including some that detail the phases of the nursing process as they relate to patient education. (See *Documenting patient teaching,* pages 128 and 129.) They come in two basic types that are similar to traditional and standardized care plans.
● The traditional type begins with the nursing diagnosis statement *Deficient knowledge* and an individualized *related to* statement (for example,

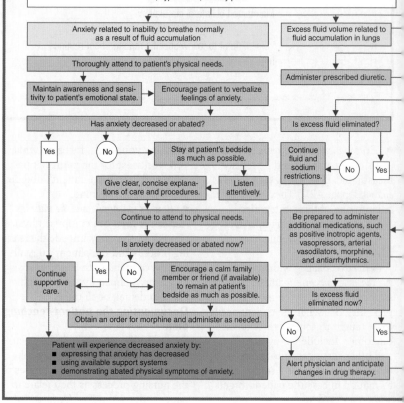

PRACTICE GUIDELINES FOR ACUTE PULMONARY EDEMA

Presence of predisposing factors, such as cardiovascular diseases, persistent cough, dyspnea on exertion, possible paroxysmal nocturnal dyspnea or orthopnea

Physical findings, including restlessness; anxiety; labored, rapid respirations; frothy, bloody sputum; decreased level of consciousness; jugular vein distention; cold, clammy skin; crepitant crackles and wheezes; diastolic (S_3) gallop; tachycardia; hypotension; thready pulse

Results of chest X-ray, arterial blood gas (ABG) analysis, pulse oximetry, pulmonary artery catheterization, electrocardiography

Anxiety related to inability to breathe normally as a result of fluid accumulation

Excess fluid volume related to fluid accumulation in lungs

Thoroughly attend to patient's physical needs.

Administer prescribed diuretic.

Maintain awareness and sensitivity to patient's emotional state.

Encourage patient to verbalize feelings of anxiety.

Has anxiety decreased or abated?

Is excess fluid eliminated?

Yes

No → Stay at patient's bedside as much as possible.

Continue fluid and sodium restrictions.

No / Yes

Give clear, concise explanations of care and procedures. ← Listen attentively.

Continue to attend to physical needs.

Be prepared to administer additional medications, such as positive inotropic agents, vasopressors, arterial vasodilators, morphine, and antiarrhythmics.

Is anxiety decreased or abated now?

Continue supportive care.

Yes / No → Encourage a calm family member or friend (if available) to remain at patient's bedside as much as possible.

Is excess fluid eliminated now?

No / Yes

Obtain an order for morphine and administer as needed.

Patient will experience decreased anxiety by:
■ expressing that anxiety has decreased
■ using available support systems
■ demonstrating abated physical symptoms of anxiety.

Alert physician and anticipate changes in drug therapy.

Deficient knowledge related to low-sodium diet). This type provides the format but requires you to come up with the plan.

● The standard type may be better for a patient who requires extensive teaching because you can check off or date steps as you complete them and add or delete information.

Traditional and standardized patient-teaching plans may include space for problems that may hinder learning, comments and evaluations, and dates and signatures.

Discharge planning

Staff nurses play a major role in preparing patients and caregivers to as-

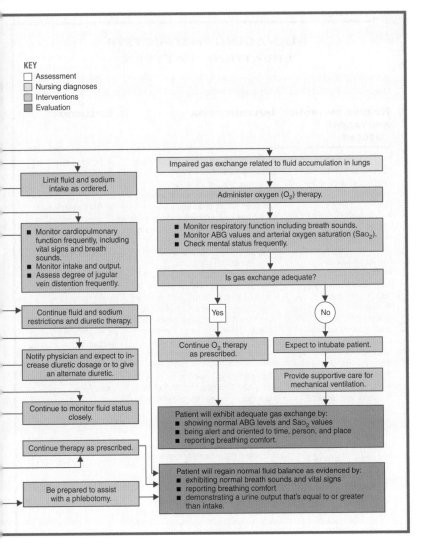

KEY
☐ Assessment
☐ Nursing diagnoses
☐ Interventions
☐ Evaluation

Limit fluid and sodium intake as ordered.

- Monitor cardiopulmonary function frequently, including vital signs and breath sounds.
- Monitor intake and output.
- Assess degree of jugular vein distention frequently.

Continue fluid and sodium restrictions and diuretic therapy.

Notify physician and expect to increase diuretic dosage or to give an alternate diuretic.

Continue to monitor fluid status closely.

Continue therapy as prescribed.

Be prepared to assist with a phlebotomy.

Impaired gas exchange related to fluid accumulation in lungs

Administer oxygen (O_2) therapy.

- Monitor respiratory function including breath sounds.
- Monitor ABG values and arterial oxygen saturation (Sao_2).
- Check mental status frequently.

Is gas exchange adequate?

Yes

No

Continue O_2 therapy as prescribed.

Expect to intubate patient.

Provide supportive care for mechanical ventilation.

Patient will exhibit adequate gas exchange by:
- showing normal ABG levels and Sao_2 values
- being alert and oriented to time, person, and place
- reporting breathing comfort.

Patient will regain normal fluid balance as evidenced by:
- exhibiting normal breath sounds and vital signs
- reporting breathing comfort
- demonstrating a urine output that's equal to or greater than intake.

---

sume responsibility for ongoing care. If you're in charge of discharge planning for a patient, begin your planning the day the patient is admitted—or sooner for a planned admission.

Components of the plan

Although discharge planning differs for each patient, the discharge plan should contain these elements:

- anticipated length of stay
- teaching content, such as instructions on diet, medications, treatments, physical activity restrictions, signs and symptoms to report to the physician, follow-up medical care, equipment, and appropriate community resources

MANAGING INEFFECTIVE BREATHING PATTERN

Below you'll find a portion of a practice guideline for a patient who has chronic obstructive pulmonary disease (COPD) and a nursing diagnosis of ineffective breathing pattern.

NURSING DIAGNOSIS AND PATIENT OUTCOME	IMPLEMENTATION	EVALUATION
Ineffective breathing pattern related to decreased lung compliance and air trapping By _1/10/07_ the patient will: ■ demonstrate a respiratory rate within 5 breaths/minute of baseline ■ maintain arterial blood gas (ABG) levels within acceptable ranges ■ verbalize understanding of the disease process, including its causes and risk factors ■ demonstrate diaphragmatic pursed-lip breathing ■ take all medication as prescribed ■ use oxygen as prescribed.	■ Monitor respiratory function. Auscultate for breath sounds, noting improvement or deterioration. ■ Obtain ABG levels and pulmonary function tests as ordered. ■ Explain lung anatomy and physiology, using illustrated teaching materials, if possible. ■ Explain COPD, its physiologic effects, and its complications. ■ Review the most common signs and symptoms associated with the disease: dyspnea, especially with exertion; fatigue; cough; occasional mucus production; weight loss; rapid heart rate; irregular pulse; and use of accessory muscles to help with breathing because of limited diaphragm function. ■ Explain the purpose of diaphragmatic pursed-lip breathing for patients with COPD; demonstrate the correct technique, and have the patient perform a return demonstration. ■ If the patient smokes, provide information about smoking-cessation groups in the community. ■ Explain the importance of avoiding fumes, respiratory irritants, temperature extremes, and exposure to upper respiratory tract infections. ■ Review the patient's medications, and explain the rationale for their use, their dosages, and possible adverse effects. Advise him to report any adverse reactions to the physician immediately. ■ For the patient receiving oxygen, explain the rationale for therapy and the safe use of equipment. Explain that the oxygen flow rate should never be increased above the prescribed target.	■ Patient's respiratory rate remains within 5 breaths/minute of baseline. ■ ABG levels return to and remain within established limits. ■ Patient verbalizes an understanding of his disease. ■ Patient properly demonstrates diaphragmatic pursed-lip breathing. ■ Patient takes all medication as prescribed. ■ Patient demonstrates the appropriate use of oxygen as prescribed.

● an instruction sheet to reinforce what the patient learns and what he needs to remember about follow-up care

● future care, including its setting, the patient's intended caregiver and support systems, actual or potential barriers to care, and any referrals.

WRITING CLEAR LEARNING OUTCOMES

The patient's learning behaviors fall into three categories: cognitive, psychomotor, and affective. With these categories in mind, you can write clear, concise, expected learning outcomes. Remember, your outcomes should clarify what you're going to teach, indicate the behavior you expect to see, and set criteria for evaluating what the patient has learned.

Review the two sets of sample learning outcomes for a patient with chronic renal failure. Notice that the outcomes in the well-phrased set start with a precise action verb, confine themselves to one task, and describe measurable and observable learning. In contrast, the poorly phrased outcomes may encompass many tasks and describe learning that's difficult or even impossible to measure.

WELL-PHRASED LEARNING OUTCOMES	POORLY PHRASED LEARNING OUTCOMES
Cognitive domain The patient with chronic renal failure will be able to: ■ state when to take each prescribed drug ■ describe symptoms of elevated blood pressure ■ list permitted and prohibited foods on his diet.	■ know his medication schedule ■ know when his blood pressure is elevated ■ know his dietary restrictions.
Psychomotor domain The patient with chronic renal failure will be able to: ■ take his blood pressure accurately, using a stethoscope and a sphygmomanometer ■ read a thermometer correctly ■ collect a urine specimen, using sterile technique.	■ take his blood pressure ■ use a thermometer ■ bring in a urine specimen for laboratory studies.
Affective domain The patient with chronic renal failure will be able to: ■ comply with dietary restrictions to maintain normal electrolyte values ■ verbally express his feelings about adjustments to be made in the home environment ■ keep scheduled physicians' appointments.	■ appreciate the relationship of diet to renal failure ■ adjust successfully to limitations imposed by chronic renal failure ■ understand the importance of seeing his physician.

Documenting the discharge plan

How you document the discharge plan will depend on the policy at your health care facility. Some facilities:

● require an assessment of discharge needs on the initial assessment form and the discharge plan documented on a separate form

● require you to include the discharge plan as a component of the discharge summary

● use forms for discharge planning that allow several members of the health care team to include information.

(Text continues on page 130.)

DOCUMENTING PATIENT TEACHING

Below, you'll find the first page of a patient-teaching flow sheet. Such flow sheets let you quickly and easily tailor your teaching plan to fit your patient's needs.

PATIENT-TEACHING FLOW SHEET
DIABETES MELLITUS

Problems affecting learning

☐ None
☑ Fatigue or pain
☐ Communication problem
☐ Cognitive or sensory impairment

LEARNING OUTCOMES	INITIAL TEACHING				
	Date	Time	Learner	Techniques and tools	
Basic knowledge ■ Define diabetes mellitus (DM).	1/10/07	1000	P	E, W	
■ List four symptoms of DM.	1/10/07	1000	P	E, W	
Medication ■ State the action of insulin and its effects on the body.	1/10/07	1000	P	E, W	
■ List the three major classifications of insulin. Give their onsets, peaks, and durations.	1/10/07	1000	P	E, W, V	
■ Demonstrate the ability to draw up insulin in a syringe and mix the correct amount.	1/10/07	1000	P	D	

KEY

Learner

P	= patient	D1	= daughter 1	_____
S	= spouse	D2	= daughter 2	_____
M	= mother	S1	= son 1	_____
F	= father	S2	= son 2	_____
		O	= other	_____

Teaching techniques

D = demonstration
E = explanation
R = role-playing

☐ Other _____

_____

		REINFORCEMENT					
Evaluation	Initials	Date	Time	Learner	Techniques and tools	Evaluation	Initials
S	JM	1/11/07	1000	P	E,W	S	JM
S	JM	1/11/07	1000	P	E,W	S	JM
S	JM						
S	JM						
Dp	JM						

Teaching tools
F = filmstrip
P = physical model
S = slide
V = videotape
W = written material

Evaluation
S = states understanding
D = demonstrates understanding
Dp = demonstrates understanding with physical coaching

Dv = demonstrates understanding with verbal coaching
T = passes written test
N = no indication of learning
NE = not evaluated

When a patient is assigned a particular diagnosis-related group (DRG), he's also assigned a case manager. (In some facilities, a patient isn't assigned a DRG until after discharge—in which case, you'll make an educated guess about which DRG will be assigned to him.) Each DRG case management plan has standard outcome criteria and includes medical and nursing interventions as well as interventions from other disciplines.

The case manager discusses outcomes with the patient and family, using the established time line for the DRG. This time line should cover all the processes that must occur for the patient to reach the expected outcome—including tests, procedures, and patient teaching—and the resources the patient will need such as social services. If it doesn't, it's adapted as necessary to fit the patient's needs. If possible, all this is done before the patient is even admitted, but it must be completed within the time limit set by your facility—usually 24 hours.

After the patient is admitted, the multidisciplinary team evaluates his progress and suggests necessary revisions, keeping in mind the need for continuity of care and the best use of resources. The case manager documents variations in the time line, processes, or outcomes, along with the reasons for the changes. The case manager also keeps a lookout for duplication of services and medical orders.

An assessment of the patient's discharge needs is started at or before admission. Home health care services—including obtaining personnel and equipment—are planned well before discharge.

TYPES OF CASE MANAGEMENT SYSTEMS

Several case management systems and various adaptations exist, but most facilities pattern their systems after the one developed at the New England Medical Center, one of the first centers to use case management in an acute care setting. Facilities typically adapt this system to meet their own needs and philosophy of care.

CASE MANAGEMENT

Case management is a method of delivering health care that controls costs while still ensuring quality care. (See *How case management works.*) In this system, Medicare pays the facility based on the patient's diagnosis—not on his length of stay or the number or types of services he receives, which means that the facility loses money if the patient has a lengthy stay or develops complications. This, in turn, forces facilities to deliver cost-effective care—without compromising the quality of care.

Tools for case management

Most facilities pattern their case management tools after the ones developed at the New England Medical Center. Called the *case management plan* and the *clinical pathway,* they allow you to direct, evaluate, and revise patient progress and outcomes.

Case management plan

The basic tool of case management systems, the case management plan spells out the standardized care that a patient with a specific diagnosis-related group (DRG) should receive. The plan covers:
- nursing-related problems
- patient outcomes
- intermediate patient outcomes
- nursing interventions
- medical interventions
- target times.

Each subsection of the plan covers a care unit to which the patient may be admitted during his illness.

Clinical pathway

Because of the length of case management plans, you probably won't use them on a daily basis. Instead, you'll turn to an abbreviated form of the plan: the clinical pathway (also known as the health care map), which covers only the key events that must occur for the patient to be discharged by the target date. Such events include:
- consultations
- diagnostic tests
- physical activities the patient must perform
- treatments
- diet
- medications
- discharge planning
- patient teaching. (For more details and a completed sample of a clinical pathway, see chapter 6, Documentation in acute care.)

After you've established a clinical pathway, follow these guidelines:
- Document variances from the pathway, grouping them by cause. Variances may result from the system, the caregivers, or a problem the patient develops.
- At shift report each day, review the clinical pathway with the other nurses. Document changes in the expected length of stay, and point out critical events scheduled for the next shift to the nurses coming on duty. Also, discuss variances that may have occurred during your shift.

Drawbacks of case management
- It can be difficult establishing a time line for some patients.
- The expected course of treatment and length of stay will likely change for a patient with several variances.

- Documentation can become lengthy and complicated for a patient with variances.

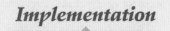

Implementation

Documenting nursing interventions has changed dramatically over the years, mainly because of frustration with tedious traditional methods and the urgent economic need to streamline hospital operations. Narrative notes are no longer a necessity. In many cases, you can use flow sheets or refer to practice guidelines instead. (See *Performing interventions,* page 132.)

DOCUMENTING INTERVENTIONS

When you document your interventions, make sure that the documentation's focus is outcome-oriented by following these guidelines:
- Document that you performed an intervention, the time that you performed it, the patient's response to it, and any additional interventions that you took based on his response.
- Follow your facility's policies when it comes to the exact style, format, and location of your documentation.
- If available, use graphic records, such as a patient care flow sheet that integrates all nurses' notes for a 1-day period, integrated or separate nurses' progress notes, or other specialized documentation forms when documenting your interventions.
- Be sure to document interventions when you give routine care, observe changes in the patient's condition, provide emergency care, and administer medications. (See chapter 1, Documenting everyday events, and chapter

4, Legally perilous documentation, for more information on documenting specific interventions.)

Patient teaching

With each patient, you'll need to implement the teaching plan you've created, evaluate its effectiveness, and clearly and completely document the results. In many facilities, you'll document patient teaching on preprinted forms that become part of the clinical record. Using these forms not only makes documentation quicker, but it also ensures that it's complete.

Whether you use a preprinted form or narrative notes, follow these guidelines:
- Check your facility's policies and procedures regarding when, where, and how to document your teaching.
- Each shift, ask yourself, "What part of the teaching plan did I complete?" and "What other teaching have I given this patient or his family members?" Then document your answers.
- Make sure that your documentation indicates that the patient's ongoing education needs are being met.

- Before discharge, document the patient's remaining learning needs.

Benefits of patient-teaching documentation

Documenting exactly what you've taught:
- provides a permanent legal record of the extent and success of teaching
- strengthens your defense against charges of insufficient patient care—even years later
- helps administrators gauge the overall worth of a specific patient-education program
- helps motivate your patient as you can show him the record of his learning successes and encourage him to continue
- saves time by preventing duplication of patient-teaching efforts by other staff members
- allows for communication between staff members by documenting what they've taught and how well the patient has learned.

Patient discharge

Patient safety *JCAHO requirements specify that when preparing a patient for discharge, you must document*

DISCHARGE SUMMARIES

By combining the patient's discharge summary with instructions for care after discharge, you can fulfill two requirements with a single form. When using this documentation method, be sure to give one copy to the patient and keep one for the record.

DISCHARGE INSTRUCTIONS

1. **Summary** *Tara Nicholas is a 55-year-old woman admitted with complaints of severe headache and hypertensive crisis.*
   Treatment: Nipride gtt for 24 hours
   Started Lopressor for hypertension
   Recommendation: Lose 10-15 lbs
   Follow low-sodium, low-cholesterol diet

2. **Allergies** *penicillin*

3. **Medications (drug, dose time)** *Lopressor 25 mg at 6am and 6pm*
   Temazepam 15 mg at 10pm

4. **Diet** *Low-sodium, low-cholesterol*

5. **Activity** *As tolerated*

6. **Discharged to** *Home*

7. **If questions arise, contact Dr.** *James Pritchett*
   Telephone No. *(555) 525-1448*

8. **Special instructions**

9. **Return visit Dr.** *Pritchett*
   Place *Health Care Clinic*
   On Date *1/19/07*   **Time** *8:45 am*

   Tara Nicholas   *JE Pritchett*
   _____   _____
   Signature of patient for receipt of in-   **Signature of physician**
   structions from physicians   **giving instructions**

---

your assessment of his continuing care needs as well as referrals for such care. To facilitate this documentation (and to save documentation time), many facilities have developed forms that combine discharge summaries and patient instructions. (See Discharge summaries.)

Not all facilities use these forms; some still require a narrative discharge summary. If you must write a narrative, include:
- the patient's status on admission and discharge
- significant highlights of the hospitalization
- outcomes of your interventions
- resolved and unresolved patient problems, continuing care needs for unresolved problems, and specific referrals for continuing care
- instructions given to the patient or family member about medications, treatments, activity, diet, referrals, and follow-up appointments as well as other special instructions.

Evaluation

Progress notes must include an assessment of your patient's progress toward the expected outcomes you established in the care plan. This method, called outcomes and evaluation documentation, focuses on the patient's response to nursing care and enables the nurse to provide high-quality, cost-effective care. It also forces you to focus on patient responses and ensure that your plan is working. (See *Writing clear evaluation statements*. Also see *Performing evaluations*.)

WRITING CLEAR EVALUATION STATEMENTS

Below, you'll find examples of clear evaluation statements describing common outcomes. Note that they include specific details of care provided and objective evidence of the patient's response to care.

RESPONSE TO P.R.N. MEDICATION WITHIN 1 HOUR OF ADMINISTRATION
- "Pt. states pain decreased from 8 to 4 (on a scale of 0 to 10) 10 minutes after receiving I.V. morphine."
- "Vomiting subsided 1 hr after 25 mg P.O. of prochlorperazine."

RESPONSE TO PATIENT EDUCATION
- "Able to describe the signs and symptoms of a postoperative wound infection.'"
- "Despite repeated attempts, pt. couldn't identify signs of hypoglycemia."

TOLERANCE OF CHANGE OR INCREASE IN ACTIVITY
- "Able to walk across the room, approximately 15 feet, without dyspnea."
- "Became fatigued after 5 minutes of assisted ambulation."

ABILITY TO PERFORM ACTIVITIES OF DAILY LIVING, PARTICULARLY THOSE THAT MAY INFLUENCE DISCHARGE PLANNING
- "Unable to wash self independently because of left-sided weakness."
- "Requires a walker to ambulate to bathroom."

TOLERANCE OF TREATMENTS
- "Consumed full liquid lunch; pt. stated she was hungry and wanted solid food."
- "Skin became pink and less dusky 15 minutes after nasal O_2 was administered at 4 L/min."
- "Unable to tolerate having head of bed lowered from 90 degrees to 45 degrees; became dyspneic."

Performing Evaluations

When you evaluate the results of your interventions, you help ensure that the care plan is working. It also gives you a chance to:
- determine if your original assessment findings still apply
- uncover complications
- analyze patterns or trends in the patient's care and his responses to it
- assess the patient's response to all aspects of care, including medications, changes in diet or activity, procedures, unusual incidents or problems, and teaching
- determine how closely care conforms to established standards
- measure how well the patient was cared for
- assess the performance of other members of the health care team
- identify opportunities to improve the quality of care.

WHEN TO PERFORM AN EVALUATION

If you work in an acute care setting, your facility's policy may require you to review care plans every 24 hours. If you work in a long-term care facility, the required interval between evaluations may be up to 30 days. In either case, you should evaluate and revise the care plan more often than required, if warranted.

EVALUATING EXPECTED OUTCOMES

Evaluation includes gathering reassessment data, comparing findings with the outcome criteria, determining the extent of outcome achievement (outcome met, partially met, or not met), writing evaluation statements, and revising the care plan.

Revision starts with determining whether the patient has achieved the expected outcomes. If they've been fully met and you decide that the problem is resolved, the plan can be discontinued. If the problem persists, the plan continues—with new target dates—until the desired status is achieved.

If outcomes have been partially met or unmet, you must identify interfering factors, such as misinterpreted information, and revise the plan accordingly. This may involve:
- clarifying or amending the database to reflect newly discovered information
- reexamining and correcting nursing diagnoses
- establishing outcome criteria that reflect new information and new or amended nursing strategies
- adding the revised nursing care plan to the original document
- recording the rationale for the revisions in the nurse's progress notes.

When documenting an evaluation, follow these guidelines:
- Make sure that your evaluation statements indicate whether expected outcomes were achieved. List evidence supporting this conclusion.
- Base statements on outcome criteria from the care plan.
- Use active verbs, such as "demonstrate" or "ambulate."
- Include the patient's response to specific treatments, such as medication administration or physical therapy.
- Describe the conditions under which the response occurred or failed to occur.
- Document patient teaching and palliative or preventive care as well.
- After evaluating the outcome, be sure to document it in the patient's chart with clear statements that demonstrate the patient's progress toward meeting the expected outcomes.

3
LEGAL AND ETHICAL IMPLICATIONS

The scope of your professional responsibility is set out by your state's Nurse Practice Act and by other state and federal regulations. Documenting the nursing care that you provide in the patient's medical record is one way of accepting that responsibility. When filling out your documentation, consider that:

● you protect your patient's interests—as well as your own—by completing your documentation in an acceptable and timely manner and in accordance with the appropriate standard of nursing care

● the failure to document appropriately has been a pivotal issue in many malpractice cases

● although the actual medical record, X-rays, laboratory reports, and other records belong to the facility, the *information* contained in them belongs to the patient, who has a right to obtain a copy of the materials.

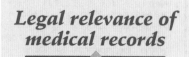 *In court* *In* Deford and Thompson v. Westwood Hills Health Care Center, Inc., Doctors Regional Medical Center and Barnes Hospital, *St. Louis City, Missouri Circuit Court, Case No. 922-9564 (1992), a patient died after a nurse attempted to insert* a feeding tube. Seven months later, when the family requested the patient's records, Westwood Hills staff mistakenly believed they weren't authorized to release them and so refused. Copies of the records were finally released more than 1 year later. The case resulted in an $80,000 verdict against Westwood Hills on a wrongful death claim.

Legal relevance of medical records

Accurately and completely documenting the nature and quality of nursing care is important because it:

● helps other members of the health care team confirm their impressions of the patient's condition and progress

● may signal the need for adjustments in the therapeutic regimen

● is used as evidence in the courtroom in malpractice suits, workers' compensation litigation, personal injury cases, and criminal cases.

STANDARDS OF DOCUMENTATION

The type of nursing information that appears in the medical record is governed by standards developed by the nursing profession and state laws. Professional organizations, such as the American Nurses Association (ANA), and regulatory agencies, such as the Joint Commission on Accreditation of Healthcare Organizations (JCAHO) and the Centers for Medicare and Medicaid Services, have established that documentation must include:

- ongoing assessment
- variations from the assessment
- nursing care
- patient's status
- relevant statements made by the patient
- responses to therapy
- medical treatment
- patient teaching.

TIMELY COMMUNICATION

The purpose of documentation is communication, with an emphasis on timeliness. Follow these guidelines when the patient's condition deteriorates or when changes in therapy are clearly indicated:

- Document the patient's status.
- Document that you contacted the physician and the time the contact was made. (If the physician didn't respond appropriately in your opinion, contact the next person in the chain of command and document this action and why you felt it necessary.)

In court When notification isn't documented, it's nearly impossible to prove that the physician was called in a timely manner and that all critical information was communicated. In a California case, Malovec v. Santa Monica Hospital, Los Angeles County, California Superior Court, Case No. SC 019-167 (1994), a woman in labor repeatedly asked the charge nurse to call the chief of obstetrics because her obstetrician refused to perform a cesarean delivery despite guarded fetal heart tracings. The charge nurse refused, and the baby was born with cerebral palsy and spastic quadriplegia. A confidential settlement was reached.

ERRORS OR OMISSIONS

Errors or omissions can severely undermine your credibility in court. A jury could reasonably conclude that you didn't perform a function if it wasn't documented. If you failed to document something and need to enter a late entry, follow your facility's guidelines and:

- add the entry to the first available line, and label it "late entry" to indicate that it's out of sequence
- record the time and date of the entry and, in the body of the entry, record the time and date it should have been made.

In court In the case of Anonymous v. Anonymous, Suffolk Superior Court, Boston (1993), failure to document led to a $1 million settlement. A 2-year-old was admitted to Children's Hospital for correction of a congenital urinary defect. Postoperative orders required blood pressure, pulse, and temperature readings to be taken every 4 hours, and respiratory rate and reaction to analgesia every hour. However, the child's care wasn't documented for 5 hours. The child was found in cardiorespiratory arrest and died from an overdose of an opioid infusion. The responsible nurse admitted failing to assess the child strictly according to the orders; she also claimed that she had as-

sessed the child adequately but had been "too busy" to document her observations.

CORRECTIONS AND ALTERATIONS

When you make a mistake in your documentation, correct it promptly. (See *Correcting a charting error,* page 64.) If it ends up in court, the plaintiff's attorney will be looking for anything that may cast doubt on the documentation's accuracy.

Alert *Never try to make the record "better" after you learn a malpractice case has been filed. Attorneys have methods for analyzing papers and inks and can easily detect discrepancies.*

Malpractice and documentation

Never lose sight of documentation's legal importance. Depending on how well you administer care and document your activities and observations, the documentation may or may not support a plaintiff's accusation of nursing malpractice. Legally, malpractice focuses on four elements:

- *Duty*—Duty is your obligation to provide patient care and to follow appropriate standards. The courts have ruled that a nurse has a duty to provide care after a nurse-patient relationship is established.
- *Breach of duty*—Breach of duty is a failure to fulfill your nursing obligations. Breach of duty can be difficult to prove because nursing responsibilities typically overlap those of physicians and other health care providers. A key question asked when a possible breach of duty is being investigated is,

"How would a reasonable, prudent nurse with comparable training and experience have acted in the same or similar circumstances?"

In court *In judging a nurse to have breached her duty, the courts must prove that the nurse failed to provide the appropriate care—as they did in* Collins v. Westlake Community Hospital, 312 N.E. 2d 614 (Ill. 1974). *A boy was hospitalized for a fractured leg, which was put in a cast and placed in traction. Although the physician ordered the nurse on duty to monitor the condition of the boy's toes, the medical record lacked documentation that she did so. In fact, 7 hours elapsed between documented nursing entries in the medical record. The boy's leg was later amputated, and the parents sued on behalf of their son. Because a nurse is responsible for continually assessing patients and because documentation of these assessments didn't appear in the record, the nurse was found to have breached her duty to this child.*

- *Causation*—The plaintiff must prove that the breach caused the injury. For the nurse to be liable, she must have *proximately caused* the injury by an act or an oversight. (See *Understanding proximity.*)
- *Damages*—Damages represent the amount of money the court orders the defendant to pay the plaintiff when a case is decided in the plaintiff's favor. To collect damages, the patient's attorney must prove that his client's injury was the result of malpractice. Usually, the injury must be physical, not just emotional or mental.

UNDERSTANDING PROXIMITY

The principle of proximity is important because, in a typical health care facility, many caregivers are involved in a patient's care. Even if a nurse did commit malpractice, it's conceivable that the patient's injury was caused by something other than the nursing intervention. For instance, even if a nurse gave a patient an overdose of a medication, and the patient later vomited blood, the cause of the vomiting might actually be a surgical error and have nothing to do with the medication.

Policies and documentation

Although most discussions about documentation center on the patient's chart, policies and procedures contained in health care facility employee and nursing manuals are also an important aspect of documentation. When dealing with policies and procedures, keep this very important point in mind:

● Deviation from a facility's policies and procedures suggests that an employee failed to meet the facility's standards of care.

In court *In a case related to a health care facility's policies, the court was pressed to distinguish between a facility's policies and its "goals." In H.C.A. Health Services v. National Bank, 745 S.W. 2d 120 (Ark. 1988), three nurses were working in a nursery composed of three connecting rooms. One nurse cared for a baby in the first (admissions) room. The other two nurses went into the second room, which housed 11 babies (two of whom were premature and one of whom was jaundiced). There was no documentation that for 1½ hours any of the nurses went into the third room, which had six babies. Documentation did show that when the first nurse finally entered the third room, she found that one of the infants had stopped breathing and had no heartbeat.*

Both the facility's executive director and the nurse who found the baby testified that, according to the facility's manual, no infant is ever to be left alone without a member of the nursery staff present. However, they also testified that this was a goal—not a policy. Another physician testified that the baby's problem would have been avoided if a nurse had been present. The court disagreed with the distinction between policies and goals and ruled against the facility and nurses and in favor of the plaintiff.

Risk management and documentation

To reduce injuries and accidents, minimize financial loss, and meet the guidelines of the JCAHO and other regulatory agencies, health care facilities have instituted risk management programs. The primary objectives of a risk management program are to:

● ensure optimal patient care
● reduce the frequency of preventable injuries and accidents leading to liability claims by maintaining or improving quality of care
● decrease the chance of a claim being filed by promptly identifying and

following up on adverse events (incidents)

- help control costs related to claims by identifying trouble spots early and intervening with the patient and his family. (See *Coordinating risk management and performance improvement*.)

Three important aspects of risk management include identifying sentinel events, identifying adverse events, and managing adverse events.

IDENTIFYING SENTINEL EVENTS

JCAHO requires health care facilities to identify and manage sentinel events, which are unexpected occurrences involving death or serious physical or psychological injury. When a sentinel event is identified, the facility must initiate an analysis of the situation. The facility should also initiate an analysis whenever there's a:

- confirmed transfusion reaction
- significant adverse drug reaction
- significant medication error.

IDENTIFYING ADVERSE EVENTS

A key part of a risk management program involves developing a system for identifying adverse events—events, such as patient falls, that would be considered an abnormal consequence of a patient's condition or treatment. These events may or may not be caused by a health care provider's breach of duty or the standard of care, which is why it's important that you have reliable sources of information and a reliable system for identifying adverse effects. (See *Primary sources of information*.) The most common "early-warning systems" are:

- *Incident reporting*—Certain criteria are used to define events that must be reported by physicians, nurses, or other health care staff, either when they're observed or shortly after. *All errors must be reported* because it's impossible to predict which ones will require intervention.
- *Occurrence screening*—Flags adverse events through a review of all or some of the medical charts. These reviews use generic criteria, but more specific reviews may focus on specialty or service-specific criteria.

Incident reporting and occurrence screening are crucial because they:

- permit early investigation and intervention
- help minimize additional adverse consequences and legal action

- provide valuable databases for building strategies to prevent repeated incidents.

MANAGING ADVERSE EVENTS

When the facility's risk manager learns of a potential or actual lawsuit:
- The risk manager notifies the medical records department and the facility's insurance carrier or attorney (or both).
- The medical records department makes copies of the patient's chart and files the original in a secure place to prevent tampering.

A claim notice also triggers a performance improvement peer review of the medical record. This review:
- may be conducted by the chairperson of the department involved, the risk management or performance improvement department, or an external reviewer to measure the health care provider's conduct against the professional standards of conduct for the particular situation.
- helps the risk manager determine the claim's merit and also helps to define the facility's responsibility for care in particular situations.
- identifies areas where changes are needed, such as policy, training, staffing, or equipment.

Completing incident reports

An incident report is a formal report, written by physicians, nurses, or other staff members, that informs facility administrators about an adverse event suffered by a patient. They're continually being revised, and some may be computerized. (See *Completing an incident report,* pages 142 and 143.) If you're filing an incident report, follow these guidelines:
- Write objectively. Record the details of the incident in objective terms, describing exactly what you saw and heard.

COMPLETING AN INCIDENT REPORT

When you witness or discover a reportable event, you must fill out an incident report. Forms vary, but most include the following information.

INCIDENT REPORT

Name _Greta Manning_

DATE OF INCIDENT
_1-20-07_

Address _7 Worth Way, Boston, MA_

TIME OF INCIDENT
_1442_

Phone _(617) 555-1122_

Addressograph if patient _____

EXACT LOCATION OF INCIDENT
(Bldg, Floor, Room No, Area)   _4-Main, Rm. 447_

TYPE OF INCIDENT (CHECK ONE ONLY)
☐ PATIENT   ☐ EMPLOYEE   ☑ VISITOR   ☐ VOLUNTEER   ☐ OTHER (specify)

DESCRIPTION OF THE INCIDENT (WHO, WHAT, WHEN, WHERE, HOW, WHY)
(Use back of form if necessary)

Patient's wife found on floor next to bed. States, "I was trying to put the siderail of the bed down to sit on it and I fell down."

Patient fall incidents	FLOOR CONDITIONS ☐ OTHER _____ ☑ CLEAN & SMOOTH ☐ SLIPPERY (WET)	
	FRAME OF BED ☐ HIGH ☑ LOW	
	NIGHT LIGHT ☐ YES ☑ NO	
	WERE BED RAILS PRESENT? ☐ NO ☐ 1 UP ☐ 2 UP ☐ 3 UP ☑ 4 UP	
	OTHER RESTRAINTS (TYPE AND EXTENT) _N/A_	
	AMBULATION PRIVILEGE ☐ UNLIMITED ☐ LIMITED WITH ASSISTANCE ☐ COMPLETE BEDREST ☐ OTHER _____	
	WERE NARCOTICS, ANALGESICS, HYPNOTICS, SEDATIVES, DIURETICS, ANTIHYPERTENSIVES, OR ANTICONVULSANTS GIVEN DURING LAST 4 HOURS? ☐ YES ☑ NO	

DRUG   AMOUNT   TIME

Patient incidents	PHYSICIAN NOTIFIED Name of Physician _J. Reynolds, MD_	DATE _1-20-07_	TIME COMPLETE IF APPLICABLE _1445_

Employee incidents	DEPARTMENT	JOB TITLE	SOCIAL SECURITY #
	MARITAL STATUS		

All incidents	NOTIFIED _C. Jones, RN_	DATE _1-20-07_	TIME _1500_
	LOCATION WHERE TREATMENT WAS RENDERED		
	NAME, ADDRESS, AND TELEPHONE NUMBERS OF WITNESS(ES) OR PERSONS FAMILIAR WITH INCIDENT - WITNESS OR NOT _Janet Adams (617) 555-0912 1 Main St., Boston, MA_		

SIGNATURE OF PERSON PREPARING REPORT	TITLE	DATE OF REPORT
Connie Smith, RN	_RN_	_1-20-07_

COMPLETING AN INCIDENT REPORT (CONTINUED)

PHYSICIAN'S REPORT — To be completed for all cases involving injury or illness
(DO NOT USE ABBREVIATIONS) (Use back if necessary)

DIAGNOSIS AND TREATMENT

Received patient in Emergency Department after reported fall in husband's room. 12 cm x 12 cm ecchymotic area noted on right hip. X-rays negative for fracture. Good range of motion, no c/o pain. VAS 0/10. Ice pack applied.———————— J. Reynolds, MD

DISPOSITION

sent home, written instructions provided

PERSON NOTIFIED OTHER THAN HOSPITAL PERSONNEL	DATE	TIME
NAME AND ADDRESS		
R. Manning (daughter), address same as pt	*1-20-07*	*1500*

PHYSICIAN'S SIGNATURE	DATE
J. Reynolds, MD	*1-20-01*

● Include only essential information. Document the time and place of the incident, the name of the physician who was notified, and the time of the notification.

● Avoid opinions. If you must express an opinion on how a similar incident may be avoided in the future, verbally share it with your supervisor and risk manager. Don't write it in the incident report.

● Assign no blame. Don't admit to liability, and don't blame or point your finger at colleagues or administrators.

● Avoid hearsay and assumptions. Don't write an incident report for an injury that occurred in another department—even if the patient who was injured is yours. The staff members in that department are responsible for documenting the details of the accident.

● File the report properly. Don't file the incident report with the medical record; instead, send it to the person designated to review it according to your facility's policy.

Documenting an incident in the medical record

When documenting an incident in the patient's medical record, keep these guidelines in mind:

● Write a factual account of the incident, including the treatment and follow-up care provided and the patient's response. This documentation shows that the patient was closely monitored after the incident, which

will help your case should it go to court.

- Include in the progress notes and in the incident report anything the patient or his family says about their role in the incident, for example, "Patient stated, "The nurse told me to ask for help before I went to the bathroom, but I decided to go on my own.'" This kind of statement helps the defense attorney prove that the patient was guilty of contributory or comparative negligence. Contributory negligence is conduct that contributed to the patient's injuries. Comparative negligence involves determining the percentage of each party's fault.

Bioethical dilemmas and documentation

As a nurse, you routinely take part in decisions involving ethical dilemmas. Some dilemmas may be more serious than others, but they all present some kind of risk. Thankfully, you aren't short on guidelines:

- JCAHO mandates that health care facilities address ethical issues in providing patient care by listing specific patient rights and maintaining a code of ethical behavior.
- A few states have incorporated patient rights into their state statutes, and most have codified statutes for nursing home patients.
- The ANA and other nursing organizations have their own ethical codes of conduct for nurses. (See *Ethical codes for nurses.*)

Bioethical issues involving documentation include:

- informed consent (including witnessing informed consent and informed refusal)
- advance directives (also known as *living wills*)
- power of attorney
- do-not-resuscitate orders
- confidentiality of the medical record.

INFORMED CONSENT

Informed consent means that the patient understands the proposed therapy and its risks and agrees to undergo it by signing a consent form. Informed consent has two elements, the information and the consent. (See *The two elements of informed consent,* page 147.) Important aspects of informed consent to remember include that:

- it's required before most treatments and procedures

In court *In life-threatening emergencies, informed consent may not be required. In such cases, the law assumes that every individual wants to live and allows the physician to intervene to save life without obtaining consent.*

- the physician (or other practitioner) who will perform the procedure is legally responsible for obtaining it, even if he delegates the duty to a nurse
- you may be asked to witness the patient's signature, depending on your facility's policy. (See *Witnessing informed consent,* pages 148 and 149.)

Legal requirements

For informed consent to be legally binding, the patient must be mentally competent and the physician must:

- explain the patient's diagnosis as well as the nature, purpose, and likeli-

Ethical codes for nurses

One of the most important ethical codes for registered nurses is the American Nurses Association (ANA) code. Licensed practical and vocational nurses (LPNs and LVNs) also have an ethical code, which is set forth in each state by the state's nurses association. The National Federation of Licensed Practical Nurses also has a code of ethics for its members. In addition, the International Council of Nurses, an organization based in Geneva, Switzerland, that seeks to improve the standards and status of nursing worldwide, has published a code of ethics. Summaries of these codes appear here.

ANA CODE OF ETHICS

The ANA views nurses and patients as individuals who possess basic rights and responsibilities and who should command respect for their values and circumstances at all times. The ANA code provides guidance for carrying out nursing responsibilities consistent with the ethical obligations of the profession. According to the ANA code, the nurse is responsible for these actions:

- Provide services with respect for human dignity and the uniqueness of the patient unrestricted by considerations of social or economic status, personal attributes, or the nature of health problems.
- Safeguard the patient's right to privacy by judiciously protecting information of a confidential nature.
- Act to safeguard the patient and the public when health care and safety are affected by the incompetent, unethical, or illegal practice of any person.
- Assume responsibility and accountability for individual nursing judgments and actions.
- Maintain competence in nursing.
- Exercise informed judgment, and use individual competence and qualifications as criteria in seeking consultation, accepting responsibilities, and delegating nursing activities to others.
- Cooperate in activities that contribute to the ongoing development of the profession's body of knowledge.
- Participate in the profession's efforts to implement and improve standards of nursing.
- Take part in the profession's efforts to establish and maintain conditions of employment conducive to high-quality nursing care.
- Share in the profession's efforts to protect the public from misinformation and misrepresentation and to maintain the integrity of nursing.
- Collaborate with members of the health care professions and other citizens in promoting community and national efforts to meet the health needs of the public.

CODE FOR LPNs AND LVNs

The code for LPNs and LVNs seeks to provide a motivation for establishing, maintaining, and elevating professional standards. It includes these imperatives:

- Know the scope of maximum utilization of the LPN and LVN, as specified by the nurse practice act, and function within this scope.
- Safeguard the confidential information acquired from any source about the patient.
- Provide health care to all patients regardless of race, creed, cultural background, disease, or lifestyle.
- Refuse to give endorsement to the sale and promotion of commercial products or services.
- Uphold the highest standards in personal appearance, language, dress, and demeanor.
- Stay informed about issues affecting the practice of nursing and delivery of health care and, where appropriate, participate in government and policy decisions.
- Accept the responsibility for safe nursing by keeping oneself mentally and physically fit and educationally prepared to practice.
- Accept responsibility for membership in the National Federation of Licensed Practical Nurses, and participate in its efforts to maintain the established standards of nursing practice and employment policies that lead to quality patient care.

(continued)

hood of success of the treatment or procedure

● describe the risks and benefits associated with the treatment or procedure

● explain the possible consequences of not undergoing the treatment or procedure

● describe alternative treatments and procedures

● inform the patient that he has the right to refuse the treatment or pro-

cedure without having other care or support withdrawn; this includes withdrawing his consent after giving it

● identify who will perform the procedure

● identify who's responsible for the patient's care

● obtain consent without coercing the patient.

Nursing responsibilities

Even if the physician obtains the informed consent himself, you aren't free from responsibilities. Before a procedure is performed:

● Make sure that the patient's record contains a signed informed consent form.

● If the patient appears to be concerned about the procedure or the physician's explanation of it, notify your supervisor or the physician. Document your notification and the time of the notification.

● If the patient wants to change his mind, notify the physician as soon as possible. Document the patient's comments, your notification of the physician and the time of the notification, and the physician's response.

INFORMED REFUSAL

JCAHO requires (and federal statutes mandate) that health care facilities (acute and long-term care) inform patients soon after admission about their treatment options. The patient has the right to refuse treatment based on knowledge of the outcomes and risks. (See *Understanding informed refusal,* page 149.) When documenting a patient's informed refusal, document that:

● you informed the patient about his treatment options

● you discussed the patient's wishes with him, which may be referred to if the patient becomes unable to participate in decision making

● the patient refused treatment and the time and date of his refusal. (See *Witnessing refusal of treatment,* page 150.)

ADVANCE DIRECTIVES

The U.S. Constitution and case law have established that the patient has the right to determine what happens to his body. JCAHO mandates that:

WITNESSING INFORMED CONSENT

When you witness the patient signing an informed consent document, you're *not* witnessing that he received or understood the information. You're simply witnessing that the person who signed the consent form is in fact the person he says he is. For this, check the patient's armband to ensure that he is in fact the correct patient. Here's a typical form.

CONSENT FOR OPERATION AND RENDERING OF OTHER MEDICAL SERVICES

1. I hereby authorize Dr. *Wesley* _____ to perform upon *Joseph Smith* _____ (Patient name), the following surgical and/or medical procedures: (State specific nature of the procedures to be performed) _____ *Exploratory laparotomy* _____

2. I understand that the procedure(s) will be performed at Valley Medical Center by or under the supervision of Dr. *Wesley* _____, who is authorized to utilize the services of other physicians, or members of the house staff as he or she deems necessary or advisable.

3. It has been explained to me that during the course of the operation, unforeseen conditions may be revealed that necessitate an extension of the original procedure(s) or different procedure(s) than those set forth in Paragraph 1; I therefore authorize and request that the above named physician, and his or her associates or assistants, perform such medical surgical procedures as are necessary and desirable in the exercise of professional judgment.

4. I understand the nature and purpose of the procedure(s), possible alternative methods of diagnosis or treatment, the risks involved, the possibility of complications, and the consequences of the procedure(s). I acknowledge that no guarantee or assurance has been made as to the results that may be obtained.

5. I authorize the above named physician to administer local or regional anesthesia (for all other anesthesia management, a separate consent must be signed by the patient or patient's authorized representative).

6. I understand that if it is necessary for me to receive a blood transfusion during this procedure or this hospitalization, the blood will be supplied by sources available to the hospital and tested in accordance with national and regional regulations. I understand that there are risks in transfusion, including but not limited to allergic, febrile, and hemolytic transfusion reactions, and the transmission of infectious diseases, such as hepatitis and AIDS (Acquired Immunodeficiency Syndrome). I hereby consent to blood transfusion(s) and blood derivative(s).

7. I hereby authorize representatives from Valley to photograph or videotape me for the purpose of research or medical education. It is understood and agreed that patient confidentiality shall be preserved.

8. I authorize the physician named above and his or her associates and assistants and Valley Medical Center to preserve for scientific purposes or to dispose of any tissue, organs, or other body parts removed during surgery or other diagnostic procedures in accordance with customary medical practice.

9. I certify that I have read and fully understand the above consent statement. In addition, I have been afforded an opportunity to ask whatever questions I might have regarding the procedure(s) to be performed, and they have been answered to my satisfaction.

Joseph Smith	*01/21/01*	*C. Gurney, RN*
Legal Patient or Authorized Representative (State Relationship to Patient)	Date	Witness

If the patient is unable to consent on his or her own behalf, complete the following:

Patient _____ is unable to consent because

_____

_____

Legally Responsible Person _____

Physician Obtaining Consent   *M. Wesley, MD*

- patients have the right to participate in decisions regarding their care
- health care facilities have a policy or procedure in place addressing how they'll implement the requirement
- facilities address forgoing or withdrawing life-sustaining treatment and withholding resuscitative services and care at the end of life.

An advance directive (sometimes referred to as a *living will*) allows the patient to decide before he becomes terminally ill the type of care he'll be given at the end of his life. The directive becomes effective only when the patient becomes terminally ill, and most state statutes require it to be written. When caring for a patient with an advance directive, follow these guidelines:

UNDERSTANDING INFORMED REFUSAL

With a few exceptions, a *competent* patient has a right to refuse mechanical ventilation, tube feedings, antibiotics, fluids, and other treatments that will clearly result in his death if they're withheld. However, it's important to remember that legal competence differs from the medical or psychiatric concept of competence. The law presumes all individuals to be competent unless deemed otherwise through a court proceeding. The patient must also have *capacity*—that is, be legally considered an adult for consent purposes under state law.

Exceptions to the right to informed refusal may include pregnant women (because the life of the unborn child is at risk) and parents wishing to withhold treatment from their child.

WITNESSING REFUSAL OF TREATMENT

If a patient refuses treatment, the physician must first explain the risks involved in making this choice. Then the physician asks the patient to sign a refusal-of-treatment release form, such as the one shown here, which you may be asked to sign as a witness. Your signature only validates the identity of the patient signing the form—not that the patient received sufficient information or understood that information.

Refusal-of-treatment release form

I, _____Brenda Lyndstrom_____, refuse to allow anyone to
      (patient's name)

_____administer parenteral nutrition_____
      (insert treatment)

The risks attendant to my refusal have been fully explained to me, and I fully understand the benefits of this treatment. I also understand that my refusal of treatment seriously reduces my chances for regaining normal health and may endanger my life.

I hereby release _____Mercy General_____
      (name of hospital)

its nurses and employees, together with all physicians in any way connected with me as a patient, from liability for respecting and following my express wishes and direction.

_____Susan Reynolds, RN_____
(witness's signature)

_____01/12/07_____
(date)

_____Brenda Lyndstrom_____
(patient's or legal guardian's signature)

_____76_____
(patient's age)

● Document the patient's current wishes in the medical record.

● If a competent patient says that he wants to revoke his advance directive, contact the physician and document exactly what he said and the time and date he said it.

   In court Some state statutes have guidelines for revoking a directive, but the patient's oral wishes will suffice until those requirements can be met.

● If the patient's request differs from what the family or physician wants,

document discrepancies carefully. Use social services or the legal department for advice on how to proceed. (See *Advance directive checklist.*)

   In court If an advance directive is in effect and the nurse or other health care provider fails to honor it, any subsequent care provided may be considered unconsented touching, assault and battery, negligence, or intentional infliction of emotional, physical, and financial distress and, as such, grounds for a malpractice suit.

ADVANCE DIRECTIVE CHECKLIST

The Joint Commission on Accreditation of Healthcare Organizations requires that information on advance directives be documented on the admission assessment form. However, many facilities also use a checklist like this one.

ADVANCE DIRECTIVE CHECKLIST

I. DISTRIBUTION OF ADVANCE DIRECTIVE INFORMATION

    A. Advance directive information was presented to the patient: . . . . ☑

        1. At the time of preadmission testing . . . . ☑

        2. Upon inpatient admission . . . . ☐

        3. Interpretive services contacted . . . . ☐

        4. Information was read to the patient . . . . ☐

    B. Advance directive information was presented to the next of kin as
the patient is incapacitated . . . . ☐

    C. Advance directive information was not distributed as the patient is
incapacitated and no relative or next of kin was available . . . . ☐

Mary Barren, RN	_01/10/07_
RN	**DATE**

	Upon admission		Upon transfer to Intensive Care Unit	
II. ASSESSMENT OF ADVANCE DIRECTIVE UPON ADMISSION	**YES**	**NO**	**YES**	**NO**
A. Does the patient have an advance directive?	☐	☑	☐	☐
If yes, was the attending physician notified?	☐		☐	
B. If no advance directive, does the patient want to execute an advance directive?	☑	☐	☐	☐
If yes, was the attending physician notified?	☑		☐	
Was the patient referred to resources?	☑		☐	
	Mary Barren, RN			
	RN		**RN**	
	_01/10/01_			
	DATE		**DATE**	

III. RECEIPT OF AN ADVANCE DIRECTIVE AFTER ADMISSION

    A. The patient has presented an advance directive after admission
and the attending physician has been notified.

RN	**DATE**

Patient Self-Determination Act

The Patient Self-Determination Act of 1990 allows patients to use advance directives and to appoint a surrogate to make decisions if the patient loses the ability to do so. This act:

● mandates that on admission, each patient be informed of his right to create an advance directive

● mandates this information be documented in the medical record

● allows the patient to create an advance directive and have this document placed in the medical record and honored.

POWER OF ATTORNEY

Power of attorney is a legal document in which a competent person designates another to act or conduct legally binding transactions on his behalf. It may encompass all of a person's affairs, including health and financial matters, or it may be limited to one specific area. It ceases if the patient becomes incompetent or revokes the document, unless he has executed a durable power of attorney. (See *Durable power of attorney.*)

When caring for a patient with a power of attorney, follow these guidelines:

● Place a copy of the written power of attorney in a conspicuous place in the patient record.

● If a competent patient says that he wants to revoke his power of attorney, contact the physician and document exactly what he said and the time and date he said it.

DO-NOT-RESUSCITATE ORDERS

The physician writes a do-not-resuscitate (DNR) order when it's medically indicated—that is, when a patient is terminally ill and expected to die. In spite of the patient's autonomy and the requirement to honor the patient's wishes, the patient can't mandate that a facility provide futile treatment.

When caring for a patient with a DNR order, remember these points:

● DNR orders should be reviewed as policy dictates or whenever a significant change occurs in the patient's clinical status.

● Some facilities temporarily suspend DNR orders during surgery. Although the patient and physician aren't seeking heroic measures at the end of life, they won't allow the patient to bleed to death if he should hemorrhage during a palliative surgical procedure.

In court *Another exception is the concept of partial or "à la carte" resuscitation codes. These are legally precarious because the standard of care is to attempt full resuscitation through all means available, not partial resuscitation.*

● The patient's family members or friends don't have the legal authority to write an advance directive or to advise the physician regarding a DNR order unless they have a legal power of attorney or durable power of attorney.

● The patient is presumed to be competent and has the sole right to state what care he wishes, unless that care isn't indicated from a medical standpoint.

DURABLE POWER OF ATTORNEY

A durable power of attorney is a legal document in which a competent person designates another person to act on his behalf if he should become incapable of managing his own affairs. Some states have created one specifically for health care. It ensures that the patient's wishes regarding treatment will be carried out if he should ever become incompetent or unable to make decisions because of illness.

CONFIDENTIALITY

One of your documentation responsibilities includes protecting the confidentiality of the patient's medical record. Usually, you can't reveal confidential information without the patient's permission. (See *Patient rights under HIPAA,* page 154.)

Nurse's role

Nurses assume a primary role in maintaining confidentiality and in safeguarding the privacy of medical records. Breaches in confidentiality can result from unintentional release of information, unauthorized entry into a patient's record, or even a casual conversation that's overheard by others. To prevent breaches:
● avoid discussing patient concerns in areas where you can be overheard
● make sure that computer passwords are protected
● make sure that computer screens aren't in public view
● keep patient charts closed when not in use
● immediately file loose patient records
● properly dispose of unneeded patient information in accordance with the facility's procedure
● don't leave faxes and computer printouts unattended

● don't release the record without the documented consent of a competent patient; release of certain information—for example, mental health records as well as information about drug and alcohol abuse and infectious diseases—is further constrained by state statutes.

In court *In the case of* Anonymous v. Chino Valley Medical Center, *San Bernardino County, California Superior Court (1997), a 35-year-old disabled inpatient underwent a blood test for human immunodeficiency virus (HIV). He specifically told the physician that he didn't want the results to be given to anyone but him. On the day of discharge, his sister was present in the hospital room. A nurse asked the sister to come into the hall so she could tell her about the patient's diet instructions upon discharge. When in the hallway, the nurse told the sister that the patient had a positive HIV test. A few moments later, the physician approached them and also conveyed the test results. No action was filed against the physician. The nurse denied releasing the information. A trial court imposed a $5,000 statutory civil penalty against the medical center.*

In the case of Hobbs v. Lopes, *645 N.E.2d 1261, Ohio App. 4 DST. (1994), a 21-year-old Ohio woman was found to be pregnant after consulting a physician for another medical problem. Options, includ-*

PATIENT RIGHTS UNDER HIPAA

The goal of the Health Insurance Portability and Accountability Act (HIPAA) is to provide safeguards against the inappropriate use and release of personal medical information, including all medical records and identifiable health information in any form (electronic, on paper, or oral).

Patients are the beneficiaries of this privacy rule, which includes these six rights:
- the right to give consent before information is released for treatment, payment, or health care operations
- the right to be educated to the provider's policy on privacy protection
- the right to access their medical records
- the right to request that their medical records be amended for accuracy
- the right to access the history of non-routine disclosures (those disclosures that didn't occur in the course of treatment, payment, or health care operations, or those not specifically authorized by the patient)
- the right to request that the provider restrict the use and routine disclosure of information he has (providers aren't required to grant this request, especially if they think the information is important to the quality of care for the patient, such as disclosing human immunodeficiency virus status to another medical provider who's providing treatment).

ENFORCEMENT OF HIPAA

Enforcement of HIPAA regulation resides with the U.S. Department of Health and Human Services (HHS) (and within the HSS, the office of Civil Rights) and is based primarily on significant financial fines. HHS can impose civil penalties up to $25,000 per year per plan for unintentional violations. With hundreds of requirements, fines could quickly add up. Criminal penalties can also be imposed for intentional violations, including fines of up to $250,000, 10 years of imprisonment, or both.

IMPACT ON NURSING PRACTICE

Keep in mind that HIPAA regulations aren't intended to prohibit health care providers from talking to one another or to patients. Instead, they exist to help ease the communication process. The regulations require organizations to make "reasonable" accommodations to protect patient privacy and to employ "reasonable" safeguards to prevent inappropriate disclosure. Changes in nursing practice will likely be needed to meet these reasonable accommodations and safeguards.

Employers must provide education to nurses regarding the policies and procedures to be followed at their individual facilities. Nurses should be aware of how infractions will be handled because they, as well as the facility, face penalties for violations.

---

ing abortion, were discussed. The physician instructed a nurse to call the woman to find out what option she had chosen. The nurse called the woman's parents' home and disclosed the fact that their daughter was pregnant and had sought advice about an abortion. The daughter sued for medical malpractice, invasion of privacy, breach of privilege, and infliction of emotional distress.

Remember: The law requires you to disclose confidential information in certain situations—for example, in instances of alleged child abuse, matters of public health and safety, and criminal cases.

4

LEGALLY PERILOUS DOCUMENTATION

If you're ever named in a malpractice suit that proceeds to court, your documentation may be your best defense. It provides a running record of your patient care. How and what you documented—and even what you didn't document—will heavily influence the outcome of the trial.

Credible evidence

Typically, the outcome of every malpractice trial boils down to one question: Whom will the jury believe? The answer usually depends on the credibility of the evidence. Here's what occurs in a malpractice suit:

- The plaintiff presents evidence designed to show that he was harmed

or injured because care provided by the defendant (in this case, the nurse) failed to meet accepted standards of care.

- The nurse strives to present evidence demonstrating that she provided an acceptable standard of care.
- If the nurse can't offer believable evidence, the jury may have no choice but to accept the plaintiff's evidence. Even worse, if the nurse's evidence—including the medical record—is discredited, the plaintiff's attorney may convince a jury of her negligence. (See *Negligent or not.*)

By knowing how to document, what to document, when to document, and even who should document, you'll create a solid record. Knowing how to handle legally sensitive situations, such as difficult and

In court

NEGLIGENT OR NOT

If you've actually been negligent and have truthfully documented the care given, the medical record will naturally be the plaintiff's best evidence in a malpractice case. In such instances, the case will probably be settled out of court. If you haven't been negligent, the medical record should be your best defense, providing the best evidence of quality care. If the record makes you seem negligent, however, the jurors may conclude that you were negligent because they base their decision on the evidence.

The lesson: A "bad" medical record can be used to make a good nurse look bad. A "good" medical record should defend those who wrote it.

nonconforming patients, offers additional safeguards.

How to document

Documentation is a craft that's refined with experience. A skilled nurse knows that she needs to document that the standard of care was delivered, keeping in mind that it isn't only *what* she documents but *how* she documents that's important.

DOCUMENT OBJECTIVELY
The medical record should contain descriptive, objective information: what you see, hear, feel, smell, measure, and count—not what you suppose, infer, conclude, or assume. It may also contain subjective information, but only when it's supported by documented facts.

Stick to the facts
● Document only what you see and hear. Don't document that a patient

pulled out his I.V. line if you didn't witness him doing so. Instead, describe your findings—for example, "Found pt., arm board, and bed linens covered with blood. I.V. line and venipuncture device were untaped and hanging free." (See *Avoiding assumptions*.) Here's an example of how to document a patient's fall:

1/28/07	0600	Heard pt. scream. Found pt. lying beside bed. Pt. has laceration 2 cm long on forehead. Side rails up. Pt. stated he climbed over side rails to go to the bathroom. BP 184/92, P 96, R 24. Dr. Phillips notified by telephone at 0600 and ordered X-ray. Pt. c/o pain in ® hip. Pt. taken for X-ray of ® hip. ———————— Ann Barrow, RN

● Describe—don't label—events and behavior. Expressions such as "appears spaced out," "exhibiting bizarre

In court

AVOIDING ASSUMPTIONS

Always aim to record the facts about a situation—not your assumptions or conclusions. In this example, a nurse failed to document the facts and instead documented her assumptions about a patient's fall. As a result, she had to endure this damaging cross-examination by the plaintiff's attorney.

ATTORNEY: Would you read your fifth entry for January 6, please?

NURSE: Patient fell out of bed...

ATTORNEY: Thank you. Did you actually see the patient fall out of bed?

NURSE: Actually, no.

ATTORNEY: Did the patient tell you he fell out of bed?

NURSE: No.

ATTORNEY: Did anyone actually see the patient fall out of bed?

NURSE: Not that I know of.

ATTORNEY: So these notes reflect nothing more than conjecture on your part. Is that correct?

NURSE: I guess so.

ATTORNEY: Is it fair to say then, that you documented something as fact even though you didn't know it was?

NURSE: I suppose so.

ATTORNEY: Thank you.

behavior," or "using obscenities," mean different things to different people. They also reflect poorly on your professionalism and force you into the uncomfortable position of having to defend your own words, which hurts your credibility and distracts the jury from the fact that you provided the standard of care to the patient.

- Be specific. Describe facts clearly and concisely. Use only approved abbreviations and express your observations in quantifiable terms. Avoid catchall phrases such as "Pt. comfortable." Instead, describe his comfort. Is he resting, reading, or sleeping? Is he in pain?

1/18/07	1400	Dressing removed from
		® mastectomy site.
		Incision is pink. No
		drainage. Measures
		12.5 cm long and 2 cm
		wide. Slight bruising
		noted near center of
		incision. Dressing dry.
		Drain site below mast-
		ectomy incision
		measures 2 cm x 2 cm.
		Bloody, dime-sized
		drainage noted on
		drain dressing. No
		edema noted. Betadine
		dressings applied. Pt.
		complaining of mild
		incisional pain, 3 on a
		scale of 0 to 10. 2
		Tylox P.O. given at
		1330 hours. Pt. re-
		ports relief at 1355.
		———— Joan Delaney, RN

Avoid bias

- Document a patient's difficult or uncooperative behavior objectively. That way, the jurors will draw their own conclusions.

1/19/07	1400	I attempted to give pt.
		medication, but he said,
		"I've had enough pills.
		Now leave me alone."
		Explained the importance
		of the medication and
		attempted to determine
		why he would not take
		it Pt. refused to talk.
		Dr. J. Ellis notified by
		telephone at 1400 that
		medication was refused.
		———— Anne Curry, RN

- Don't use unprofessional adjectives, such as *obstinate, drunk, obnoxious, bizarre,* or *abusive,* that suggest a negative attitude toward the patient. This type of documentation:
  – invites the plaintiff's attorney to attack your professionalism
  – leads to bad feelings—and possibly more—between you and your patient.

Remember: The patient has a legal right to see his medical record. If he spots a derogatory reference, he'll be hurt, angry, and more likely to sue.

KEEP THE MEDICAL RECORD INTACT

The patient's medical record includes documentation about all aspects of his care. Sometimes, it can get rather big and bulky. Whatever you do, don't take this as a sign to get rid of older or less critical documents because every piece of documentation in the patient's record is important. You never know when you may have to refer back to it or rely on it during a malpractice case.

Take special care to keep the patient's record complete and intact by following these guidelines:

CONSEQUENCES OF MISSING RECORDS

The case of *Keene v. Brigham and Women's Hospital* 786 N.E.2d 824 (2003) underscores the significance of keeping the medical record intact.

A neonate developed respiratory distress within hours of birth. As a result of cyanosis, he was transferred to the neonatal intensive care unit. Blood tests, including a complete blood count (CBC) and a blood culture, were performed. Afterward, he was transferred back to the regular nursery for "routine care" with instructions to watch for signs and symptoms of sepsis and to withhold the antibiotic therapy pending the results of the CBC.

Approximately 20 hours after the neonate was transferred back to the nursery, the neonate was found in septic shock. He was also having seizures. It wasn't until this time that antibiotics were administered. Subsequent testing revealed that the neonate had contracted neonatal sepsis and meningitis. The results of the blood tests revealed the presence of group B beta-hemolytic streptococcus. However, the identity of the person to whom this information was conveyed and what actions were taken or not taken couldn't be determined because approximately 18 hours of records, including the records relating to these events, couldn't be found.

COURT'S DECISION

Pursuant to the doctrine of spoliation, the court held the health care facility accountable for prejudice resulting from loss of evidence. Therefore, the court allowed an adverse inference to be drawn that said without evidence to the contrary, the missing records would likely contain proof that the antibiotics should have been administered sooner and that the defendant's failure to do so caused the neonate's injuries.

- Don't discard pages from the medical record, even for innocent reasons. It's likely to raise doubt in the jury's mind about the record's reliability. (See *Consequences of missing records.*)
- If you replace an original sheet with a copy, cross reference it with lines such as, "Recopied from page 4" or "Recopied on page 6," and be sure to attach the original.
- If a page is damaged, note "Reconstructed documentation," and attach the damaged page.

What to document

Juries believe that incomplete documentation suggests incomplete nursing care—which is why malpractice attorneys are fond of saying, "If it wasn't documented, it wasn't done." This isn't literally true, of course, but it's an easy conclusion for a jury to draw, which is why precise documentation is of utmost importance. (See *Documenting precisely.*) Areas of documentation that are frequently reviewed in malpractice cases include:

- timely vital signs
- reporting changes in the patient's condition
- medications given
- patient responses
- discharge teaching.

DOCUMENT CRITICAL AND EXTRAORDINARY INFORMATION

The documentation of critical and extraordinary information is of utmost

DOCUMENTING PRECISELY

Patients or their families may believe a bad outcome is due to poor care. As you know, this isn't always the case. Here's an example of how precise documentation saved the day for one nurse.

A son wanted to sue a hospital and nurse for an incident involving his elderly father, who had been hospitalized for a cholecystectomy. Several days after surgery, his father became disoriented and disorderly, fell out of bed, and broke both hips. He never walked again.

In talking with his attorney, the son claimed, "That nurse either didn't know or didn't care that Dad was confused and agitated. She did nothing to protect him from harm. I want to sue."

The son's description of the father's care sounded like nursing negligence—until the attorney reviewed the patient's record and the nurse's notes. The nurse provided a detailed account of the events preceding the fall. Clearly, she knew about the pa-

tient's problem and did everything she could to protect him. Specifically, she:
- confined him to bed with a Posey restraint in compliance with the physician's order
- assigned an aide to stay with him when he became agitated
- made sure that the side rails were always up
- notified coworkers and asked them to watch the patient (his bed was visible from the nurses' station)
- documented all times that the patient and restraint were checked.

The record established that the nurse acted properly and showed concern for the patient. The patient's son was convinced that this unfortunate accident was just that—an accident.

Even if the case had gone to court, that nurse would have been well prepared to meet any challenge to her memory. The details were all there, in black and white.

---

importance and can't be overlooked. Whenever documenting such information, follow these guidelines:

● Whenever you encounter a critical or an extraordinary situation, document the details thoroughly. Failure to document details can have serious repercussions. (See *What you don't document can hurt you,* page 160. Also see *Documenting critical information: A case in point,* page 161.)

● Never document some things, such as conflicts among the staff. (See *Keeping the record clean,* pages 162 and 163.)

Here's an example to show how to document extraordinary information correctly:

1/2/07	0900	Digoxin 0.125 mg P.O. not given because of nausea and vomiting. Dr. T. Kelly notified that digoxin not given. Dr. T. Kelly gave order for digoxin 0.125 mg I.V. Administered at 0915 hours ———— ———— Ruth Bullock, RN

DOCUMENT FULL ASSESSMENT DATA

Failing to document an adequate physical assessment is a key factor in many malpractice suits. When performing a physical assessment, follow these guidelines:

● When initially assessing your patient, focus your documentation on

WHAT YOU DON'T DOCUMENT CAN HURT YOU

Only careful documentation can substantiate your version of events. Consider the situations here.

THE CASE OF THE SUPPOSED PHONE CALL

A patient was admitted to the health care facility for surgery for epicondylitis (tennis elbow). After the surgery, a heavy cast was applied to his arm. The patient complained to the nurse of severe pain, for which the nurse repeatedly gave pain medication.

The next morning, when the surgeon visited, he split the patient's cast. By that time, the ulnar nerve was completely paralyzed, and the patient was left with a permanently useless, clawed hand.

The patient subsequently sued the nurse for failing to notify the surgeon about his pain. At the deposition, the dialogue between the nurse and the plaintiff's attorney sounded like this:

ATTORNEY: Did you call the doctor?
NURSE: I must have called him.
ATTORNEY: Do you remember calling him?
NURSE: Not exactly, but I must have.
ATTORNEY: Do you have a record of making that call?
NURSE: No, I don't.
ATTORNEY: If you had made such a call, shouldn't there be a record of it?
NURSE: Yes, I guess so.
ATTORNEY: "Guess" is right; you can't really say that you made that call. You can only "guess" that you "must have."

THE CASE OF THE DOCUMENTATION DEFICIT

In the case of *Sweeney v. Purvis*, 665 So. 2d 926 (Ala., 1995), a 42-year-old woman was transferred to a rehabilitation facility 10 days after being admitted to another facility with a brain infarction. On her first day there, she attended therapy sessions without a problem.

The next day, after therapy, she had cramping in her left leg that wasn't relieved by analgesics. She also complained of pain in her left heel. The nursing staff called the physician, who ordered a heating pad applied to the affected leg.

The patient reported little pain that evening, but the next day her left leg appeared swollen, so she stayed in bed. When she tried to get out of bed, she again had pain. The licensed practical nurse caring for her noted a positive Homans' sign, which may indicate the presence of a blood clot. The registered nurse (RN) on duty also got a positive response and reported it to her manager. Believing that the manager would notify the physician, the RN didn't document the positive Homans' sign or tell the next shift about it.

The next morning, a nurse practitioner and an RN examined the patient. Because her left calf appeared enlarged, the nurses were concerned about her undergoing therapy—if a clot were present, movement could cause it to move to her lung. When told about her condition, the physician told the nurses to get her up for therapy.

That afternoon at lunch, the patient shook, turned blue, and developed pinpoint pupils. Then her breathing and pulse stopped. Paramedics transported her to the hospital, where she died.

The administrator of the patient's estate sued the physician and his professional corporation for wrongful death. In court, the RN who noted the positive Homans' sign testified that she told her manager about it, and the manager told her she would contact the physician.

The nurse-manager testified that she didn't recall the RN telling her about the patient's condition, and she didn't remember contacting the physician. The physician testified that he didn't recall the nurse-manager notifying him of the positive Homans' sign. Additionally, no documentation in the nurses' notes, the physician's orders, or the interdisciplinary progress notes supported the RN's claim that the physician was notified.

The jury decided in favor of the plaintiff and awarded $500,000 in damages.

The lesson? Appropriate nursing assessments aren't enough if you don't document your findings. This patient's death might have been averted if the nurse had written "positive Homans' sign" in the medical record.

DOCUMENTING CRITICAL INFORMATION: A CASE IN POINT

This case illustrates the significance of documenting critical information accurately as proof that you provided the accepted standard of care.

FAILURE TO DOCUMENT

Patti Bailey was admitted to the health care facility to deliver her third child. During her pregnancy, she had gained 63 lb, her blood pressure had risen from 100/70 mm Hg in her first trimester to 140/80 mm Hg at term, and an ultrasound done at 22 weeks showed possible placenta previa.

In the 4 hours after her admission, she received 10 units of oxytocin in 500 ml of dextrose 5% in lactated Ringer's solution. Documentation during this period was scant—her blood pressure was never documented, and there were only single notations of the fetal heart rate and how labor was progressing. The nurses failed to document the baby's reaction to the drug as well as the nature of the mother's contractions.

Suddenly, after complaining of nausea and epigastric pain, Mrs. Bailey suffered a generalized tonic-clonic seizure. Because her condition was so unstable, she couldn't undergo a cesarean section, and her baby

girl was delivered by low forceps. Mrs. Bailey developed disseminated intravascular coagulation and required 20 units of whole blood, platelets, and packed red blood cells within 8 hours of delivery.

Incredibly, Mrs. Bailey's nurse had documented nothing in the labor or delivery records or the progress notes.

DEFICIENT POLICY AND PROCEDURE MANUALS

When the unit's policy and procedure manuals were reviewed, no protocol for administering oxytocin and assessing the patient was included. At the very least, the manuals should have recommended using an oxytocin flow sheet to document vital signs, labor progress, fetal status, and changes in the drug administration rate.

THE RESULT

Although Mrs. Bailey recovered, her daughter has seizures and is developmentally disabled. Now age 15, the daughter can't walk or talk and has a gastrostomy tube for nutrition. The case was settled out of court for $450,000; the nurse and hospital were held responsible for one-third of the judgment, and the physician paid the rest.

---

his chief complaint, but also document all his concerns and your findings.
- After completing the initial assessment, establish your nursing care plan. A well-written care plan provides a clear approach to the patient's problems and can assist in your defense—*if* it was carried out.
- Phrase each patient problem statement clearly, and don't be afraid to modify the statement as you gather new assessment data.
- State the care plan for solving each problem, and then identify the actions you intend to implement. (See

Using good interview techniques to improve documentation, page 163.)

DOCUMENT DISCHARGE INSTRUCTIONS

The responsibility for giving discharge instructions is usually yours. If a patient receives improper instructions, and an injury results, you could be held liable. When documenting discharge instructions, follow these guidelines:
- Document that you distributed printed instruction sheets describing treatments and home care procedures that the patient will have to perform.

KEEPING THE RECORD CLEAN

What you say and how you say it are of utmost importance in documentation. Keeping the patient's record free from negative, inappropriate information—potential legal bombshells—can be quite a challenge when you're writing detailed narrative notes. Here are some guidelines to help you sidestep documentation pitfalls and document an accurate account of your patient's care and status.

AVOID DOCUMENTING STAFFING PROBLEMS

Even though staff shortages may affect patient care or contribute to an incident, you shouldn't refer to staffing problems in a patient's record. Instead, discuss them in a forum that can help resolve the problem. Call the situation to the attention of the appropriate personnel, such as your nurse-manager, in a confidential memo or an incident report. Also, review your facility's policy and procedure manuals to determine how you're expected to handle this situation.

KEEP STAFF CONFLICTS AND RIVALRIES OUT OF THE RECORD

Entries about disputes with nursing colleagues (including characterization and criticism of care provided), questions about a physician's treatment decisions, or reports of a colleague's rude or abusive behavior reflect personality clashes and don't belong in the medical record. They aren't legitimate concerns about patient care.

As with staffing problems, address concerns about a colleague's judgment or competence in the appropriate setting. After making sure that you have the facts, talk with your nurse-manager. Consult with the physician directly if an order concerns you. Share your opinions, observations, or reservations about colleagues with your nurse-manager only; avoid mentioning them in a patient's record.

If you discover personal accusations or charges of incompetence in a patient's record, discuss this with your supervisor.

HANDLING INCIDENT REPORTS

An incident report is a confidential, administrative communication that's filed separately from the patient's record. Some facilities require the notation, "Incident form completed," while others require you not to document in the record that an incident report was filed. Be familiar with your facility's policy, so you'll know how to accurately document this.

You should always document the facts of an incident in the patient's chart. For example, "Found pt. lying on the floor at 1250 hours. No visible bleeding or trauma. Pt. returned to bed with all side rails up and bed in low position. Vital signs: BP 120/80, P 76, T 98.2°. Notified Dr. Gary Dietrich at 1253 hours, and he saw pt. at 1300 hours" is a sufficient and accurate statement of the facts.

STEER CLEAR OF WORDS ASSOCIATED WITH ERRORS

Terms such as *mistake, accidentally, somehow, unintentionally, miscalculated,* and *confusing* can be interpreted as admissions of wrongdoing. Instead, let the facts speak for themselves—for example, "Pt. was given Demerol 100 mg I.M. at 1300 hours for abdominal pain VAS 7/10. Dr. T. Smith was notified at 1305 and gave no new orders. Pt.'s vital signs are BP 120/82, P 80, R 20, T 98.4°."

If the ordered drug dose was 50 mg, this entry will let other health care providers know that the patient was overmedicated.

AVOID NAMING NAMES

Naming another patient in someone else's record violates confidentiality. Use the word roommate, initials, or a room and bed number to describe the other patient.

Make sure that your documentation indicates which instructional materials were given and to whom, as the courts typically consider teaching materials as evidence that instruction took place.

● Document that the instructions given were tailored to the patient's specific needs and that they included verbal or written instructions that were provided.

● If caregivers practice procedures with the patient and family in the health care facility, document this, along with the results.

USING GOOD INTERVIEW TECHNIQUES TO IMPROVE DOCUMENTATION

Assessing a patient's condition adequately is part of your professional and legal responsibility. That means following up and documenting each of the patient's complaints. Documenting your data can be easier when you know how to ask questions that elicit the most information from your patient. Here's an example of an open-ended interview with a patient being assessed for abdominal pain.

NURSE: How would you describe the pain in your abdomen?

PATIENT: It's dull but constant. Actually, it doesn't bother me as much as my blurry eyesight.

NURSE: Tell me about your blurry eyesight.

PATIENT: When I work long hours at my computer, all the words and lines seem to blend together. Sometimes it also happens when I watch television. I probably should see my eye doctor, but I haven't had the time.

NURSE: We'll be sure to follow up on your blurred vision. Now, how about that abdominal pain. How does it affect your daily routine and your sleep?

Here's what went right in this interview.

■ First, the nurse didn't dismiss the patient's vision problem. If she had and it turned out to be serious, she might have been judged negligent.

■ Second, she asked open-ended questions so that the patient could explain his answers rather than simply saying "yes" or "no."

■ Third, she didn't put words in the patient's mouth. For example, she avoided saying, "The abdominal pain bothers you when you try to sleep, doesn't it?" That would have been a leading question. And the patient, assuming the nurse knows the right answer because she's a nurse, might have answered "yes"—even if the correct answer was "no."

UNDERSTANDING THE IMPORTANCE
OF TIMELY DOCUMENTATION

Although you would never document care before providing it, you may wait until the end of your shift or until your dinner break to complete your nurse's notes. That's what one nurse did. Some time later, she was summoned to court as a witness in a malpractice suit. She took the witness stand, answered the attorney's questions, and regularly referred to and read from the record while doing so. She relied heavily on it for her defense and, in the process, implicitly asked the jury to do the same.

The plaintiff's attorney began his crossexamination by asking the nurse to read from her entries. After a few minutes, here's what happened:

ATTORNEY: Excuse me, may I interrupt? As I listened to you read these entries, a question occurred to me. Maybe it occurred to the jury, too. Would you tell us whether you made the entries you are reading at the time of the events they describe?

NURSE: Well, no, I would have made them sometime later.

ATTORNEY: You're sure?

NURSE: Yes.

ATTORNEY: Thank you. Now, I'd like you to look at the record and tell the jury whether you noted the time that you actually gave the patient his medication.

NURSE: No, I didn't.

ATTORNEY: Now, I'd like you to look at the chart again and tell the jury whether you indicated the time that you made the entry.

NURSE: No.

ATTORNEY: Given the absence of those two pieces of information, how could you so promptly and confidently respond to my original question? How can you remember so clearly now that you made the entry sometime after the event it describes? Is it because your regular practice is to wait until the end of your shift to record each and every detail of every event that transpired over your entire shift, and that you rely solely on your memory when making all these entries?

NURSE: Well, yes, that's true.

ATTORNEY: Would you tell the jury how long a shift you worked that day?

NURSE: A 10-hour shift.

ATTORNEY: And how many patients did you see over that 10-hour period?

NURSE: About 15.

ATTORNEY: Now, each of these 15 patients was different, correct? Each had his own individualized care plan that corresponded to his particular health problems, isn't that right?

NURSE: That's right.

ATTORNEY: And how many different times did you see each of these different patients over the 10-hour period?

NURSE: I probably saw each one, on average, about once an hour.

ATTORNEY: In other words, you probably had 150 patient contacts on that shift alone, is that correct?

NURSE: I suppose so.

ATTORNEY: Now, during the course of your shift, do unexpected events sometimes develop? Unanticipated developments that must be attended to?

NURSE: Sometimes, yes.

ATTORNEY: And when these situations occur, do they distract you from things you had planned to do?

NURSE: Sometimes.

ATTORNEY: After working such a long shift, do you sometimes feel tired?

NURSE: Yes.

ATTORNEY: And at the end of a shift, are you sometimes in a hurry? With things to do, places to go, people to see?

NURSE: Yes.

ATTORNEY: Now, would you tell the jury the purpose of the record you keep for each patient?

NURSE: Well, we want to communicate information about the patient to others on the health care team, and we want to develop a historic account of the patient's problems, what has been done for him, and his progress.

ATTORNEY: So, other people rely on the information in this record when they make their own decisions about the patient's care?

NURSE: Yes, that's true.

ATTORNEY: So you would agree that the record must be reliable?

NURSE: Yes.

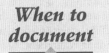

When to document

Finding the time to document can be a problem during a busy shift. But timely entries are crucial in malpractice suits. Here are some tips:

● Document your nursing care and other relevant activity when you perform it or not long after.
● Don't document ahead of time. Documenting before performing an intervention makes your notes inaccurate and also omits information about the patient's response to intervention. (See *Understanding the importance of timely documentation.*)

Who should document

You, and only you, should document your nursing care and observations. At times, because of understaffing or other circumstances, you may be tempted to ask another nurse to complete your portion of the medical record. However, doing so is illegal and prohibited by your state's nurse practice act.

DO YOUR OWN DOCUMENTING

Do your own documenting, and refuse to do anyone else's. Having someone else document for you may:
● lead to disciplinary actions that range from a reprimand to the suspension of your nursing license

- harm your patient if your coworker makes an error or misinterprets information
- make you and your employer accountable for negligence because delegated documentation is illegal and may constitute fraud
- destroy the credibility and value of the medical record, leading reasonable nurses and physicians to doubt it's accuracy
- diminish the record's value as legal evidence.

Remember: A judge will give little, if any, weight to a medical record that contains secondhand observations or hearsay evidence.

COUNTERSIGN CAUTIOUSLY

Although countersigning doesn't imply that you performed the procedure, it does imply that you reviewed the entry and approved the care given. To act correctly and to protect yourself, review your employer's policy on countersigning and follow these guidelines:

- If your facility interprets countersigning to mean that the licensed practical nurse (LPN), graduate nurse, or nursing assistant performed the nursing actions in the countersigning registered nurse's presence, don't countersign unless you were there when the actions occurred.
- If your facility acknowledges that you don't necessarily have time to witness your coworkers' actions, your countersignature implies that the LPN or nursing assistant had the authority and competence to perform the care described. In countersigning, you verify that all required patient care procedures were carried out.

- If policy requires you to countersign a subordinate's entries, review each entry and make sure that it clearly identifies who did the procedure. If you sign off without reviewing an entry, or if you overlook a problem the entry raises, you could share liability for any patient injury that results.
- If another nurse asks you to document her care or sign her notes, don't. Your signature will make you responsible for anything written in the notes above it.

Documenting legally sensitive situations

Among the most legally charged situations are those involving dissatisfied patients, suicidal patients, violent patients, and patients who carry out "nonconforming" behavior, such as refusing treatment, leaving the health care facility against medical advice, or mishandling equipment.

HANDLE DIFFICULT PATIENTS WITH CARE

No doubt you've cared for dissatisfied patients and heard remarks such as these: "I've been ringing and ringing for a nurse. I could have died before you got here!" or "This food is terrible—take it away!" If you tend to dismiss these remarks, you may be increasing your risk of a lawsuit. (See *How to handle a difficult patient situation.*) If a patient suggests that he's going to sue you and other caregivers:
- document this on the progress notes

- report it to your nurse-manager or your employer's legal department or attorney.

1/8/07	1000	Pt. stated that he plans to file suit against this facility for causing his bed sores. ———— Dave Bevins, RN

ASSESS INTENT TO COMMIT SUICIDE

Take all self-destructive behaviors and comments about suicide seriously. A person with suicidal intent not only has thoughts about committing suicide, he also has a concrete plan. If you suspect a patient is at risk for self-destructive behavior or a suicide attempt, follow your facility's policy and document that you:

- immediately notified the physician
- assessed the patient for suicide clues
- instituted suicide precautions, according to facility policy
- notified the nursing supervisor, other members of the health care team, and the risk manager
- updated the patient's care plan.

1/21/07	1100	Pt. reports that she lost her job yesterday. 3 months ago she had a miscarriage. She states, "I don't think I'm supposed to be here." Speaks with a low-toned voice, appears sad, avoids eye contact, and has an unkempt appearance. Reports getting no more than 3 hours of sleep per night for several weeks and states, "That's why I lost my job—I couldn't stay awake at work." Pt. reports having thoughts about suicide but declares, "I would never kill myself." She denies having a suicide plan. Has no history of previous suicide attempts. Pt. lives alone with no family nearby. Doesn't belong to a church and denies having any close friends. Denies having a history of drug or alcohol abuse or psychiatric illness. Dr. W. Patterson called at 1045 and told of this conversation with pt. She will see pt. for further evaluation at 1130. Will maintain suicide precautions until evaluated by dr. ——— Roger C. Trapley, RN

SAFELY RESPOND TO VIOLENT PATIENTS

When a patient demonstrates violent behavior, quick action is needed to protect him, other patients, and the staff from harm. Depending on their policies, some facilities prepare to handle a violent individual by mobilizing personnel. (See *Mobilizing staff for a violent patient.*) When responding to a violent patient, follow your facility's policy and document that you:

● called for help immediately and contacted security

● informed the physician, nursing supervisor, and risk manager of the patient's violence

● remained with the patient, but without crowding him and with a coworker, if necessary

● used your communication skills and a calm, nonthreatening tone of voice and stance to try to calm the patient

● listened to the patient and acknowledged his anger

● removed dangerous objects from the area.

Remember: Never challenge or argue with a violent patient.

MOBILIZING STAFF FOR A VIOLENT PATIENT

If you're caring for a patient who becomes violent, you may be required to call a specific code through the paging operator such as "code orange room 462B." Specific staff members, such as security personnel, male staff members, and individuals trained to handle volatile situations, would respond to the call. The patient would then be approached and physically subdued and restrained enough to ensure safety without harming himself, staff, or other patients, after which he'll need to be closely monitored and assessed, and the cause of the episode will need to be determined. He may also require continued chemical or physical restraints if his behavior persists and no physical causation is determined.

| 1/6/07 | 1715 | Heard shouts and a crash from pt.'s room at 1645. Upon entering room, saw dinner tray and broken dishes on floor. Pt. was standing, red-faced, with fist in air yelling, "My dog gets better food than this." Called for help and maintained a distance of approx. 5' from pt. When other nurses arrived, I told them to wait in hall. Pt. was throwing books and other items from nightstand to floor. Firmly told pt. to stop throwing things and that I wanted to help him. I stated, "I can see you're angry. How can I help you?" Pt. responded, "Try getting me some decent food." Asked a nurse in the hall to call dietary office to see what other choices were on menu for tonight. Told pt. I would try to get him other food choices. Asked pt. to sit down with me to talk. Pt. sat on edge of his bed and I sat on chair approx. 4' from pt. Pt. started to cry and said, "I'm so scared. I don't want to die." Listened to pt. verbalize his fears for several minutes. ————— — Kristen Burger, RN |

1/6/07 continued	1715	When asked, pt. stated he would like to speak with chaplain and would agree to talk with a counselor. He apologized for his behavior and stated he was embarrassed. Contacted Dr. A. Hartwell by telephone at 1705 and told him of pt.'s behavior. Doctor approved of psych. consult and gave verbal order. On-call psychiatrist paged at 1708. Hasn't yet returned call. Nursing supervisor, Jack Fox, RN, also notified of incident. ———— ———— Kristen Burger, RN

DOCUMENT PATIENT'S NONCONFORMING BEHAVIOR

When a patient does something—or fails to do something—that may contribute to an injury or explain why he hasn't responded to nursing and medical care, follow your facility's policy and document:

- patient's behaviors
- that you informed the patient of the possible consequences of his actions
- outcomes resulting from the patient's noncompliance.

Failure to provide information

When you encounter a patient who refuses to provide accurate or complete information about his health history, current medications, or treatments, follow your facility's policy and document:

- that you tried to obtain the information from other sources or forms

- any trouble you've had in communicating with the patient.

1/5/07	0830	When asked for a list of his current medications, the pt. said, "Why do you want to know? What business is it of yours? I don't know why I have to answer that question." ———— Nora Martin, RN

Unusual possessions

- Document unauthorized personal belongings discovered in the patient's possession (including alcoholic beverages, tobacco, heating pads, medications, vitamins, and other items that should be checked by the biomedical department before use).
- In your documentation, describe the object and how you disposed of it.

1/9/07	1100	Found 3 cans of unopened beer in pt.'s bedside table when checking his soap supply. Explained to pt. that beer was not allowed in the hospital. Took beer to nurse's station to be sent home with family. Dr. A. Kennedy notified by telephone at 1140 hours. He stated he would discuss this with pt. on rounds later today. Pt. denied having drunk any alcohol during hospitalization. No alcohol odor on breath. No empty cans in the trash or room. ———— Elaine Kasmer, RN

Firearms at bedside

If you observe or have reason to believe that your patient has a firearm

in his possession, follow these guidelines:

- Contact security and your nursing supervisor immediately, making sure that you follow your facility's guidelines.
- Keep other patients, staff, and visitors away from the area.
- Let the security guard deal with the firearm.

Here's an example of what to document:

1/18/07	1000	When reaching in bed-
		side table at 0930 to
		retrieve basin to assist
		pt. with a.m. care, noted
		black gun, approx. 6"
		long. Closed bedside
		table door, pushing
		table back out of reach
		of bed, left room and
		closed door. Called
		security at 0931 and
		reported gun in bed-
		side table of Rm. 312
		to Officer Halliday,
		who responded that a
		security guard would
		be sent up immediately,
		to keep out of pt.'s
		room, and to keep
		staff, visitors, and
		other patients away
		from area. Called Mary
		Delaney, RN, nursing
		supervisor, at 0933,
		who reported she's on
		her way to the floor
		immediately. Security
		officer Moore spoke
		with pt., who produced
		license to carry gun
		and turned unloaded
		gun over to the officer
		to be locked in hospital
		safe until discharge.
		Ms. Delaney reinforced
		hospital policy on fire-
		arms to pt. who stated
		he understood. ———
		——— Tom O'Brien, RN

Misuse of equipment

If you witness your patient misusing equipment, follow these guidelines:

- Explain to the patient that such misuse can harm him.
- Tell him to call for the nurse if he feels that equipment isn't working properly, is causing him discomfort, or if he has other concerns.
- Document in the progress notes what you saw the patient do (or what he told you he did) and what you did about the problem.

1/6/07	0930	I.V. rate set at 60
		ml/hr, 1,000 ml D5W
		1,000 ml in bag. ———
		——— K. Comerford, RN
1/6/07	1020	Checked I.V. at 1000
		840 ml left in bag. Pt.
		stated, "I flicked the
		switch because I didn't
		see anything happening.
		Then I pressed the
		green button and the
		arrow." BP 110/82, P
		80, T 98.4°. No signs
		of fluid overload.
		Breath sounds clear
		bilaterally. Instructed
		pt. not to touch the
		pump or I.V. Reposi-
		tioned pump to limit
		pt. access. Dr. T. Huang
		notified at 1015 hours.
		——— K. Comerford, RN

AMA discharges and elopements

If your patient wants to be discharged against medical advice (AMA), follow these guidelines:

- Notify your nurse-manager, the patient's physician, and possibly a member of the patient's family, who may be able to persuade the patient to stay. (Expect the patient's physician to inform the patient of the risks posed by refusing further treatment.)

- If the patient still intends to leave, complete the paperwork required by your facility, and document the time and the patient's condition in the record.
- Document the patient's desire for leaving AMA and any reason he gave.
- Document how he left, such as by cab, with a friend or family member, or by wheelchair. (For more information on documenting AMA discharges, see chapter 1, Documenting everyday events.)

If your patient elopes from the health care facility without having said anything about leaving, follow these guidelines:
- Look for him on your unit immediately, and notify security, your nurse-manager, and the patient's physician and family.
- Notify the police if the patient is at risk for harming himself or others.
- Document the time you discovered the patient missing, your attempts to find him, and the times and people notified. The legal consequences of a patient leaving the facility without medical permission can be particularly severe if he's confused or mentally incompetent, especially if he's injured or dies of exposure as a result of his absence.

5

COMPUTERIZED PATIENT RECORDS

The computerized patient record is the patient-centered product of a complex, interconnected set of clinical software applications that processes, inputs, and sends data. The computerized patient record:

● formats and categorizes information, making it readily available to provide guidance to clinicians and act as a record of the patient's care

● provides a longitudinal record of the patient's health care history in a particular facility and beyond

● includes ambulatory and in-patient records that can be accessed in many ways to fill information needs.

Whether you're a seasoned advanced practice nurse or a nursing student tackling your first clinical assignment, it's up to you to learn how to incorporate the computerized patient record into your daily practice, even as its importance becomes infused with new relevance and character thanks to other emerging technologies, such as:

● computerized order entry

● nurse-clinician documentation systems

● real-time clinical and operational report writing

● Internet-based self scheduling

● diagnostic test results and reports

● nursing care plan

● bar-coding of medications to help prevent medication errors.

The move toward computerized documentation

An increase in patient mortality due to medication and other procedural errors combined with the problems created by the nursing shortage has lead the health care industry to accelerate the development and implementation of computerized documentation systems. Other factors behind this move toward increased implementation include:

● more accurate standardization of health care billing transactions demands far more accurate documentation to satisfy third-party payers (see *Documentation: Headed for change*)

● the increasing complexity of health care facility business functions.

The most compelling reason for the development of a proficient electronic medical record (EMR) system, however, is better patient care.

A WORK IN PROGRESS

Definitions and parameters for workable computerized patient records, EMRs, and other computerized patient records remain a work in progress. However, informatics—the merging of medical and nursing science with computer science to better manage data—continues to see its role expand in all health care environments. (See *Raising the standards and value of documentation*.) Several medical and nursing informatics organizations are working to create standards, such as the:

- American Medical Informatics Association
- American Nursing Informatics Association
- Healthcare Information and Management Systems Society
- North American Nursing Diagnosis Association-International (NANDA-I)
- Nursing Informatics Working Group.

Advantages of computerized patient records

Today, there are more reasons for all clinical documentation to be incorporated into a computerized patient record than not. (See *Computerized patient record: Key advantages*.) Advantages include:

- Improved standardization—Standardization of clinical data and reporting has been pushed to the forefront by the Health Insurance Portability and Accountability Act, which requires accurate and timely reports required for accrediting, regulatory, and third-party payers. This increased demand for reports requires computerization of the report writer, which, in turn, requires clinical data input.
- Improved quality of the medical record—With a properly designed and implemented clinical information system, computerized patient record documentation improves the overall caliber of clinical information. It also returns the focus of nurses to providing nursing care.
- Improved legibility—In 1999, the Institute of Medicine published a report that recommended the move toward a universal system of computerized order entry because medication errors were commonly caused by the inability to properly decipher handwritten orders. With computerized physician order entry, legibility is a nonissue.
- Increased access to information—Accessing patient data is quick and painless by filing clinical information in the same location from patient to patient and department to department. Across the board universality also saves time and contributes to more accurate assessment of recorded data. Mobile workstations allow access to information closer to the point of care.
- Quicker retrieval—Typically, you can retrieve information more quickly with computers than with traditional documentation systems. Most systems allow you to print a patient medication administration record each shift that contains information to guide your care. (See *Computer-generated medication administration record*.)

COMPUTERIZED PATIENT RECORD: KEY ADVANTAGES

This list highlights the key benefits of using a computerized patient record:
- ability for all providers to see each other's documentation
- access by different providers at different locations
- access by different providers at the same time
- access to clinical information
- access to computerized patient records at appropriate workstations
- automated reports for quality indicators
- clinical decision making easier and more accurate
- ease in auditing documentation
- ease of access—"where to look"
- increased quality of documentation
- legibility
- multidisciplinary access
- online clinical support information
- patient-driven care planning
- point-of-care documentation (no more waiting until the end of your shift)
- "real-time" diagnostic results and reports
- reduced redundant documentation
- remote access.

COMPUTER-GENERATED
MEDICATION ADMINISTRATION RECORD

The computer-generated medication administration record contains vital information to help guide your nursing care throughout your shift. It may be necessary to print out a new record at various times throughout your shift, so new physician's orders are reflected.

```
Medical ICU-4321                  Patient Care Hospital
1/14/07      07:00                PAGE 001
==============================================================

WILLIAMS, HENRY                   64   MWMC
MR#: 5555555       DOB 10/26/40   MICU 302
FIN#: 1010101010                  Admitted: 1/12/07
DR: Daniel Smith                  Service: Internal Medicine
==============================================================


Summary: 1/14 07:00 to 15:00

ALLERGIES AND CODE STATUS
1/12/07       MED ALLERGY: NO KNOWN DRUG ALLERGY
              NO INTUBATION

PATIENT INFORMATION:
1/12/07       Admit Dx: TIA
1/12/07       Final Dx: Stroke
1/12/07       Patient condition: Fair
1/12/07       Clinical guideline: Stroke
1/12/07       Language: English
1/12/07       PMH: No problems respiratory, HTN, No prob-
              lems GI, No problems GU, Type 2 diabetes, No
              problems skin, No problems blood, No prob-
              lems musculoskeletal, No problems psych, No
              problems hearing, glasses, cholecystectomy
              1982, Tobacco use: denies, Alcohol use: cur-
              rent, 1 beer/day, Illicit drug use: denies,
              Immunizations: Flu vaccine: 2004
1/12/07       Living will: yes, on chart
1/12/07       Durable power of attorney: yes, Name of
              DPOA: June Smith, Phone number 5555551234
1/12/07       Organ donor: yes, card on chart

CONSULTS:
1/12/07       Consult Westside Neurological Associates to
              see patient regarding flaccid left side and
              expressive aphasia**Nurses, call consult
              now**

ISF NOTES:
1/12/07       Care plan: General care of the adult
1/12/07       Nursing protocol: Falls prevention
1/12/07       Nursing protocol: Skin breakdown (preven-
              tion)
1/12/07       Goal: Patient will tolerate a progressive
              increase in activity level.
```

(continued)

COMPUTER-GENERATED MEDICATION
ADMINISTRATION RECORD (CONTINUED)

```
Medical ICU-4321                    Patient Care Hospital
1/14/07       07:00      PAGE 002
===============================================================

WILLIAMS, HENRY                    66   MWMC
MR#: 5555555        DOB 10/26/40   MICU 302
FIN#: 1010101010                   Admitted: 1/12/07
DR: Daniel Smith                   Service: Internal Medicine
===============================================================

Summary: 1/14 07:00 to 15:00

NURSE COMMUNICATIONS:
1/12/07        IV site RA2, #20 inserted, restart on
               1/15/07

ALL CURRENT MEDICAL ORDERS
Doctor to Nurse Orders:
1/12/07        Blood cultures x 2 if temperature > 101  F,
               Nurse please enter as a secondary order,
               when necessary.
1/12/07        Cardiology: ECG 12 lead Stat, prn chest
               pain, Nurse please enter as a secondary
               order, when necessary.
1/12/07        Sequential Teds: Patient to wear continuous-
               ly while in bed.
1/12/07        Foley catheter to urometer, measure output
               q 1 hour, notify MD if UO < 30 ml/hour or
               > 300 ml/hour x 2 hours.
1/12/07        Notify MD for SBP > 180 mm Hg or < 110 mm Hg
1/12/07        Notify MD for change in mental status
1/12/07        Accucheck q 6 hours

Vital Sign Orders:
1/12/07        VS: q 1 hour with neurological checks

Diet:
1/12/07        Diet: NPO

I&O Orders:
1/12/07        Per ICU routine

Activity:
1/12/07        Activity: Bedrest with HOB elevated 30 de-
               grees
IVS:
1/12/07        IV line Dextrose 5% & Sodium Chloride 0.45%
               1000 ml, Rate: 80 ml/hour, x 2 bags

Scheduled Medications:
1/12/07        Decadron Dexamethasone Inj 4 mg, IV, q 6
               hours
                     09        15
1/12/07        Lopressor Metoprolol Inj 5 mg, IV, q 6 hours
```

COMPUTER-GENERATED MEDICATION ADMINISTRATION RECORD *(CONTINUED)*

```
Medical ICU-4321              Patient Care Hospital
1/14/07      07:00            PAGE 003
============================================================

WILLIAMS, HENRY                    64  MWMC
MR#: 5555555      DOB 10/26/40     MICU 302
FIN#: 1010101010                   Admitted: 1/12/07
DR: Daniel Smith                   Service: Internal Medicine
============================================================

Summary: 1/14 07:00 to 15:00

                    09       15
1/12/07       Heparin inj 5,000 units, SC, q 12 hours
                    09

Miscellaneous Medications:
1/12/07       Lasix Furosemide Inj 40 mg, IV, Now

PRN Medications:
1/12/07       Tylenol Acetaminophen Supp 650 mg, #1, PR,
              q  4 hour prn pain or temperature > 101 F

Laboratory:
1/14/07       Basic metabolic panel tomorrow, collect at
              05:00
1/14/07       CBC/Diff/Plts tomorrow, collect at 05:00
1/14/07       Cardiac troponin, tomorrow, collect at 05:00

Radiology:
1/12/07       Computed tomography: CT scan of the head
              without contrast STAT

Ancillary:
1/12/07       Respiratory care: Oxygen via nasal cannula
              at 2L/minute.
1/12/07       Physical therapy: Patient evaluation and
              treatment
                        Last page
```

Disadvantages of computerized records

Every day, we learn how to improve computerized patient records. However, if we're to make use of them fully, we must become proficient in their strengths, and adapt to their weaknesses, such as:

● Computer downtime—Systems can crash or break down, making information temporarily unavailable. Downtimes will happen and, in fact, they're occasionally necessary.

PREVENTING BREACHES IN PATIENT CONFIDENTIALITY

This chart provides specific measures you can take to ensure that information about your patients remains confidential.

TYPE OF BREACH	HOW TO PREVENT IT
COMPUTERS	
Displays Displaying information on a screen that's viewed by unauthorized users (especially for handheld computers)	Make sure that display screens don't face public areas. For portable devices, install encryption software that makes information unreadable or inaccessible.
E-mail Sending confidential messages via public networks such as the Internet, where they can be read by unauthorized users	Use encryption software when sending e-mail over public networks.
Printers Sharing printers among units with differing functions and information (unauthorized people can read printouts)	Request that your unit have a separate printer not shared with another unit.
COPIERS	
Discarded copies of patient health information in trash cans adjacent to copiers	Use secure disposal containers adjacent to copiers for future paper shredding.
CORDLESS AND CELLULAR PHONES	
Holding conversations vulnerable to eavesdropping by outsiders with scanning equipment	Use phones with built-in encryption technology.
FAX MACHINES	
Faxing confidential information to unauthorized persons	Before transmission, verify the fax number and that the recipient is authorized to receive confidential information.
VOICE PAGERS	
Sending confidential messages that can be overheard on the pager	Restrict use of voice pagers to nonconfidential messages.

● Unfamiliarity—There are still segments of the nursing population that aren't comfortable with computer usage. Used improperly, computerized systems can threaten a patient's right to privacy. (See *Preventing breaches in patient confidentiality.*) They can also yield inaccurate or incomplete information if multiple operating systems aren't integrated within a health care system.

MAINTAINING CONFIDENTIALITY WITH COMPUTERIZED DOCUMENTATION

The American Nurses Association (ANA) and the American Medical Records Association offer these guidelines for maintaining the confidentiality of computerized medical records:

● *Never share your password or computer signature.* Never give your personal password or computer signature to anyone—including another nurse in the unit, a nurse serving temporarily in the unit, or a physician. Your health care facility can issue a short-term password authorizing access to certain records for infrequent users.

● *Be aware of your surroundings.* Don't display confidential patient information on a monitor where it can be seen by others or leave print versions or excerpts of the patient's medical record unattended. Keep a log that accounts for every copy of a computer file that you've printed.

● *Log off if not using your terminal.* Don't leave a computer terminal unattended after you've logged on. (Some computers have a timing device that shuts down a terminal after a certain period of inactivity.)

● *Follow your facility's policy for correcting errors.* Computer entries are part of the patient's permanent record and, as such, can't be deleted. In most cases, you can correct an entry error before storing the entry. To correct an error after storage, mark the entry "error" or "mistaken entry," add the correct information, and date and sign the entry.

● *Make backup files.* Make sure that stored records have backup files—an important safety feature. If you inadvertently delete part of the permanent record (even though there are safeguards against this), type an explanation into the file along with the date, the time, and your initials. Submit an explanation in writing to your nurse-manager, and keep a copy for your records.

How computerized systems work

In addition to having a mainframe computer, most health care facilities have personal computers or terminals at workstations throughout the facility, so departmental staff have quick access to vital information and can easily enter patient care orders. Some facilities have bedside terminals that make data even more accessible. Here's a quick overview of how these systems work:

● Before entering a patient's clinical record onto a computer, you must first enter your password, which is usually your personal computer identification number. Passwords commonly specify the type of information that a particular team member can access. For example, a dietitian may be assigned a code that allows her to see dietary orders but not physical therapy orders.

● The patient's name, account number, medical record number, and other demographic data are then entered.

● The physician can log into the system and access the physician's order screens. When he chooses the appropriate orders, the computer system transmits the orders to the patient's nursing department and the other appropriate departments. For example, if the physician orders medications for the patient, the order is transmit-

the patient's electronic chart to the screen. This will allow her to scan the record to compare data on vital signs, laboratory test results, or intake and output; enter new data on the care plan or progress notes; and sign out medications that she's administered. Bar code technology is simplifying medication administration even further. (See *Bar code technology.*)

Systems and functions

Depending on which type of computer hardware and software your health care facility has, you may access information by using a keyboard, light pen, touch-sensitive screen, mouse, or voice activation. Currently used systems include the Nursing Information System (NIS), the Nursing Minimum Data Set (NMDS), the Nursing Outcomes Classification (NOC) system, and voice-activated systems.

NURSING INFORMATION SYSTEM

The NIS makes nursing documentation easier by reflecting most or all of the components of the nursing process, so they can meet the standards of the ANA and Joint Commission on Accreditation of Healthcare Organizations.

Nursing benefits
● Provides different features and can be customized to conform to a facility's documentation forms and formats (see *Computers and the nursing process*)
● Manages information either passively or actively

ted to the patient's nursing department and the pharmacy. This type of direct-order transmittal helps prevent dosing errors and cuts down on medication errors by eliminating order transcription errors.
● After the physician's orders are entered, the nurse can log into the system and enter the patient's name (or choose his name from a patient census list) or account number to bring

COMPUTERS AND THE NURSING PROCESS

Nursing information systems (NISs) can increase efficiency and accuracy in all phases of the nursing process—assessment, nursing diagnosis, planning, implementation, and evaluation—and can help nurses meet the standards established by the American Nurses Association and the Joint Commission on Accreditation of Healthcare Organizations. In addition, an NIS can help you spend more time meeting the patient's needs. Consider the following uses of computers in the nursing process.

ASSESSMENT

Use the computer terminal to document admission information. As data are collected, enter further information as prompted by the computer's software program. Enter data about the patient's health status, history, chief complaint, and other assessment factors. Some software programs prompt you to ask specific questions and then offer pathways to gather further information. In some systems, if you enter an assessment value that's outside the usual acceptable range, the computer will flag the entry to call your attention to it.

NURSING DIAGNOSIS

Most current programs list standard nursing diagnoses with associated signs and symptoms as references; you must still use clinical judgment to determine a nursing diagnosis for each patient. With this information, you can rapidly obtain diagnostic information. For example, the computer can generate a list of possible diagnoses for a patient with selected signs and symptoms, or it may enable you to retrieve and review the patient's records according to the nursing diagnosis.

PLANNING

To help nurses begin writing a care plan, newer computer programs display recommended expected outcomes and interventions for the selected diagnoses. Computers can also track outcomes for large patient populations and general information to help you select patient outcomes. You can use computers to compare large amounts of patient data, help identify outcomes the patient is likely to achieve based on individual problems and needs, and estimate the time frame for reaching outcome goals.

IMPLEMENTATION

Use the computer to document actual interventions and patient-processing information, such as transfer and discharge instructions, and to communicate this information to other departments. Computer-generated progress notes automatically sort and print out patient data, such as medication administration, treatments, and vital signs, making documentation more efficient and accurate.

EVALUATION

During evaluation, use the computer to document and store observations, patient responses to nursing interventions, and your own evaluation statements. You may also use information from other members of the health care team to determine future actions and discharge planning. If a desired patient outcome hasn't been achieved, document interventions taken to ensure such desired outcomes. Then re-evaluate the second set of interventions.

- *Passive systems* collect, transmit, organize, format, print, and display information that you can use to make a decision, but they don't suggest decisions for you.
- *Active systems* suggest nursing diagnoses based on predefined assessment data that you enter.

- Provides standardized patient status and nursing intervention phrases that you can use to construct your progress notes; these more sophisticated systems let you change the standardized phrases, if necessary, allowing room for you to add your own documentation

The most recent NISs are interactive, meaning they prompt you with questions and suggestions that are in accordance with the information you enter. These systems prove especially helpful because they:
- require only a brief narrative, and the questioning and diagnostic suggestions that the systems provide ensure quick but thorough documentation
- allow you to add or change information so that you can tailor your documentation to fit each patient.

NURSING MINIMUM DATA SET

The NMDS attempts to standardize nursing information into three categories of data:
- nursing care
- patient demographics
- service elements. (See *Elements of the Nursing Minimum Data Set.*)

Nursing benefits
- Allows you to collect nursing diagnosis and intervention data and identify the nursing needs of various patient populations
- Lets you track patient outcomes and describe nursing care in various settings, including the patient's home
- Helps establish accurate estimates for nursing service costs and provides data about nursing care that may influence health care policy and decision making
- Helps you provide better patient care by allowing you to compare nursing trends locally, regionally, and nationally, and to compare nursing data from various clinical settings, patient populations, and geographic areas
- Encourages more consistent nursing documentation
- Makes documentation and information retrieval faster and easier (Currently, NANDA-I assigns numeric

codes to all nursing diagnoses so they can be used with the NMDS.)

NURSING OUTCOMES CLASSIFICATION

The NOC system provides the first comprehensive, standardized method of measuring nursing-sensitive patient outcomes.

Nursing benefits

- Allows you to compare your patients' outcomes to the outcomes of larger groups according to such parameters as age, diagnosis, or health care setting
- Is essential to support ongoing nursing research
- Makes possible the inclusion of patient data-related outcomes that have been absent from computerized medical information databases in the past

VOICE-ACTIVATED SYSTEMS

Voice-activated systems are most useful in departments that have a high volume of structured reports such as the operating room. The software program uses a specialized knowledge base—nursing words, phrases, and report forms, combined with automated speech recognition technology—that allows the user to record, prompt, and complete nurses' notes by voice.

Nursing benefits

- Require little or no keyboard use
- Include information on the nursing process, nursing theory, nursing standards of practice, report forms, and a logical format
- Use trigger phrases that cue the system to display passages of report text and also allow word-for-word dictation and editing
- Increase the speed of reporting and free the nurse from paperwork so that she can spend more time with patients

6

DOCUMENTATION IN ACUTE CARE

A medical record with well-organized, completed forms will help you communicate patient information to the health care team, garner accreditation and reimbursements, and protect you and your employer legally. It will also allow you to spend more time providing direct patient care.

Nursing admission assessment form

Also known as a *nursing database,* the nursing admission assessment form contains your initial patient assessment data. In order to complete the form, you'll have to collect relevant information from various sources and analyze it to assemble a complete picture of the patient. Keep these points in mind when using an admission assessment form:

- It's meant to be a record of your nursing observations, the patient's health history, and your physical examination findings.
- It may be organized by body system or by patient responses, such as relating, choosing, exchanging, and communicating.
- It may include data about:
  - the patient's medications
  - the patient's known allergies to foods, medications, and other substances
  - nursing findings related to activities of daily living (ADLs)
  - the patient's current pain level
  - your impressions of the patient's support systems
  - documentation of the patient's advance directives, if any.

Patient safety *To comply with the Joint Commission on Accreditation of Healthcare Organizations' (JCAHO) Patient Safety Goals, the admission record should also include a current list of the patient's medications.*

- When completing the form, you may have to fill in blanks, check off boxes, or write narrative notes. (See *Completing the nursing admission assessment.*)

ADVANTAGES

- Carefully completed, provides pertinent physiologic, psychosocial, and cultural information
- Contains subjective and objective data about the patient's current health

(Text continues on page 188.)

COMPLETING THE NURSING ADMISSION ASSESSMENT

Most health care facilities use a combined checklist and narrative admission form such as the one shown here. The nursing admission assessment becomes a part of the patient's permanent medical record.

ADMISSION DOCUMENT
(To be completed on or before admission by admitting RN)

Name: *Raymond Bergstrom*   Hospital I.D. No.: *4227*

Age: *71*   Insurer: *Aetna*

Birth date: *4/15/33*   Policy No.: *605310P*

Address: *3401 Elmhurst Ave.,*   Physician: *Joseph Milstein*

Jenkintown, PA 19046   Admission date: *1/28/07*

          Unit: *3N*

Preoperative teaching according to standard? ☑ Yes ☐ No

Preoperative teaching completed on _____ *1/28/07*

If no,   ☐ Surgery not planned   ☐ Emergency surgery

Signature *Kate McCauley, RN*

Admitted from: **Mode:**

☐ Emergency room   ☐ Ambulatory

☐ Home   ☑ Wheelchair

☑ Physician's office   ☐ Stretcher

☐ Transfer from   Accompanied by:

          Wife

T *101° F*   P *120*   R *24*   **Pulses:**

BP (Lying/sitting)   L: *P* Radial *P* DP *P* PT

Left: _____   R: *P* Radial *P* DP *P* PT

Right: *120 / 68*   Apical pulse *120*

Height *5'7"*   ☑ Regular   ☐ Irregular

Weight *160 lb.*   P = Palpable   D = Doppler   O = Absent

Pain:

⓪ 1 2 3 4 5 6 7 8 9 10 (small: "0" indicates no pain; "10" indicates worst pain imaginable)

Signature *K. McCauley, RN*

(continued)

MEDICAL & SURGICAL HISTORY

Check (P) if patient or (R) if a blood relative has had any of the following. Check (H) if patient has ever been hospitalized. If it isn't appropriate to question patient because of age or gender, cross out option, e.g., ~~infertility~~.

	(H)	(P)	(R)	Interviewer comments		(H)	(P)	(R)	Interviewer comments
Addictions (e.g., alcohol, drugs)	☐	☐	☐		Hepatitis	☐	☐	☐	
					High cholesterol	☐	☑	☐	
Angina	☐	☐	☐		Hypertension	☐	☐	☐	
Arthritis	☐	☐	☐		~~Infertility~~	☐	☐	☐	
Asthma	☐	☑	☑		Kidney disease/ stones	☐	☐	☐	
Bleeding problems	☐	☐	☐						
Blood clot	☐	☐	☐		Leukemia	☐	☐	☐	
Cancer	☐	☐	☐		Memory loss	☐	☐	☐	
Counseling	☐	☐	☐		Mood swings	☐	☐	☐	
CVA	☐	☐	☐		Myocardial infarction	☐	☐	☐	
Depression	☐	☐	☐		Prostate problems	☐	☐	☐	
Diabetes	☐	☐	☑		Rheumatic fever	☐	☐	☐	
Eating disorders	☐	☐	☐		Sexually trans. disease	☐	☐	☐	
Epilepsy	☐	☐	☐		Thyroid problems	☐	☐	☐	
Eye problems (not glasses)	☐	☐	☐		TB or positive test	☐	☐	☐	
					Other	☐	☐	☐	
Fainting	☐	☐	☐		**List any surgeries the patient has had:**				
Fractures	☐	☐	☐		**Date**	**Type of surgery**			
Genetic condition	☐	☐	☐						
Glaucoma	☐	☐	☐		Has the patient ever had a blood				
Gout	☐	☐	☐		transfusion: ☐ Y ☑ N				
Headaches	☐	☐	☐		reaction: ☐ Y ☐ N				

UNIT INTRODUCTION

Patient rights given to patient: ☑ Y ☐ N

Patient verbalizes understanding: ☑ Y ☐ N

☑ Patient ☑ Family oriented to:

Nurse call system/unit policies: ☑ Y ☐ N

Smoking/visiting policy/intercom/

side rails/TV channels: ☑ Y ☐ N

Patient valuables:

☑ Sent home

☐ Placed in safe

☐ None on admission

Patient meds:

☑ Sent home

☐ Placed in pharmacy

☐ None on admission

COMPLETING THE NURSING ADMISSION ASSESSMENT (CONTINUED)

ALLERGIES OR REACTIONS

Medications/dyes	☑ Y ☐ N	*PCN – rash*
Anesthesia drugs	☐ Y ☑ N	
Foods	☐ Y ☑ N	
Environmental (e.g., tape, latex, bee stings, dust, pollen, animals, etc.)	☑ Y ☐ N	*Dust, pollen, cats*

ADVANCE DIRECTIVE INFORMATION

1. Does patient have health care power of attorney? ☐ Y ☑ N
   Name: _____ Phone: _____
   If yes, request copy from patient/family and place in chart.
   Date done: _____ Init. _____
2. Does patient have a living will? ☑ Y ☐ N
3. Educational booklet given to patient/family? ☑ Y ☐ N
4. Advise attending physician if there is a living will or power of attorney. ☑ Y ☐ N

ORGAN & TISSUE DONATION

1. Has patient signed an organ and/or tissue donor card? ☐ Y ☑ N
   If yes, request information and place in chart. Date done: _1/28/07_
   If no, would patient like to know more about the subject of donation? ☑ Y ☐ N
2. Has patient discussed his wishes with family? ☑ Y ☐ N

MEDICATIONS

Does patient use any over-the-counter medications?

Aspirin ☐ Y ☑ N Laxatives ☑ Y ☐ N
Vitamins ☑ Y ☐ N Weight loss ☐ Y ☑ N

What does the patient usually take for minor pain relief? _Acetaminophen_

Prescribed medication (presently in use)	Reason	Dose and frequency	Last time taken
1. *Proventil*	*asthma*	*2 puffs q 4 hr*	*1/21/07*
2.			

Herbal remedies

1. _____
2. _____

Signature _Kate McCauley, RN_ Date _1/28/07_

status and clues about actual or potential health problems

- Reveals the patient's expectations for treatment, his ability to comply with treatment, and details about his lifestyle, family relationships, and cultural influences
- Guides you through the nursing process by helping you readily formulate nursing diagnoses, create patient problem lists, construct care plans, and begin discharge planning
- Useful in describing the patient's living arrangement, caregivers, resources, support groups, and other relevant information needed for discharge planning
- Used by JCAHO, quality improvement groups, and other parties to continue accreditation, justify requests for reimbursement, and maintain or improve the standards of quality patient care
- Serves as a baseline for later comparison with the patient's progress

DISADVANTAGES

- May be unable to complete the nursing admission assessment form if the patient is too sick to answer questions or a family member can't answer for him

DOCUMENTATION STYLE

Admission assessment forms follow a medical format, emphasizing initial symptoms and a comprehensive review of body systems or a nursing process format. (See chapter 2, Documenting from admission to discharge.) Regardless of which format you use, document admission assessments in one or a combination of three styles: open-ended, closed-ended, and narrative. (See *Writing a narrative admission assessment.*)

Standard open-ended style

- Uses standard fill-in-the-blank pages with preprinted headings and questions
- Uses phrases and approved abbreviations
- Organized into specific categories, so you can easily document information and retrieve it

Standard closed-ended style

- Arranged categorically with preprinted headings, checklists, and questions
- Calls for you to simply check off the appropriate responses
- Eliminates the problem of illegible handwriting and makes reviewing documented information easy
- Clearly establishes the type and amount of information required by the health care facility

Narrative notes

- Handwritten or computer-generated
- Summarize information obtained by general observation, the health history interview, and a physical examination
- Allows you to list your findings in order of importance

Alert *The current trend in health care facilities is to avoid writing long narrative note entries because they're time-consuming to write and read, require you to remember and document all significant information in a detailed, logical sequence, and interfere with efficient data retrieval. If using narrative notes, make sure that you keep them concise, pertinent, and based on your evaluations.*

(Text continues on page 194.)

WRITING A NARRATIVE ADMISSION ASSESSMENT

Here's an example of a nursing admission assessment form documented in narrative style. The data begin with the patient's health history.

Patient's name: _James McGee_

Address: _20 Tomlinson Road, Elgin, IL 60120_

Home phone: _(555) 203-0704_

Work phone: _(555) 389-2050_

Sex: _Male_

Age: _55_

Birth date: _5/11/50_

Social Security no.: _189-30-2415_

Place of birth: _Waterbury, CT_

Race: _Caucasian_

Nationality: _American_

Culture: _Irish-American_

Marital status: _Married, Susan, age 48_

Dependents: _James, age 16; Gretchen, age 14_

Contact person: _Wife (same address as patient) or Clare Hennigan, sister (1214 Ridge Road, De Kalb, IL 60115; phone [555] 203-1212)_

Religion: _Roman Catholic_

Education: _M.S. Degree_

Occupation: _Chemistry teacher, Schawnburg High School_

Chief health complaint

States, "I've had several episodes of gnawing pain in my stomach, and I feel very tired. My doctor examined me and told me I should have some tests to find out what's wrong."

Health history

Has been feeling unusually tired for about a month. States he lost 12 lb last month and about 5 lb before that without trying. States that he's busier at work than usual. He thinks his fatigue may be caused more by his schedule than by physical problems.

(continued)

Past health: *Had measles, mumps, chickenpox as child. Hospitalized at age 6 for tonsillectomy and adenoidectomy. Had a concussion and a fractured left leg at age 17 from a football accident. Has had no complications from that. Immunizations are up-to-date. Last tetanus shot 5 years ago; received hepatitis B vaccine 1 year ago.*

Functional health: *Describes himself as having a good sense of humor. Feels good about himself; feels he gets along fairly well with people and has many friends.*

Cultural and religious influences: *Says he has strong religious background, goes to church regularly —important part of his life.*

Family relationships: *Because he's enrolled in a doctorate program at night, pt. regrets he doesn't get to spend much time with wife and children. Jimmy and Gretchen get along well together, but sometimes compete for time with him.*
Pt. says he's usually easygoing but lately blows up at the kids when stress and deadlines from school have him tied in knots.
Describes relationship with wife, father, and sister as good (mother deceased).

Sexuality: *Says he and wife had a "decent [adequate] sex life" before he started work toward PhD. Now he's too tired.*

Social support: *Has many close friends who live in his neighborhood. Would like to socialize more with friends but schoolwork claims most of his time.*

Other:

Personal health perception and behaviors: *Smokes cigarettes — between 1 and 2 packs/day. Never used illicit drugs. Takes vitamin and mineral supplements and occasional nonprescription cold medicines. Diet is eat and run — usually goes to fast-food place for dinner before night class. Drinks 1 or 2 glasses of beer a week when he has time for dinner at home. Drinks 6 to 8 cups black coffee daily.*

Rest and sleep: *Describes himself as a morning person. Gets up at 6:30 a.m., goes to bed between 11:30 p.m. and midnight. Likes to get about 8 hours of sleep, but rarely does. Needs to study at night after kids are asleep.*

Exercise and activity: *Says he'd like to be more active but can't find the time. Occasionally takes a walk in the evening but has no regular exercise regimen.*

Nutrition: *24-hour recall indicates deficiency in iron, protein, and calcium. Takes vitamin and mineral supplements. Skips lunch often. States he's been losing weight without trying.*

Recreation: *Likes swimming, hiking, and camping. Tries to take family camping at least once each summer. Wishes he had more time for recreation.*

Coping: *Describes his way of coping as avoiding problems until they get too big. Feels he copes with day-to-day stresses O.K. Says job is busy and stressful most days. Says he's feeling a lot of pressure trying to juggle family, career, and educational responsibilities.*

Socioeconomic: *Earns around $57,000 a year. Has health insurance and retirement benefits through job. Wife Susan is a secretary earning $25,000.*

(continued)

Environmental: *No known environmental hazards. Lives in 3-bedroom house in town.*

Occupational: *Works 7 hours a day with ¹/₂ hr for lunch. Gets along well with coworkers. Feels pressure to attain doctorate to advance his career into educational administration. Has had present position for 12 years.*

Family health history

Maternal and paternal grandfathers are deceased. Both grandmothers are alive and well at ages 87 and 94. Father is alive and well at age 75; mother is deceased (at age 59, of breast cancer). Younger sister is alive and well.

Physical status

General health: *Complains of recent stomach pain and fatigue. Had two head colds last winter. No other illnesses or complaints.*

Skin, hair, and nails: *Pallor, no skin lesions. Hair receding, pale nails*

Head and neck: *Headaches occasionally, relieved by aspirin. No history of seizures. Reports no pain or limited movement*

Nose and sinuses: *No rhinorrhea, has occasional sinus infections, no history of nosebleeds*

Mouth and throat: *Last dental exam and cleaning 6 months ago*

Eyes: *Last eye exam 1 year ago. Reports 20/20 vision.*

Ears: *Reports no hearing problems. No history of ear infections. Last hearing evaluation 2 years ago.*

Respiratory system: No history of pneumonia, bronchitis, asthma, or dyspnea.

Cardiovascular system: No history of murmurs or palpitations. No history of heart disease or hypertension.

Breasts: Flat

GI system: Frequent episodes of indigestion, sometimes relieved by several doses of an antacid (usually Mylanta). Currently complains of gnawing stomach pain. Rates pain as 5 on a scale of 0 (no pain) to 10 (worst pain imaginable). Regular bowel movements but recently noticed dark, tarry stools.

Urinary system: No history of kidney stones or urinary tract infections. Voids clear yellow urine several times a day without difficulty.

Reproductive system: No history of sexually transmitted disease. Is currently sexually active, though tired. States that sexual relationship with marriage partner is "fine."

Nervous system: Reports no numbness, tingling, or burning in extremities

Musculoskeletal: Reports no muscle or joint pains or stiffness

Immune and hematologic systems: Pt. says doctor told him his hemoglobin was low. Reports no lymph gland swelling.

Endocrine system: No history of thyroid disease

DOCUMENTATION GUIDELINES

● Before completing the admission assessment form, consider the patient's ability and readiness to participate.

● Perform an in-depth interview later if the patient is too ill to answer questions.

● Find secondary sources (family members or past medical records, for example) to provide needed information if the patient is too ill to answer questions, and document your source of information.

● During your interview, try to alleviate as much of the patient's discomfort and anxiety as possible.

● Create a quiet, private environment for your talk.

If you're unable to conduct a thorough initial interview:

● ask the patient to complete a questionnaire about his past and present health status, and use this to document his health history, or base your initial assessment on your observations and physical examination (if the patient is too ill to be interviewed and family members aren't available)

● document on the admission form why you couldn't obtain complete data

● conduct an interview and document the complete information on the admission form or progress notes as soon as possible, noting the date and time of the entry; new information may require you to revise the care plan accordingly.

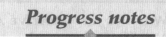

Progress notes

Use progress notes to document the patient's status and track changes in his condition. Progress notes describe, in chronological order:

● patient problems and needs

● pertinent nursing observations

● nursing reassessments and interventions

● patient responses to interventions

● progress toward meeting expected outcomes.

ADVANTAGES

● Promote effective communication among all members of the health care team and continuity of care

● Contain a column for the date and time and a column for detailed comments (see *Keeping standard progress notes*)

● Usually reflect the patient's problems (the nursing diagnoses)

● Ease information retrieval

● Contain information that doesn't fit into the space or format of other forms

DISADVANTAGES

● If disorganized, may require reading through the entire form to find needed information

● May waste time by making you document information that has already been documented on other forms

● May contain insignificant information because the documenter feels compelled to fill in space

DOCUMENTATION GUIDELINES

● When writing progress notes, include the date and time of the care

KEEPING STANDARD PROGRESS NOTES

Use the following example as a guide for completing your progress notes.

PROGRESS NOTES

Date	Time	Comments
1/20/07	0900	Notified Dr. T. Watts re Ⓛ lower lobe crackles and ineffective cough. R 40 and shallow. Skin pale. Nebulizer treatment ordered. _____ Ruth Bullock, RN
1/20/07	1030	Skin slightly pink after nebulizer treatment. Lungs clear. R 24. Showed pt. how to do pursed-lip and abdominal breathing. _____ Ruth Bullock, RN
1/20/07	1400	Ⓛ leg wound 3 cm x 1 cm wide x 1 cm deep. Small amount of pink-yellow, non-odorous drainage noted on dressing. Surrounding skin reddened and tender. Wound irrigated and dressed as ordered. _____ _____ Ruth Bullock, RN
1/20/07	1930	Pt. instructed about upper GI test. Related correct understanding of test purpose and procedure. _____ —Ann Barrow, RN

given or your observations, what prompted the entry, and other pertinent data, such as contact with the physician or other health care providers.

● If your facility uses progress notes designed to focus on nursing diagnoses, be sure to document each nursing diagnosis, problem, goal, or expected outcome that relates to your entry. (See *Using nursing diagnoses to write progress notes,* page 196.)

● Don't repeat yourself. Avoid including information that's already on the flow sheet, unless there's a sudden change in the patient's condition.

● Be specific. Avoid vague wording, such as "appears to be," "no problems," and "had a good day." Instead, document specifics. State exactly what the patient said, using quotations marks.

1/6/07	1000	Pt. ate 80% of breakfast and 75% of lunch; OOB to bathroom and walked in hallway 3 times for a distance of 10 feet with no shortness of breath. — _____ K. Comerford, RN

USING NURSING DIAGNOSES TO WRITE PROGRESS NOTES

Progress notes can be written using a nursing diagnosis, as the example below shows.

Patient identification information		**County Hospital, Van Nuys, CA**
John Adams		
111 Oak St.		
Van Nuys, CA 91388		
(202) 123-4560		

PROGRESS NOTES

Date and time	Nursing diagnosis and related problems	Notes
1/9/07 —2300	Acute pain related to pressure ulcer on Ⓛ elbow.	Pt. rates pain an 8 on a scale of 0 to 10, with 0 being no pain and 10 being the worst pain ever experienced. Pt. frowning when pointing to wound. BP 130/84; P 96. Pain aggravated by dressing change at 2200. Percocet ῑ given P.O. and pt. repositioned on Ⓡ side. ——— ———————— *Anne Curry, RN*
1/9/07 —2330	Acute pain related to pressure ulcer on Ⓛ elbow.	States that pain is relieved (0/10 on pain scale). Will give Percocet ½ hour before next dressing change and before future dressing changes. ———————— *Anne Curry, RN*

● Make sure that all progress notes have the specific date and time of the care given or observation noted.

Alert *Don't document entries in blocks of time ("1500 to 2330 hours," for example). Be specific with your times and dates whenever possible.*

● Document new patient problems, resolutions of old problems, and deteriorations in the patient's condition.

● Avoid using unapproved abbreviations.

● Document your observations of the patient's response to the care plan. If behaviors are similar to agreed-upon objectives, document that the goals are being met. If the goals aren't being met, document what the patient can or can't do to meet them.

1/9/07	1600	Dyspnea resolving. Pt.
		can perform ADLs and
		ambulate 20 feet $\bar{s}$
		SOB.——— Lois Cahn, RN

1/9/07	2000	Dyspnea unrelieved. Con-
		tinues to have tachypnea
		and tachycardia 1 hr
		after receiving O_2 by
		rebreather mask. Blood
		drawn for ABG analysis
		shows PO_2, 70; PCO_2,
		32; pH, 7.40 ———
		——— Carol Davis, RN

● Outline your interventions clearly—how and when you notified the physician, what his orders were, and when you followed through with them.

1/9/07	2000	Wants to know when
		he'll be getting chemo-
		therapy. Dr. J Milstein
		notified. Pt. informed
		that Dr. J. Milstein
		ordered chemotherapy
		to start this afternoon.
		——— Esther Blake, RN

Kardex

The patient care Kardex (sometimes called the *nursing Kardex*) gives a quick overview of basic patient care information. It typically contains boxes for you to check off what applies to each patient as well as current orders for medications, patient care activities, treatments, and tests. (See *Components of a patient care Kardex,* pages 198 to 200.) It can come in various shapes, sizes, and types, and may also be computer-generated. (See *Characteristics of a computer-generated Kardex,* pages 201 and 202.) A Kardex includes:

● patient's name, age, marital status, and religion (usually on the address stamp)
● allergies
● medical diagnoses, listed by priority
● nursing diagnoses, listed by priority
● current physicians' orders for medication, treatments, diet, I.V. therapy, diagnostic tests, procedures, and other measures
● do-not-resuscitate status
● consultations
● results of diagnostic tests and procedures
● permitted activities, functional limitations, assistance needed, and safety precautions
● emergency contact numbers
● discharge plans and goals.

ADVANTAGES
● Provides quick access to data about task-oriented interventions, such as medication administration, I.V. therapy, and other treatments
● If combined with the care plan, provides all necessary data for patient care

DISADVANTAGES
● Won't be effective if:
  – it doesn't have enough space for appropriate data
  – it isn't updated frequently
  – it isn't completed
  – nurse doesn't read it before giving patient care.

(Text continues on page 200.)

COMPONENTS OF A PATIENT CARE KARDEX

Here you'll find the kind of information that might be included on the cover sheet of a patient care Kardex for a medical-surgical unit. Inside the Kardex, which is folded in half horizontally, you'll find additional patient care information.

Keep in mind that the categories, words, and phrases on a Kardex are brief and intended to quickly trigger images of special circumstances, procedures, activities, or patient conditions.

Care status
Self-care	☐
Partial care with assistance	☐
Complete care	☑
Shower with assistance	☐
Tub	☐
Active exercises	☑
Passive exercises	☑

Special care
Back care	☑
Mouth care	☑
Foot care	☐
Perineal care	☑
Catheter care	☑
Tracheostomy care	☐
Other (specify): _____

Condition
Satisfactory	☐
Fair	☑
Guarded	☐
Critical	☐
No code	☑
Advance directive	
Yes	☑
No	☐
Date: _1/18/07_	

Prosthesis
Dentures	
upper	☑
lower	☑
Contact lenses	☐
Glasses	☑
Hearing aid	☐
Other (specify): _____

Isolation
Strict	☐
Contact	☐
Airborne	☐
Neutropenic	☐
Droplet	☐
Other (specify): _____

Diet
Type: _2 gm Na_	
Force fluids	☐
NPO	☐
Assist with feeding	☑
Isolation tray	☐
Calorie count	☐
Supplements: _____

Tube feedings ☐
Type:
Rate:
Route:
NG tube	☐
G tube	☐
J tube	☐

Admission
Height: _6'1"_
Weight: _161 lb. (73 kg)_
BP: _118/84_
Temp: _99.6° F_
Pulse: _101_
Resp.: _21_

Frequency
BP: _q 4 hr._
TPR: _q shift_
Apical pulses: _____
Peripheral
  pulses: _q shift_
Weight: _daily_
Neuro check: _____
Monitor: _____
Strips: _____
Turn: _q 2 hr._
Cough: _q 1 hr._
Deep breathe: _q 1 hr._
Central venous
  pressure: _____
Other (specify): _____

GI tubes
Salem sump ☐
Levin tube ☐
Feeding tube ☐
Type (specify): _____

Other (specify): _____
_____

Activity
Bed rest ☐
Chair *t.i.d.* ☑
Dangle ☐
Commode ☐
Commode with
   assist ☑
Ambulate ☐
BRP ☐
Fall-risk category ☑
   (specify): *# 1*
Other (specify): _____
_____

Mode of transport
Wheelchair ☑
Stretcher ☐
With oxygen ☐

I.V. devices
Heparin lock ☐
Peripheral I.V. ☑
Central line ☐
Triple-lumen CVP ☐
Hickman ☐
Jugular ☐
Peripherally inserted ☐
Parenteral nutrition ☐
Irrigations: _____
_____
_____
_____

Dressings
Type: _____
Change: _____
_____

Allergies
_____
_____
_____
_____
_____
_____

Emergency contact
Name: _____
_____
Telephone no: _____
_____

Respiratory therapy
Pulse oximetry
   Spo$_2$ level (%) _____
Oxygen ☑
   liters/minute *2 L/min*
Method
   Nasal cannula ☑
   Face mask ☐
   Venturi mask ☐
   Partial rebreather
     mask ☐
   Nonrebreather mask ☐
   Trach collar ☐
Nebulizer ☐
Chest PT ☑
Incentive spirometry ☑
T-piece ☐
Ventilator ☐
   Type: _____
   Settings: _____
   Other (specify): _____
_____
_____

Drains
Type: _____
Number: _____
Location: _____

Urine output
I & O ☑
Strain urine ☐
Indwelling catheter ☐
   Date inserted: _____
   Size: _____
Intermittent catheter ☐
   Frequency: _____

Side rails
Constant ☐
PRN ☐
Nights ☐

Restraints
Date: _____
Type: _____
_____

Specimens and tests
BGM q 6 h
24-hour collection ☐
Other (specify): _____
_____

Stools
*Stools negative
for occult blood*

Special notes
*Evaluate pain level
q 1 h*

Social services
Consulted 1/18/07

(continued)

The format and specific information on a Kardex will vary with the needs of the patient population. For instance, the cover sheet of a patient care Kardex on a critical care unit would include the same basic information already shown plus information specific to the unit, including:

Monitoring
Hardwire ☐
Telemetry ☐
Arterial line ☐

Pulmonary artery
catheter ☐
  Pulmonary artery
  pressure:
  Pulmonary artery wedge
  pressure:
Other (specify): _____
_____

Mechanical ventilation
Type: _____
Tidal volume: _____
F_{IO_2}: _____
Mode: _____
Rate: _____

On an obstetrics unit, you might find this additional information on the Kardex cover sheet:

Delivery
Date: _____
Time: _____
Type of delivery: _____
_____

Special procedures
Perianal rinse ☐
Sitz bath ☐
Witch hazel compress ☐
Breast binders ☐
Ice ☐
Abdominal binders ☐
Other (specify): _____
_____

Mother
Due date: _____
Gravida: _____
Para: _____
Rh: _____
Blood type: _____
Membranes ruptured:
_____
Episiotomy ☐
Lacerations ☐
RhoGAM studies?
  Yes ☐ No ☐
Rubella titer?
  Yes ☐ No ☐

Infant
Male ☐
Female ☐
Full term ☐
Premature ☐
  Weeks: _____
Apgar score ☐
Nursing ☐
Formula ☐
Condition (specify): _____
_____
_____
Other (specify): _____
_____
_____

● May erroneously become the working care plan
● At most facilities, isn't part of the permanent record and is discarded after the patient is discharged

DOCUMENTATION GUIDELINES
● Make the Kardex more effective by tailoring the information to the needs of your particular setting. Make sure that it's designed for specific units and reflects the needs of the patients on those units.
● Document information that helps nurses plan daily interventions (for example, the time a particular patient prefers to bathe, his food preferences before and during chemotherapy, and

CHARACTERISTICS OF A
COMPUTER-GENERATED KARDEX

Typically used to record laboratory or diagnostic test results and X-ray findings, a computerized Kardex commonly includes information regarding medical orders, referrals, consultants, specimens, vital signs, diet, activity restrictions, and other pertinent patient information.

```
1/10/07      05:39                          PAGE 001
================================================================

Stevens, James                   M 65
MR#: 000310593           Acct#: 9400037290
DR: J. Carrio                    2/W 204-01
DX: Unstable angina      Date:  1/10/07
================================================================

SUMMARY: 1/10      0701 to 1501

PATIENT INFORMATION
1/10          ADVANCE DIRECTIVE: No.
              Advance directive does not exist.
1/10          ORGAN DONOR: Yes
1/10          ADMIT DX: Unstable angina
1/10          MED ALLERGY: None known
1/10          ISOLATION: Standard precautions

MISC. PATIENT DATA

NURSING CARE PLAN PROBLEMS
1/10          Acute pain R/T: anginal pain

ALL CURRENT MEDICAL ORDERS

NURSING ORDERS:
1/10          Activity, OOB, up as tol.
1/10          Routine V/S q 8 h
1/10          Telemetry
1/10          If 1800 PTT < 50, increase heparin drip to
              1200 units/hr. If 50 to 100, maintain 1000
              units/hr. If >100, reduce to 900 units/hr.
1/10          Please contact M. Sweeney to see pt. regard-
              ing diabetic management and insulin treat-
              ment.
DIET:
1/10          Diabetic: 1600 cal., start with lunch today

I.V.s.:
SCHEDULED MEDICATIONS:
1/10          Nitroglycerin oint 2%, 1-1/2 inches, apply
              to chest wall q 8 h, starting on 3/10, 1800
              hrs.
1/10          Diltiazem tab 90 mg, #1, P.O., q 6 h 0800,
              1400, 2000, 0200
1/10          Furosemide tab 40 mg, #1, P.O., daily 0900
```

(continued)

```
1/10/07    05:39                              PAGE 001
===============================================================

Stevens, James                    M 65
MR#: 000310593            Acct#: 9400037290
DR: J. Carrio                     2/W 204-01
DX: Unstable angina       Date:  1/10/07
===============================================================

SUMMARY: 1/10    0701 to 1501

1/10            Potassium chloride tab 10 mEq, #1, P.O. dai-
                ly 0900
1/10            Labetalol tab 100 mg, #1/2, P.O. bid 0900,
                1800

STAT/NOW MEDICATIONS:
1/10            Furosemide tab 40 mg, #1, P.O., now
1/10            Potassium chloride tab 10 mEq, #1, P.O., now

PRN MEDICATIONS:
1/10            Procardia nifedipine cap 10 mg, #1, subling.
                q 6 h, prn SBP >170 or DSBP >105
1/10            Acetaminophen tab 325 mg, #2, P.O., q 4 h,
                prn for pain
1/10            Temazepam cap 15 mg, #1, P.O., q HS, prn
1/10            Alprazolam tab 0.25 mg, #1/2, P.O., q 8 h,
                prn

LABORATORY:
1/10            CK & MB 1800 today
1/10            CK & MB 0200 tomorrow
1/10            Urinalysis floor to collect
1/10            PTT 1800 today

ANCILLARY:
1/10            Stress test persantine, prep H1, Patient
                handling: wheelchair, Schedule: tomorrow

                        Last page
```

which analgesics or positions are usually required to ease pain).

If you're documenting on a medication administration record (MAR)—formerly known as a *medication Kardex*—follow these guidelines:

● Be sure to document the date and time of the administration, the medication dose and route, and your initials.

● Indicate when you administer a stat dose and, if appropriate, the specific number of doses ordered or the stop date.

● Write legibly, using only standard abbreviations accepted or approved by your facility. When in doubt about how to abbreviate a term, spell it out.

● After giving the first dose of a medication, sign your full name, your licensure status, and your initials in the appropriate space.

● After withholding a medication dose, document which dose wasn't given (usually by circling the time it was scheduled or by drawing an asterisk) and the reason it was omitted (for example, withholding oral medications from a patient the morning of scheduled surgery).

● If your MAR doesn't have space for information, such as the parenteral administration site, the patient's response to medications given as needed, or deviations from the medication order, record this information in the progress notes.

1/12/07	0800	Withheld Procardia per
		order of Dr. S. Patel
		because pt.'s BP: 98/58.
		——— Dave Bevins, RN

Graphic forms

Used for 24-hour assessments, graphic forms usually have a column of data printed on the left side of the page, times and dates printed across the top, and open blocks within the side and top borders. You'll use graphic forms to plot various changes—in the patient's vital signs, weight, intake and output, blood glucose, appetite, and activity level, for instance.

ADVANTAGES

● Present information at a glance
● Allow the nurse to trend data and identify patterns
● Save registered nurses valuable time because of the ability of health care personnel, such as licensed practical nurses, to document measurements on graphic forms

DISADVANTAGES

● May be difficult to read if data placed on graphic forms isn't accurate, legible, and complete
● Lose value if needed information isn't documented
● Demand the double-checking of transcription entries to ensure accuracy
● Must be combined with narrative documentation

    Alert Don't use the information on graphic forms alone because these forms don't present a complete picture of the patient's clinical condition.

Chart right

Using a graphic form

Plotting information on a graphic form, such as the sample shown here, helps you visualize changes in your patient's temperature, blood pressure, heart rate, weight, and intake and output.

GRAPHIC FORM

Instructions: Indicate temperature in "O" and pulse in "X"

DATE	1/5/07	1/6/07			
POSTOP. DAY	2	3			

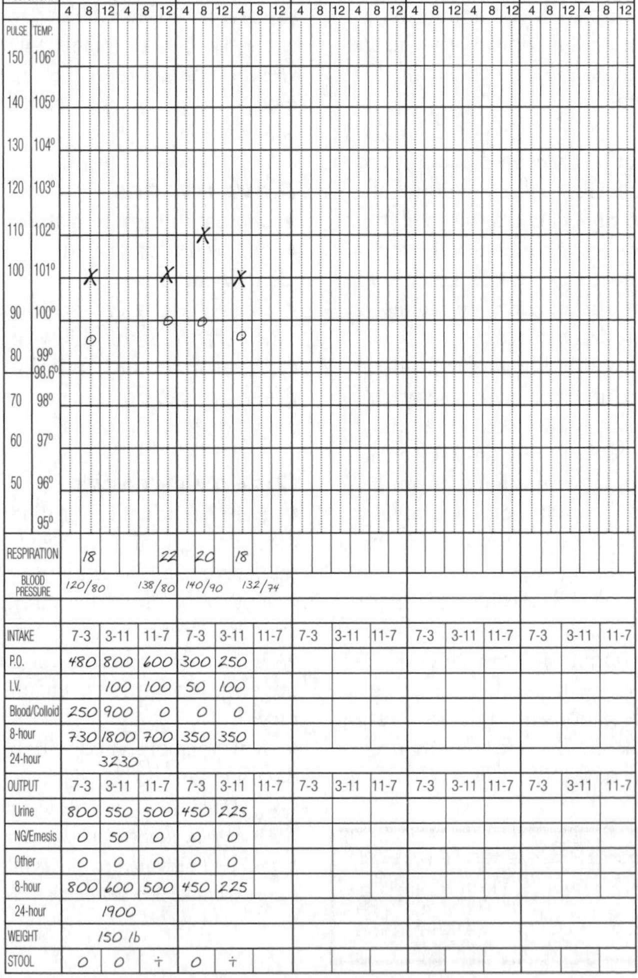
4 8 12 4 8 12
PULSE TEMP.
150 106°
140 105°
130 104°
120 103°
110 102°
100 101°
90 100°
80 99°
98.6°
70 98°
60 97°
50 96°
95°
X
O

	1/5/07	1/6/07			
RESPIRATION	18, 22	20, 18			
BLOOD PRESSURE	120/80, 138/80	140/90, 132/74			

INTAKE	7-3	3-11	11-7	7-3	3-11	11-7	7-3	3-11	11-7	7-3	3-11	11-7	7-3	3-11	11-7
P.O.	480	800	600	300	250										
I.V.		100	100	50	100										
Blood/Colloid	250	900	0	0	0										
8-hour	730	1800	700	350	350										
24-hour		3230													
OUTPUT	7-3	3-11	11-7	7-3	3-11	11-7	7-3	3-11	11-7	7-3	3-11	11-7	7-3	3-11	11-7
Urine	800	550	500	450	225										
NG/Emesis	0	50	0	0	0										
Other	0	0	0	0	0										
8-hour	800	600	500	450	225										
24-hour		1900													
WEIGHT		150 lb													
STOOL	0	0	÷	0	÷										

DOCUMENTATION GUIDELINES

- For greater accuracy, document on graphic forms at the same time each day.
- Document the patient's vital signs on both the graphic form and the progress notes when you administer medications, such as an analgesic, antihypertensive, or antipyretic. This provides a record of the patient's response to a drug that may produce a change in a particular vital sign.
- Document vital signs on both forms for such events as chest pain, chemotherapy, a seizure, or a diagnostic test, to indicate the patient's condition at that time.
- Be sure to document legibly, to put data in the appropriate time line, and to make the dots on the graph large enough to be seen easily.
- Connect the dots if your facility requires you to do so. (See *Using a graphic form.*)

Flow sheets

Flow sheets have vertical or horizontal columns for documenting dates, times, and interventions. You can insert nursing data quickly and concisely, preferably at the time you give care or observe a change in the patient's condition. Because flow sheets provide an easy-to-read record of changes in the patient's condition over time, they allow all members of the health care team to compare data and assess the patient's progress. They have several uses:

- Flow sheets are handy for documenting data related to a patient's

ADLs, fluid balance, nutrition, pain management, and skin integrity.
- Flow sheets are also useful for documenting nursing interventions.
- In response to a request by JCAHO, nurses are using these forms to document basic assessment findings and wound care, hygiene, and routine care interventions. (See *Using a flow sheet to document routine care,* pages 206 to 211.)

   Alert *If using a flow sheet to document, make sure that you don't ignore your other documentation responsibilities. Using a flow sheet doesn't exempt you from narrative documentation, patient teaching, patient responses, detailed interventions, and attending to unusual circumstances.*

ADVANTAGES

- Allow you to evaluate patient trends at a glance
- Reinforce nursing standards of care and allows precise nursing documentation

DISADVANTAGES

- Aren't well-suited for documenting unusual events
- Can lead to incomplete or fragmented documentation
- May fail to reflect the needs of the patients and the documentation needs of the nurses on each unit
- Adds bulk to the medical record, causing handling and storage problems and duplication of documentation
- May cause legal problems if inconsistent with the progress notes

   In court *To avoid legal trouble with inconsistency between the flow sheet and the progress notes, make sure*

(Text continues on page 212.)

USING A FLOW SHEET TO DOCUMENT ROUTINE CARE

As this sample shows, a patient care flow sheet lets you quickly document your routine interventions.

PATIENT CARE FLOW SHEET

Date *1/22/07*	2300–0700	
Respiratory		
Breath sounds	*Clear 2330 PW*	
Treatments/results	——	
Cough/results	——	
O₂ therapy	*Nasal cannula @ 2 L/min PW*	
Cardiac		
Chest pain	*c̄ PW*	
Heart sounds	*Normal S₁ and S₂ PW*	
Telemetry	*N/A*	
Pain		
Type and location	*Ⓛ flank 0400 PW*	
Intervention	*Morphine 0415 PW*	
Pt. response	*Improved from #9 to #3 in 1/2 hr PW*	
Nutrition		
Type	——	
Toleration %	——	
Supplement	——	
Elimination		
Stool appearance	*c̄ PW*	
Enema	*N/A*	
Results	——	
Bowel sounds	*Present all quadrants 2330 PW*	
Urine appearance	*Clear, amber 0400 PW*	
Indwelling urinary catheter	*N/A*	
Catheter irrigations	——	

0700–1500	1500–2300
Crackles @LL 0800 GR	Clear 1600 MLF
Nebulizer 0830 GR	———
Mod. amt. tenacious yellow mucus, 0900 GR	———
Nasal cannula @ 2 L/min GR	Nasal cannula @ 2 L/min MLF
ō GR	ō MLF
Normal S_1 and S_2 GR	Normal S_1 and S_2 MLF
N/A	N/A
@ flank 1000 GR	@ flank 1600 MLF
Repositioned and morphine 1010 GR	Morphine 1615 MLF
Improved from #8 to #2 in 45 min. GR	Complete relief in 1 hr MLF
Regular GR	Regular MLF
90% GR	80% MLF
1 can Ensure GR	———
ō GR	↑ soft dark brown MLF
N/A	N/A
———	———
Present all quadrants 0800 GR	Hyperactive all quadrants 1600 MLF
Clear, amber 1000 GR	Dark yellow 1500 MLF
N/A	N/A
———	———

(continued)

PATIENT CARE FLOW SHEET

Date 1/22/07	2300–0700	
I.V. therapy		
Tubing change	————	
Dressing change	————	
Site appearance	No edema, no redness 2330 PW	
Wound		
Type	Ⓛ flank incision 2330 PW	
Dressing change	Dressing dry and intact 2330 PW	
Appearance	Wound not observed PW	
Tubes		
Type	N/A	
Irrigation	————	
Drainage appearance	————	
Hygiene		
Self/partial/complete	————	
Oral care	————	
Back care	0400 PW	
Foot care	————	
Remove / reapply	0400 PW	
elastic stockings		
Activity		
Type	Bed rest PW	
Toleration	Turns self PW	
Repositioned	2330 Supine PW 0400 Ⓛ side PW	
ROM	————	
Sleep		
Sleeps well	0400 PW 0600 PW	
Awake at intervals	2330 PW 0400 PW	
Awake most of the time	————	

0700–1500	1500–2300
1100 GR	————
1100 GR	————
No redness, no edema, no drainage 0800 GR	No redness, no edema 1600 MLF
Ⓛ flank incision 1200 GR	Ⓛ flank incision 2000 MLF
1200 GR	2000 MLF
See progress note. GR	See progress note. MLF
N/A	N/A
————	————
————	————
Partial 1000 GR	Partial 2100 MLF
1000 GR	2100 MLF
1000 GR	2100 MLF
1000 GR	————
1000 GR	2100 MLF
OOB to chair X 20 min. 1000 GR	OOB to chair X 20 min. 1800 MLF
Tol. well GR	Tol. well MLF
Ⓛ side 0800 GR Ⓡ side 1400 GR	Self MLF
1000 (active) GR 1400 (active) GR	1800 (active) MLF 2200 (active) MLF
N/A	N/A
————	————
————	————

(continued)

PATIENT CARE FLOW SHEET

Date 1/22/07	2300–0700	
Safety		
ID bracelet on	2330 PW 0200 PW 0400 PW	
Side rails up	2330 PW 0200 PW 0400 PW	
Call button in reach	2330 PW 0200 PW 0400 PW	
Equipment		
Type IVAC pump	Continuous 2300 PW	
Teaching		
Wound splinting	0400 PW	
Deep breathing	0400 PW	
Initials/Signature/Title	PW / Pam Watts, RN	

PROGRESS SHEET

Date	Time	Comments
1/22/01	1200	Ⓛ flank dressing saturated with serosang. drng. Dressing removed. Wound edges well-approximated except for 2-cm opening noted at lower edge of incision. Small amount serosang. drng noted oozing from this area. No redness noted along incision line. Sutures intact. Incision line painted with povidone-iodine. Five 4″ x 4″ gauze pads applied and taped in place. Dr. T. Wong notified of increased amt. of drng. ——— Susan Reynolds, RN
1/22/07	2000	Dr. T. Wong to see pt. Ⓛ flank drsg. removed. 2-cm opening noted at lower edges of incision. Otherwise, wound edges well-approximated. Dr. T. Wong sutured opening with one 3-0 silk suture. No redness or drng. noted along incision

0700–1500	1500–2300
0800 SR 1200 SR 1500 SR	1600 MLF 2200 MLF
0800 SR 1200 SR 1500 SR	1600 MLF 2200 MLF
0800 SR 1200 SR 1500 SR	1600 MLF 2200 MLF
Continuous 0800 SR	Continuous 1600 MLF
1000 SR	———
1000 SR	1600 MLF
SR / Susan Reynolds, RN	MLF / Mary La Farge, RN

PROGRESS SHEET

Date	Time	Comments
1/22/07	2000	(continued)
		line. Painted incision line with povidone-iodine and applied
		two 4" x 4" gauze pads. Taped drsg. in place. ———
		——————————— Mary La Farge, RN.

data on the flow sheet is consistent with data in your progress notes. Discrepancies can damage your credibility and increase your chance of liability.

DOCUMENTATION GUIDELINES

- Use flow sheets to document all routine assessment data and nursing interventions, such as repositioning or turning the patient, range-of-motion exercises, patient education, wound care, and medication administration.
- Progress notes need only include the patient's progress toward achieving desired outcomes and any unplanned assessments.
- If documenting the information requested isn't sufficient to give a complete picture of the patient's status, document additional information in the space provided on the flow sheet. If your flow sheet doesn't have additional space, and you need to document more information, use the progress notes. If additional information isn't necessary, draw a line through this space to indicate that further information isn't required.
- Fill out flow sheets completely, using the key symbols provided, such as a check mark, an "X," initials, circles, or the time to indicate that a parameter was observed or an intervention was carried out.

- When necessary, use the abbreviation "N/A" (not applicable) or another abbreviation approved by your facility.
- Don't leave blank spaces—they imply that an intervention wasn't completed, wasn't attempted, or wasn't recognized.
- If you have to omit something, document the reason.

Clinical pathways

A clinical pathway (also known as a *critical pathway*) integrates the principles of case management into nursing documentation. (See *Function of the clinical pathway*.) They're usually organized by categories according to the patient's diagnosis, which dictates his expected length of stay, daily care guidelines, and expected outcomes. The care guidelines specified for each day may be organized into various categories, and the structure and categories may vary from one facility to the next, depending on which are appropriate for the specific diagnosis-related group. Categories include:

- activity
- diet or nutrition
- discharge planning
- medications

FUNCTION OF THE CLINICAL PATHWAY

The clinical pathway outlines the standard of care for a specific diagnosis-related group and incorporates multidisciplinary diagnoses. It also incorporates interventions that must occur for the patient to be discharged by a target date.

Within the managed care system, clinical pathways set the standard for patient progress and provide the nursing staff with

necessary written criteria to guide and monitor patient care. In some health care facilities, the nursing diagnosis forms the clinical pathway's basis for patient care, although critics believe that structuring the pathway in this way interferes with communication and coordination of care among non-nursing members of the health care team.

- patient teaching
- treatments.

For an example of a completed clinical pathway, see *Following a clinical pathway,* pages 214 and 215.

ADVANTAGES

- Can eliminate duplicate documentation if used as a permanent documentation tool
- Allow for narrative notes to be written only when a standard on the pathway remains unmet or when the patient's condition warrants a deviation in care as planned on the pathway
- Become part of the patient's permanent record
- Allow nurses to advance the patient's activity level, diet, and treatment regimens without waiting for a physician's order as long as standardized orders or standing protocols have been determined and accepted
- Reduce phone calls to physicians because nurses have the freedom to make nursing decisions
- Improve communication among all members of the health care team because everyone works from the same plan
- Improve quality of care due to the shared accountability for patient outcomes
- Improve patient teaching and discharge planning
- May help some patients recover more quickly and go home sooner than anticipated

Alert *If your facility uses clinical pathways, check its policy to see if it allows certain adapted clinical pathways to be distributed to patients. Some facilities find that many patients feel less anxiety and cooperate more with therapy because they know what to expect.*

DISADVANTAGES

- Most effective for a patient who has only one diagnosis; less effective for a patient with several diagnoses or one who experiences complications (because of the difficulty establishing a time line for such a patient)
- Lengthy, fragmented documentation possible (if the care plan is likely to change)

DOCUMENTATION GUIDELINES

- When writing a clinical pathway, collaborate with the physician and other members of the health care team. Standardized orders for the clinical pathway require the physician's signature on admission of the patient.
- To ensure consistent documentation from shift to shift, review the clinical pathway during the change-of-shift report with the nurse who's taking over. Point out critical events, note changes in the patient's expected length of stay, and discuss variances that may have occurred during your shift.
- If an objective for a particular day remains unmet, document this fact on the appropriate form as justifiable or unjustifiable.
- When developing a clinical pathway to distribute to patients, use simple vocabulary, keep your instructions short, and avoid unapproved abbreviations and complex medical terminology. Explain the diagnosis, review tests and care the patient can expect, and inform him about activity restrictions, diet, medications, and home health care services.

FOLLOWING A CLINICAL PATHWAY

At any point in a treatment course, a glance at the clinical pathway allows you to compare the patient's progress and your performance as a caregiver with care standards. Here is a sample pathway.

	CLINICAL PATHWAY: COLON RESECTION WITHOUT COLOSTOMY			
	Patient visit	**Presurgery Day 1**	**O.R. Day**	**Postop Day 1**
Assessments	History and physical with breast, rectal, and pelvic exam Nursing assessment	Nursing admission assessment	Nursing admission assessment on TBA patients in holding area Review of systems assessment*	Review of systems assessment*
Consults	Social service consult Physical therapy consult	Notify referring physician of impending admission		
Labs and diagnostics	Complete blood count (CBC) PT/PTT ECG Chest X-ray (CXR) Chem profile CT scan ABD w/wo contrast CT scan pelvis Urinalysis Barium enema & flexible sigmoidoscopy or colonoscopy Biopsy report	Type and screen for patients with hemoglobin (Hgb) <10	Type and screen for patients in holding area with Hgb <10	CBC
Interventions	Many or all of the above labs/diagnostics will have already been done. Check all results and fax to the surgeon's office.	Admit by 8 a.m. Check for bowel prep orders Bowel prep* Antiembolism stockings Incentive spirometry Ankle exercises* I.V. access* Routine vital signs (VS)* Pneumatic inflation boots	Shave and prep in O.R. Nasogastric (NG) tube maint.* Intake and output (I/O) VS per routine* Catheter care* Incentive spirometry* Ankle exercises* I.V. site care* Head of bed (HOB) 30°* Safety measures* Wound care* Mouth care*	NG tube maintenance* I/O* VS per routine* Catheter care* Incentive spirometry* Ankle exercises* I.V. site care* HOB 30°* Safety measures* Wound care* Mouth care* Antiembolism stockings
I.V.s		I.V. fluids, D_5½ NSS	I.V. fluids, D_5LR	I.V. fluids, D_5LR
Medication	Prescribe GoLYTELY or Nulytely 10a—2p Neomycin @ 2p, 3p, and 10p Erythromycin @2p, 3p, and 10p	GoLYTELY or Nulytely 10a—2p Erythromycin @ 2p, 3p, and 10p Neomycin @ 2p, 3p and 10p	Preop antibiotics (ABX) in holding area Postop ABX × 2 doses PCA (basal rate 0.5 mg) subQ heparin	PCA (basal rate 0.5 mg) subQ heparin
Diet/GI	Clears presurgery day NPO after midnight	Clears presurgery day NPO after midnight	NPO/NG tube	NPO/NG tube
Activity			4 hours after surgery, ambulate with abdominal binder* Discontinue pneumatic inflation boots once patient ambulates	Ambulate t.i.d. with abdominal binder* May shower Physical therapy b.i.d.
KEY: * = NSG activities V = Variance N = No var. **Signatures:**	1.　2.　3. V　V　V Ⓝ　N　N 1. C. Molloy, RN 2. 3.	1.　2.　3. V　V　V Ⓝ　Ⓝ　Ⓝ 1. M. Connel, RN 2. C. Roy, RN 3. J. Kane, RN	1.　2.　3. V　V　V Ⓝ　Ⓝ　Ⓝ 1. L. Singer, RN 2. J. Smith, RN 3. P. Joseph, RN	1.　2.　3. V　V　V Ⓝ　Ⓝ　Ⓝ 1. L. Singer, RN 2. J. Smith, RN 3. P. Joseph, RN

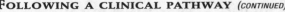

CLINICAL PATHWAY: COLON RESECTION WITHOUT COLOSTOMY

	Postop Day 2	Postop Day 3	Postop Day 4	Postop Day 5
Assessments	Review of systems assessment*	Review of systems assessment*	Review of systems assessment*	Review of systems assessment*
Consults		Dietary consult		Oncology consult if indicated (or to be done as outpatient)
Labs and diagnostics	Electrolyte 7 (EL-7) CXR	CBC EL-7	Pathology results on chart	CBC EL-7
Interventions	Discontinue NG tube if possible* (per guidelines) I/O* VS per routine* Discontinue catheter* Ambulating* Incentive spirometry* Ankle exercises* I.V. site care* HOB 30°* Safety measures* Wound care* Mouth care* Antiembolism stockings	I/O* VS per routine* Incentive spirometry* Ankle exercises* I.V. site care* Safety measures* Wound care* Antiembolism stockings	I/O* VS per routine* Incentive spirometry* Ankle exercises* I.V. site care* Safety measures* Wound care* Antiembolism stockings	Consider staple removal Replace with Steri-Strips Assess that patient has met discharge criteria*
I.V.s	I.V. fluids $D_5\frac{1}{2}$ NSS+ MVI	I.V. convert to Heplock	Heplock	Discontinue Heplock
Medication	PCA (0.5 mg basal rate)	Discontinue PCA P.O. analgesia Resume routine home meds	P.O. analgesia Preoperative meds	P.O. analgesia Preoperative meds
Diet/GI	Discontinue NG tube per guidelines: (Clamp tube at 8 a.m. if no N/V and residual <200 ml, Discontinue tube @ 12 noon)* (Check with physician first)	Clears if pt. has BM/flatus Advance to postop diet if tolerating clears (at least one tray of clears)*	House	House
Activity	Ambulate q.i.d. with abdominal binder* May shower Physical therapy b.i.d.	Ambulate at least q.i.d. with abdominal binder* May shower Physical therapy b.i.d.	Ambulate at least q.i.d. with abdominal binder* May shower Physical therapy b.i.d.	
Teaching	Reinforce preop teaching* Patient and family education p.r.n.* re: family screening	Reinforce preop teaching* Patient and family education p.r.n.* re: family screening Begin discharge teaching	Reinforce preop teaching* Patient and family education p.r.n.* Discharge teaching re: reportable s/s, F/U and wound care*	Review all discharge instructions and Rx including* follow-up appointments: with surgeon within 3 weeks, with oncologist within 1 month if indicated
KEY: * = NSG activities V = Variance N = No var. **Signatures:**	1. 2. 3. V V V Ⓝ Ⓝ Ⓝ 1. _A. McCarthy, RN_ 2. _R. Mayer, RN_ 3. _P. Drake, RN_	1. 2. 3. V V V Ⓝ Ⓝ Ⓝ 1. _A. McCarthy, RN_ 2. _R. Mayer, RN_ 3. _P. Drake, RN_	1. 2. 3. V V V Ⓝ Ⓝ Ⓝ 1. _L. Singer, RN_ 2. _J. Smith, RN_ 3. _P. Joseph, RN_	1. 2. 3. V V V Ⓝ Ⓝ Ⓝ 1. _L. Singer, RN_ 2. _J. Smith, RN_ 3. _P. Joseph, RN_

Patient-teaching plans

Standard-setting and reimbursing agencies require health care facilities to instruct patients about their condition and treatment regimen. Patient-teaching plans must meet your patient's particular needs. (See *Filing a teaching plan,* pages 216 and 217.)

(Text continues on page 218.)

FILING A TEACHING PLAN

Your teaching plan should include your assessment findings; projected learning outcomes, along with the activities, methods, and tools needed to accomplish the outcomes; and the techniques you'll use to evaluate the effectiveness of teaching.

This teaching plan was structured for Harold Harmon, a patient who has heart failure.

Assessment findings	Learning outcomes	Activities
Mr. Harmon needs to understand the action of his medication.	Mr. Harmon will: — explain the action of digoxin. — state when to take the drug.	— Present written brochures. — Discuss content. — Check Mr. Harmon's knowledge.
Mr. Harmon needs to learn how to take his pulse.	Mr. Harmon will take his pulse and come within two beats of his physician's or nurse's results.	— Show Mr. Harmon a videotape that includes instruction on how to take a pulse. — Instruct him to study printed materials. — Demonstrate the procedure. — Provide feedback and practice time. — Ask Mr. Harmon to demonstrate the procedure.
Mr. Harmon reports feeling increased anxiety. He needs to learn how to cope with this anxiety and to control stress in his life.	Mr. Harmon will explain two techniques that he'll use to help him relax.	— Invite Mr. Harmon to watch a videotape on how to control stress. — Encourage him to read printed materials (booklets, pamphlets) on techniques to reduce stress. — Demonstrate deep-breathing and progressive muscle relaxation techniques. — Role-play a guided imagery scene. — Present a case study on how other people cope with stress.

Teaching methods	Teaching tools	Evaluation methods
—One-on-one discussion	—Printed materials describing digoxin's action	—Question and answer
		—Written test
	—Patient-teaching aid on digoxin	
	—Illustration of a medication clock	
—Demonstration	—Videotape	—Question and answer
—Supervised practice sessions	—Printed materials	—Return demonstration
—One-on-one discussion	—Photographs or illustrations of key steps in the procedure	
—One-on-one discussion	—Printed materials	—Question and answer
—Group discussion (with family)	—Videotape	—Interview
		—Observation
—Role-playing		—Return demonstration of relaxation techniques
—Case study		
—Self-monitoring		

When constructing a patient-teaching plan, follow these steps:

- Assess the patient's cognitive level, any barriers to learning (such as language, hearing loss, illiteracy, cultural beliefs, or others), and what he already knows about the topic.
- Compile *learning outcomes* or *objectives*—a list of topics and strategies that the patient needs to know or perform to attain his maximum level of health and self-care.
- Devise teaching activities, methods, and tools (such as brochures, one-on-one discussions, and videotapes) to convey and reinforce the information.
- Design a way to evaluate your teaching effectiveness, such as a written quiz or an oral question-and-answer session.

Translated into reality, the instructive elements and activities should:

- define the patient's condition
- identify risk factors associated with the patient's condition
- explain what causes the patient's condition and variations of the patient's condition
- point out the importance of therapy, emphasizing, if necessary, the consequences of untreated disease
- explain the goals of treatment, and identify the components of the treatment plan
- define the patient's anticipated learning outcomes and provide a time frame.

ADVANTAGES

- Become part of the patient's care plan, which is part of the medical record
- Tell health care team members at a glance what the patient learned and what he still needs to learn and do about his health condition
- Show performance-improvement measures in progress and meets professional and accrediting requirements as well

DOCUMENTATION GUIDELINES

- Check your facility's policies and procedures to learn where you're expected to file the patient-teaching plan—for example, within the care plan, on charts, in progress notes, in the patient-education office, or elsewhere.
- When writing the patient-teaching plan, be sure to follow the nursing process.
- Keep the plan succinct and precise.
- Talk with the patient and his family about the patient-teaching plan, and agree on realistic learning outcomes. Encourage and expect his participation in the plan. Doing so usually increases his cooperation and your effectiveness.

Patient-teaching forms

Although patient-teaching forms vary according to the health care facility, most contain general information about the patient's learning abilities, goals to be met, and skills to be acquired by the time of discharge. You can document information by filling in blanks, checking boxes, or writing brief narrative notes. (See *Documenting your teaching.*)

(Text continues on page 224.)

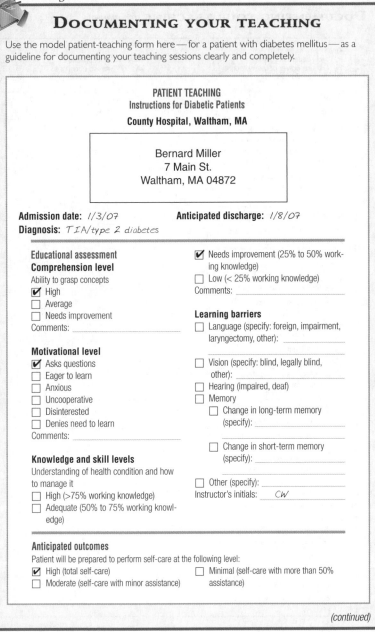

Chart right

DOCUMENTING YOUR TEACHING

Use the model patient-teaching form here—for a patient with diabetes mellitus—as a guideline for documenting your teaching sessions clearly and completely.

PATIENT TEACHING
Instructions for Diabetic Patients

County Hospital, Waltham, MA

Bernard Miller
7 Main St.
Waltham, MA 04872

Admission date: 1/3/07   **Anticipated discharge:** 1/8/07
Diagnosis: TIA/type 2 diabetes

Educational assessment
Comprehension level
Ability to grasp concepts
☑ High
☐ Average
☐ Needs improvement
Comments: _____

Motivational level
☑ Asks questions
☐ Eager to learn
☐ Anxious
☐ Uncooperative
☐ Disinterested
☐ Denies need to learn
Comments: _____

Knowledge and skill levels
Understanding of health condition and how to manage it
☐ High (>75% working knowledge)
☐ Adequate (50% to 75% working knowledge)

☑ Needs improvement (25% to 50% working knowledge)
☐ Low (< 25% working knowledge)
Comments: _____

Learning barriers
☐ Language (specify: foreign, impairment, laryngectomy, other): _____

☐ Vision (specify: blind, legally blind, other): _____
☐ Hearing (impaired, deaf)
☐ Memory
  ☐ Change in long-term memory (specify): _____

  ☐ Change in short-term memory (specify): _____

☐ Other (specify): _____
Instructor's initials: _CW_

Anticipated outcomes
Patient will be prepared to perform self-care at the following level:
☑ High (total self-care)
☐ Moderate (self-care with minor assistance)
☐ Minimal (self-care with more than 50% assistance)

(continued)

Key

P	=	patient taught	N/A	=	not applicable
F	=	caregiver or family taught	A	=	asked questions
R	=	reinforced	B	=	nonattentive, poor concentration

Date	1/4/07	1/5/07	1/5/07	
Time	1900	0800	1330	
Assessed educational needs Assessment of patient's (or caregiver's) current knowledge of disease (include medical, family, and social histories)	A/CW			
Assessment of learner's reaction to diagnosis (verbal and nonverbal responses)	A/CW			
General diabetic education goals The patient (or caregiver) will:				
■ define diabetes mellitus.	P/A/CW	R/EG	D/ME	
■ state hormone produced in the pancreas.	P/A/CW	R/EG	D/ME	
■ identify three signs and symptoms of diabetes.	P/CW	R/EG	D/ME	
■ discuss risk factors associated with the disease.	P/CW	R/EG	D/ME	
■ differentiate between type 1 and type 2 diabetes.	P/A/CW	R/EG	D/ME	
Survival skill goals The patient (or caregiver) will:				
■ identify the name, purpose, dose, and time of administration of medication ordered.		P/EG	R/ME	
■ properly administer insulin.	N/A			
– draw up insulin properly.	N/A			
– discuss and demonstrate site selection and rotation.	N/A			
– demonstrate proper injection technique with needle angled appropriately.	N/A			
– explain correct way to store insulin.	N/A			
– demonstrate correct disposal of syringes.	N/A			
■ distinguish among types of insulin.	N/A			
– species (pork, beef, recombinant DNA)	N/A			
– regular	N/A			
– NPH/Ultralente (longer acting)	N/A			
■ Properly administer mixed insulins.	N/A			
– demonstrate injecting air into vials.	N/A			

C = expressed denial, resistance
D = verbalized recall
E = demonstrated ability

1/5/07	1/6/07	1/7/07	1/7/07	1/8/07
1830	1000	0800	1830	0800
.				
				D/EG
				D/EG
				D/EG
				D/EG
				D/EG
D/LT				D/EG

(continued)

Date	1/4/07	1/5/07	1/5/07	
Time	*1900*	*0800*	*1330*	
– draw up mixed insulin properly (regular before NPH).	*N/A*			
■ demonstrate knowledge of oral antidiabetic agents.				
– identify name of medication, dose, and time of administration.		*P/EG*	*A/ME*	
– identify purpose of medication.		*P/EG*	*A/ME*	
– state possible adverse effects.		*P/EG*	*A/ME*	
■ list signs and symptoms, causes, implications, and treatments of hyperglycemia and hypoglycemia.		*P/EG*	*A/ME*	
■ monitor blood glucose levels satisfactorily.				
– demonstrate proper use of blood glucose monitoring device.				
– perform fingerstick.				
– obtain accurate blood glucose reading.				
Healthful living goals The patient (or caregiver) will:				
■ consult with the nutritionist about meal planning.			*P/ME*	
■ follow the diet recommended by the American Diabetes Association.			*P/ME*	
■ state importance of adhering to diet.			*P/ME*	
■ give verbal feedback on 1-day meal plan.			*P/ME*	
■ state the effects of stress, illness, and exercise on blood glucose levels.			*P/ME*	
■ state when to test urine for ketones and how to address results.			*P/ME*	
■ identify self-care measures for periods when illness occurs.			*P/ME*	
■ list precautions to take while exercising.			*P/ME*	
■ explain what steps to take when patient doesn't want to eat or drink on proper schedule.			*P/ME*	
■ agree to wear medical identification (for example, a MedicAlert bracelet).			*P/ME*	

1/5/07	1/6/07	1/7/07	1/7/07	1/8/07
1830	1000	0800	1830	0800
	D/EG	F/EG	R/LT	D/EG
	D/EG	F/EG	R/LT	D/EG
	D/EG	F/EG	R/LT	D/EG
		F/EG		D/EG
P/LT	E/EG	E/EG	R/LT	E/EG
P/LT	E/EG	E/EG	R/LT	E/EG
P/LT	E/EG	E/EG	R/LT	E/EG
R/LT	A/EG			D/EG
R/LT	A/EG			D/EG
R/LT	A/EG			D/EG
D/LT	A/EG			D/EG
D/LT	A/EG			D/EG
D/LT	A/EG			D/EG
D/LT	A/EG			D/EG
D/LT	A/EG			D/EG
D/LT	A/EG			D/EG
A/LT				D/EG

(continued)

DOCUMENTING YOUR TEACHING (CONTINUED)

Date	1/4/07	1/5/07	1/5/07	
Time	1900	0800	1330	
Safety goals The patient (or caregiver) will:				
■ state the possible complications of diabetes.	P/CW	R/EG		
■ explain the importance of careful, regular skin care.	P/CW	R/EG		
■ demonstrate healthful foot care.	P/CW	R/EG		
■ discuss the importance of regular eye care and examinations.	P/CW	R/EG		
■ state the importance of oral hygiene.	P/CW	R/EG		
Individual goals				
Initial Signature				
CW Carol Witt, RN, BSN				
EG Ellie Grimes, RN, MSN				
ME Marianne Evans, RN				
LT Lynn Tata, RN, BSN				

ADVANTAGES

● Make documenting patient education quicker and easier by creating a record of a patient's outcomes, responses, and level of learning
● Provide a legal defense for many years against charges of inadequate patient care
● Prevent duplication of patient-teaching efforts by other staff members
● Provide a tool for performance improvement

DOCUMENTATION GUIDELINES

● When filling out patient-teaching forms, include the patient's learning ability, his response to teaching, and the outcomes.
● Check your facility's policies and procedures regarding when, where, and how to document your patient teaching. If your facility doesn't have a preprinted form, talk to your supervisor about developing one. In the meantime, document your patient teaching in accurate, detailed progress notes.
● Each shift, ask yourself these questions: What part of the patient-teaching plan did I complete? What other instruction did I give the patient or his family? Document your answers.
● Document that the patient's ongoing educational needs are being met.

1/5/07	1/6/07	1/7/07	1/7/07	1/8/07
1830	1000	0800	1830	0800
D/LT		F/EG		D/EG
D/LT		F/EG		D/EG
D/LT		F/EG		D/EG
D/LT				
D/LT				

- Before discharge, document the patient's remaining learning needs, and note whether you provided him with printed or other patient-teaching aids.
- Evaluate your teaching. One way is by using a checklist. (See *Evaluating your teaching: The checklist method,* page 226.)

Discharge summary–patient instruction forms

To comply with JCAHO requirements related to discharge planning, you must document your assessment of a patient's continuing care needs as well as any referrals for such care. To facilitate this kind of documentation, many health care facilities combine discharge summaries and patient instructions in one form. On such forms, a narrative style coexists with open- and closed-ended styles.

Another form summarizes the discharge plans made by the different services on one page, emphasizing and documenting a team approach to discharge planning. This form is started at admission, updated during the hospital stay, and completed as discharge arrangements are finalized. (See *Using a multidisciplinary discharge document,* pages 227 and 228.)

EVALUATING YOUR TEACHING: THE CHECKLIST METHOD

A checklist is a simple, quick way of obtaining information, evaluating your teaching, and gauging your patient's progress at various learning stages. It clearly shows you and your patient which goals he has achieved and which goals remain. To devise a useful checklist, follow these tips:

- Make sure the list is concise but wide-ranging enough to cover all aspects of the skill or activity being evaluated.
- Limit the items on the checklist to a group of related activities, such as the steps in tracheostomy care or the segments of a cardiac rehabilitation plan.
- Arrange items in a logical order—sequentially, chronologically, or in order of importance.

- Identify the essential steps of the activities or behavior you're evaluating.
- Relate items on the list to the patient's learning goal and to your teaching methods.
- Use only one idea or concept for each item.
- Phrase each item succinctly and accurately.
- Test your checklist on at least two patients before adapting permanently.
- Use the checklist along with other evaluation tools to promote balance and avoid giving it undue importance.

This sample checklist might be used for evaluating how well a patient with diabetes has learned to draw up insulin.

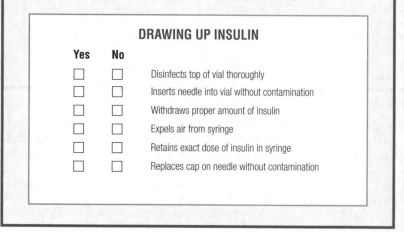

DRAWING UP INSULIN

Yes	No	
☐	☐	Disinfects top of vial thoroughly
☐	☐	Inserts needle into vial without contamination
☐	☐	Withdraws proper amount of insulin
☐	☐	Expels air from syringe
☐	☐	Retains exact dose of insulin in syringe
☐	☐	Replaces cap on needle without contamination

ADVANTAGES

The combination discharge summary-patient instruction form:
- provides useful information about additional teaching needs
- points out whether the patient has the information he needs to care for himself or get further help
- establishes compliance with JCAHO requirements

- helps to safeguard the nurse from malpractice accusations.

The multidisciplinary discharge document:
- allows all members of the health care team to reinforce information that may be discipline-specific
- eliminates second-guessing.

USING A MULTIDISCIPLINARY DISCHARGE DOCUMENT

Many health care facilities use a multidisciplinary discharge form. This sample form has spaces that can be filled in by the nurse, physician, and other health care providers.

ADMISSION/DISCHARGE DOCUMENT

Patient name: _Mary Mayer_

Address: _312 Woodlake Drive_

Philadelphia, PA 19111

Birth date: _4/12/41_   Date of admission: _1/1/07_

Patient no.: _347/9284_   HMO no.: _43217575_

Physician: _Dr. Michael Bloom_   Discharge date: _1/9/07_   Unit: _5N_

Discharged to:	Discharged by:	Accompanied by:
☑ Home	☐ Ambulatory	_husband_
☐ Transfer to:	☑ Wheelchair	
	☐ Stretcher	

Valuables w/patient ☑ Y ☐ N

Meds w/patient ☑ Y ☐ N

I.V. access DC'd ☑ Y ☐ N

Discharge planning

1. Name _Frank Mayer_   Relationship _Husband_

Phone (H) _(555)492-7342_   (W) _____

2. Name _Rose Hayes_   Relationship _Sister_

Phone (H) _(555)492-1965_   (W) _____

3. Name _____   Relationship _____

Phone (H) _____   (W) _____

4. Name _____   Relationship _____

Phone (H) _____   (W) _____

5. Name _____   Relationship _____

Phone (H) _____   (W) _____

Health team referrals

Date	Discipline contacted	Reason	Signature
1/1/07	Nutritional services	Dietary compliance	C. Weir, RN
1/5/07	Respiratory therapy	Treatments	P. Cummins, RT
1/7/07	Physical therapy	Weight bearing	L. Doyle, RN

(continued)

Supplies/Equipment needed at home

Date	Item	Provider	Signature
1/8/07	Walker	DME R US	B. Frank, MSW
1/8/07	O₂ supplies	DME R US	B. Frank, MSW

Community resources — Resource information provided (list resources)

Date		Signature
1/9/07	1. Meals On Wheels	B. Frank, MSW
	2.	
	3.	
	4.	

Education needs — Teaching topic completed
(refer from 24-hour document)

Date		Signature
1/1/07	1. Cardiac medications	C. Weir, RN
1/2/07	2. Low-salt diet restrictions	P. Brown, NT
	3.	
	4.	
	5.	
	6.	
	7.	
	8.	

Learning ability — Knowledge assessment of discharge needs

Date		Patient	Caregiver (Indicate relationship)	Signature
1/9/07	States diagnosis/disease	☑Y ☐N	☑Y ☐N husband	C. Weir, RN
1/9/07	States prognosis	☑Y ☐N	☑Y ☐N	C. Weir, RN
1/9/07	States medication regimen	☑Y ☐N	☑Y ☐N	C. Weir, RN
1/9/07	States complications	☑Y ☐N	☑Y ☐N	C. Weir, RN
1/9/07	Asks pertinent questions	☑Y ☐N	☑Y ☐N	C. Weir, RN
1/9/07	Other	☐Y ☑N	☐Y ☑N	C. Weir, RN

DOCUMENTATION GUIDELINES

● Upon discharge, give your patient a copy of his discharge instructions and document his receipt of them.
● Document a final physical assessment, including vital signs.
● Document the patient's condition from admission to discharge with interventions in a final summary located in the narrative section or another predetermined location. The summary should include the date, time, location, and mode of discharge.
● Outline the patient's care, provide useful information for further teaching and evaluation, and document that the patient has the information he needs to care for himself or to get further help.

Dictated documentation

In some situations, nurses dictate from a nursing unit or clinical setting, and clerical personnel transcribe the information for the written clinical record. This occurs commonly among visiting nurses who may dictate into a recorder or a cell phone between patient visits.

ADVANTAGES

● Convenient and highly accurate
● Can be performed without the distractions and interruptions encountered in a clinical setting
● Allows the nurse more time for patient care

● Can be done at any time of day or night
● Complies with accreditation and regulatory standards such as JCAHO standards
● May actually improve the quality of documentation

DISADVANTAGES

● If delayed, can prevent necessary documentation from being made readily available to physicians and other health care team members
● May be more costly than handwritten documentation
● May require an adjustment period for staff unaccustomed to this type of documentation

DOCUMENTATION GUIDELINES

● Refer to your health care facility's policy and procedures manual for dictation guidelines, and consult the transcriptionist if you have related questions.
● Before dictating a report, familiarize yourself with the recording equipment. Then review the existing records and the notations you made during contact with your patient.
● Prepare a brief outline of your report so that it illustrates the nursing process.
● At the beginning of your dictation, name the patient and state his identification number, if necessary.
● Tell the transcriptionist when the report begins and ends. Be sure to provide the date of the report and the date of the visit with the patient. Instruct the transcriptionist to provide the date of transcription. At the end

of the report, include a summary, evaluation, and recommendations. Discuss your plans for the next time you'll see the patient.

- Use a checklist as you dictate to make sure that you include all the necessary information. For example, state the purpose of your time with the patient, list assessments performed and findings, discuss any new or changing patient problems, list interventions and patient responses, identify future care needs, explain patient teaching provided, and describe the patient's response.
- Try to dictate the information as near to the time that you provided care as possible so that your activities and observations are fresh in your mind.
- Speak clearly and slowly, avoiding unnecessary medical terminology or uncommon abbreviations.
- If you need to add information or change something you've said, give clear and specific directions to the transcriptionist.

Patient self-documentation

Although self-documentation obviously isn't feasible or desirable for every patient, it can be effective for patients who must perform considerable self-care (diabetic patients, for example) or for patients trying to discover what precipitates a problem (such as those with chronic headaches). (See *Teaching self-documentation skills.*)

ADVANTAGES

- Can be used in inpatient and outpatient care settings
- May become a permanent part of the medical record, depending on health care facility policy
- Aids in teaching the patient about his problem and its causes, symptoms, and treatment
- Provides needed clues to the problem's precipitators and suggests solutions to the problem
- Improves therapeutic compliance by making the patient an active participant in his treatment and providing him with some control
- May be more accurate than data interpreted by someone else

DISADVANTAGES

- Takes time, patience, planning, motivation, and perseverance—on the part of both the nurse and the patient
- Requires the patient to understand how to keep careful documentation, what's important to document, and when to document; if he doesn't, the documentation won't be useful and may even adversely affect his treatment and recovery

DOCUMENTATION GUIDELINES

- Help the patient become comfortable with the documentation system he'll be using. If he's to use preprinted forms, take the time to review each aspect of a form with him. If he's to use a chart or a graph, show him how to use the form. If he's to keep journal-style documentation, tell him exactly how you want him to document and, if possible, show him examples of self-documentation. (See *Keeping a record of monitored activity,* page 232.)

TEACHING SELF-DOCUMENTATION SKILLS

For some patients, self-documentation has wide-ranging benefits. By learning to keep a log or a journal, for example, a patient may find out what triggers certain health problems (such as headaches, asthma attacks, or hypoglycemic episodes). When the trigger emerges, the patient and caregiver can implement preventive strategies.

To help a patient learn self-documentation skills, some health care facilities use individual self-documentation forms such as the sample headache log shown at right.

REVIEWING INSTRUCTIONS

Give the patient instructions and review them with him. Tell him to complete the headache log daily. Inform him that doing so may help him to identify what triggers his headaches (for example, environmental factors, foods, or stress). Explain that information collected in the log may also help him discover effective ways to relieve a headache after it starts.

Instruct the patient to describe the details of each headache in a diary, log, or small notebook.

CHECKING THE BOXES

Review these steps with the patient:
■ Using the log page at right as a guide, document the date and time of the headache and any warning signs.
■ Put a check mark in the appropriate box to indicate the headache's intensity.
■ Next, check the box to mark how long you've had the headache.
■ Check the appropriate box for other signs or symptoms that accompany your headache, such as nausea, vomiting, or sensitivity to light.
■ Continue by checking the steps you took to relieve the headache (for example, medication, biofeedback, rest) as well as the effectiveness of these measures.

HEADACHE LOG

Date and time headache began
1/25/07 – 5:00 p.m.

Warning signs
☑ Flashing lights ☐ Zigzag patterns
☐ Blind spots ☐ None
☐ Colors ☐ Other

Intensity
☐ Mild ☐ Severe
☑ Moderate ☐ Disabling

Duration
☑ Less than 4 hours ☐ 12 to 24 hours
☐ 4 to 7.5 hours ☐ More than 1 day
☐ 8 to 11.5 hours ☐ More than 2 days

Associated signs and symptoms
☐ Upset stomach ☐ Sensory, motor,
☑ Nausea or vomiting   or speech
☐ Dizziness   disturbances
☑ Sensitivity to light ☐ Other

Measures for relief
☑ Medication ☐ Ice pack
☐ Rest ☐ Relaxation
☑ Sleep   exercises
☐ Biofeedback

Extent of relief
☐ None ☐ Marked
☑ Mild ☐ Complete
☐ Moderate

Possible triggers
Caffeine and sugar

COMPLETING THE LOG

Urge the patient to think carefully about the events that occurred before the headache. For instance, was his headache triggered by emotional stress, by drinking a cup of coffee, or by something else? Tell him to write down the details of such potential triggers in his log.

KEEPING A RECORD OF MONITORED ACTIVITY

In many situations, your patient can provide additional information more accurately than a member of the health care team can. For example, a patient who wears a Holter monitor to evaluate the effect of medication on his heart and his daily activities is better acquainted with his status than a health care provider is.

Keeping this in mind, some health care facilities prepare patient instructional materials in conjunction with a diary-like chart (such as the example shown here), which the patient refers to and completes for the medical record.

Date	Time	Activity	Feelings
1/15/07	10:30 a.m.	Rode home from hospital in cab	Legs tired, felt short of breath
	11:30 a.m.	Watched TV in living room	Comfortable
	12:15 p.m.	Ate lunch, took propranolol	Indigestion
	1:30 p.m.	Walked next door to see neighbor	Felt short of breath
	2:45 p.m.	Walked home	Very tired, legs hurt
	3:00 to 4:00 p.m.	Urinated, took nap	Comfortable
	5:30 p.m.	Ate dinner slowly	Comfortable
	7:20 p.m.	Had bowel movement	Felt short of breath
	9:00 p.m.	Watched TV, drank one beer	Heart beating fast for about 1 minute, no pain
	11:00 p.m.	Took propranolol, urinated, and went to bed	Tired
1/16/07	8:15 a.m.	Woke up, urinated, washed face and arms	Very tired, rapid heartbeat for about 30 seconds
	10:30 a.m.	Returned to hospital	Felt better

- Identify the person that the patient can contact if he has questions.
- Emphasize the benefits of self-documentation to the patient (increased knowledge about his condition and increased control of his treatment, for example). By doing so, you may help boost his interest in keeping his records updated.
- Finally, show him the results of his self-documentation, pointing out how or what the data contribute to his treatment.

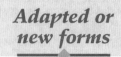

Adapted or new forms

You may find that one or several documentation forms you've been using no longer suit your needs. This may

occur because of changes in therapies, patient populations, or reimbursement criteria.

When developing a new form or adapting an old one, remember to ask yourself these questions:
- What problems exist with the old forms?
- What information is really needed?
- What changes would correct these problems?
- Which parts of the old forms remain valuable and need to be retained?

Even if your health care facility uses a computerized documentation system, ask staff members to help design the new form or reprogram the system. To develop an effective form, follow these guidelines:
- If your facility uses a specific nursing theory or framework for delivering nursing care, make sure that the nursing assessment form reflects it.
- If the old nursing assessment form reflects a medical format, change it to highlight the nursing process. For example, reorganize the form according to human response patterns or functional health care designs.
- Ask staff members who will be using the new form to evaluate possible formats and indicate which they prefer. Ask for their ideas about how best to organize and document their data.
- List all information the new form must include. Be sure to document this information to comply with professional practice standards published by such organizations as the American Nurses Association and JCAHO.
- Consider combining documentation styles in one form. Decide which style is most appropriate for each type of information included in the form. For instance, a narrative note may best suit one part of the form, whereas an open-ended style may best convey information on another part.
- After developing the new form, write procedural guidelines for its use. Provide clear explanations and completed examples for each section.
- Ask staff members not involved in developing the form to analyze both the form and the guidelines. This helps identify potentially confusing sections that require more detailed explanation or revision.
- Before adopting the new form, have staff members test it to make sure they can use it easily for entering information and retrieving it as well.
- If you expect the form will become a permanent part of the medical record, check the section devoted to form adoptions in your facility's policy and procedures manual. Some health care facilities require a form to be approved by the medical records committee or certain departments before official use.

7

DOCUMENTATION IN SELECTED CLINICAL SPECIALTY AREAS

Many nursing documentation guidelines employed in the workplace today are relevant to all nurses, regardless of their clinical specialty. There are, however, certain areas of nursing practice that utilize specialized guidelines and forms. If you work in one of these specialized areas, you need to know what to document, when to document, and what forms to document with.

Emergency department nursing

As an emergency department (ED) nurse, it's never been more incumbent upon you to keep careful and accurate documentation. Thorough documentation:

● contributes to quality patient care by providing a physical record of the care you provided
● facilitates communication between all members of the health care team
● acts as a legal safeguard against allegations of negligence and litigation, which is why EDs across the country

are developing their own specialized documentation forms and systems.

Some recent additions to routine ED nursing documentation include:
● documenting barriers to learning
● documenting nutritional risk factors
● pain assessment
● screening for domestic violence.

SPECIAL CONSIDERATIONS

As an ED nurse, you're responsible for many different facets of patient care, and no one aspect of care is more or less important than any other. The Standards of Emergency Nursing Practice influence your documentation practices by stating that the nursing plan, patient evaluation, interventions, patient assessment data, and nursing diagnoses must be documented in a retrievable form—but how you document these aspects of care greatly depends upon the patient you're caring for. Knowing what you must document and how and when to document may not prevent litigation, but proper documentation will act as a medical and legal record of your nursing care should litigation arise.

Obtaining informed consent in an emergency situation

Informed consent means that the patient understands the proposed therapy, alternate therapies, the risks, and the hazards of not undergoing treatment at all. However, in specific circumstances, emergency treatment (to save a patient's life or to prevent loss of organ, limb, or a function) may be done without first obtaining consent. The presumption is that the patient would have consented if he had been able to unless there's a reason to believe otherwise.

1/21/07	1000	Arrived in ED at 0940 via ambulance following MVA. Not responding to verbal commands, opens eyes and pushes at stimulus in response to pain, making no verbal responses. Has bruising across upper chest, labored breathing, skin pale and cool, normal heart sounds, reduced breath sounds throughout ℝ lung, normal breath sounds 𝕃 lung, no tracheal deviation. P 112, BP 88/52, RR 26. Dr. T. Mallory called at 0945 and came to see pt. I.V. line inserted in 𝕃 antecubital with 20G catheter. 1000 ml NSS infusing at 125 ml/hr. 100% oxygen given via nonrebreather mask. Stat CXR ordered to confirm pneumothorax. Pt. identified by driver's license and credit cards as Michael Brown of 123 Maple St., Valley View. Doctor called house to speak with family about need for immediate chest tube and treatment, no answer, left message on machine. Business card of Michelle Brown found in wallet. — Sandy Becker, RN

1/21/07 continued	1000	Company receptionist confirms she is wife of Michael Brown, but she's out of the office and won't return until this afternoon. Left message for wife to call doctor. — Sandy Becker, RN
1/21/07	1015	Tracheal deviation to 𝕃 side, difficulty breathing, cyanosis of lips, and mucous membranes, distended neck veins, absent breath sounds in ℝ lung, muffled heart sounds. P 120, BP 88/58, RR 32. Neurologic status unchanged. Dr. T. Mallory called pt.'s home and wife's place of business but was unable to speak with her. Again, left messages. Because of deteriorating condition, pt.'s inability to give consent, and inability to reach wife, Dr. T. Mallory has ordered chest tube to be inserted on ℝ side to relieve tension pneumothorax. — Sandy Becker, RN

When you're unable to obtain informed consent, be sure to document:
- why you weren't able to obtain informed consent
- measures that were taken to try to obtain informed consent from the patient's family, including repeated attempts to obtain the consent, if the patient is unresponsive
- interventions taken and their outcomes.

Courts will uphold emergency medical treatment as long as reasonable effort was made to obtain consent and no alternatives were available to save life and limb.

Triage

Your documentation of patient triage—deciding which patients should be treated before others and where the treatment should take

place—is crucial. When documenting patient triage, follow these guidelines:

● Document that you obtained the most important components of the initial patient assessment (such as obtaining a focused history of the patient's chief complaint, performing a limited physical examination, and classifying the patient's problem for urgency) as quickly as possible. When assessment is complete, you'll be better able to determine patient acuity, prioritize care needs, and make appropriate room placement. (See *Triage assessment principles.*) Most ED documentation forms have a triage space at the top of the form for this important information.

● If the patient must sit in the waiting room for an extended period, document that you periodically reevaluated him according to your facility's policy. Make sure to document your findings after each evaluation, even if your assessment is unchanged.

Trauma

Many EDs are designated trauma centers and must document specific data to demonstrate that they're providing the level of trauma care that they're licensed to deliver. Most trauma centers have trauma flow sheets used for patients meeting trauma alert criteria. (See *Trauma flow sheet,* pages 238 to 243.) Specific criteria that must be documented for trauma patients include:

● arrival time in the ED
● time the trauma alert was activated
● time the trauma surgeon arrived
● treatment prior to arrival
● primary survey (assessing airway, breathing, circulation, and cervical spine control)

● secondary survey (a more detailed assessment by body system).

An important consideration during the care of many trauma patients is forensics. If a patient arrives in your ED after sustaining a gunshot or stab wound and, in order to fully assess him, you need to cut the clothes off his body, follow these guidelines:

● Document why you had to cut the patient's clothes off and the precautions you took to keep from contaminating or destroying possible evidence, such as avoiding cutting through any puncture holes in the clothes.

● Document the name of the person to whom you gave the patient's clothing and other belongings. (This person will usually be a local law enforcement officer.)

Sexual assault

The term *rape* refers to nonconsensual sexual intercourse. It's a violent assault in which sex is used as a weapon. (See *Understanding rape,* page 244.) EDs commonly see and treat sexual assault victims, and while many EDs have sexual assault nurse examiners who examine these patients, some don't. When documenting the care of a sexual assault victim, follow these guidelines:

● Make sure that your documentation is clear and accurate. Criminal charges and a conviction may be dependent upon your actions and documentation.

● Document the time the patient arrived in the ED and, if she was accompanied by police officers, docu-

(Text continues on page 244.)

TRIAGE ASSESSMENT PRINCIPLES

To make triage decisions effectively, you must gather and interpret both subjective and objective data rapidly and accurately. Follow this rule: "When in doubt, triage up." That is, if you're uncertain as to the seriousness of a patient's condition, treat it as more, rather than less, serious. Triage activity consists of:

■ obtaining a focused history of the patient's chief complaint

■ performing a limited physical examination

■ classifying the patient's problem for urgency

■ reassuring the patient that he'll receive definitive medical care as soon as possible.

OBTAIN A HISTORY

Focus on the patient's chief complaint. Document it in his own words, using quotation marks, if possible. Have him qualify his complaint as precisely as he can, using the PQRST acronym (**P**rovocative/**P**alliative, **Q**uality/**Q**uantity, **R**egion/**R**adiation, **S**everity scale, **T**iming) or a similar device.

Also document the patient's age, current medications (including over-the-counter and herbal remedies as well as vitamins) and time of last dose, allergies, date of last tetanus toxoid inoculation, and any other medical history, such as height, weight, and last menstrual period.

PERFORM A PHYSICAL EXAMINATION

Observe the patient's general appearance, and assess vital signs and level of consciousness (LOC). Follow these guidelines:

■ Take oral or tympanic temperature as appropriate. Rectal temperature is the most accurate; take this as indicated and if you can ensure the patient's privacy.

■ Check radial or apical pulse. Note rate, rhythm, and quality. While assessing the pulse, check skin temperature and capillary refill time.

■ Check blood pressure as quickly and accurately as possible.

■ Note rate, depth, symmetry, and quality of respirations. Also note skin color and turgor, facial expression, accessory muscle use, and any audible breath sounds.

■ Assess LOC using a scale such as the Glasgow Coma Scale, or make a notation that the patient is oriented to time, place, and person.

CLASSIFYING EMERGENCY CONDITIONS

Classify your patient's condition as either emergent or urgent. A patient with an emergent condition will probably die or lose organ function without immediate medical attention. Emergent conditions include:

■ cardiac arrest

■ chest pain, severe, with dyspnea or cyanosis

■ coma

■ emergency childbirth or complications of pregnancy

■ head injury, severe

■ hemorrhage, severe

■ hyperpyrexia (temperature over 105° F [40.6° C])

■ multiple injuries

■ open chest or abdominal wounds

■ poisoning or drug overdose

■ profound shock

■ respiratory distress or arrest

■ seizures.

An urgent condition is a condition that doesn't immediately threaten the patient's life or organ functions. You can delay treatment for 20 minutes to 2 hours, if necessary, if you find:

■ abdominal pain, severe

■ back injury

■ bleeding from any orifice

■ chest pain not associated with respiratory symptoms

■ nausea, vomiting, or diarrhea (persistent)

■ panic

■ temperature of 102° to 105° F (38.9° to 40.6° C).

TRAUMA FLOW SHEET

This form is an example of a trauma flow sheet. Note how the Trauma Nursing Assessment section follows the primary and secondary surveys to make charting easier.

TRAUMA FLOW SHEET
Trauma Nursing Assessment

Arrival time: _1420_ Date: _1/2/07_
Mechanism of injury: _Dog bite_
Via: ☐ Ambulance   Transferred from: _____
☒ Private vehicle   Allergies: _None known_
Sex: ☒ M ☐ F   Current meds: _None_

Treatment prior to arrival (PTA):
☐ CPR   ☐ Intubation   ☐ C-spine   ☐ Oxygen
☐ Mast   ☐ Splints   ☐ IV   ☐ Other: _____
  ☐ Inflated   ☐ Chest tube   _____
  ☐ Deflated   ☐ R ☐ L   _____

Primary survey

Airway:
☒ Open
☐ Compromised

Interventions:
☐ Oral airway
☐ Endo/naso/cryco
☐ Trach
☒ None

Oxygen:
☐ Nasal canula
☐ Simple mask
☐ Nonrebreathing
☐ Ambu-bag _____ Liters

C-Spine
☐ Immobilized PTA   Type: _____
☐ Immobilized in ED
Time: _____   Type: _____

Breathing

☒ Spontaneous
☐ Bagged

Breath sounds:
☒ Clear bilateral
☐ Diminished ☐ L ☐ R
☐ Absent   ☐ L ☐ R

Respiratory effort:
☒ Unlabored
☐ Labored

Circulation
Pulse: ☒ Present/rate: _106_
         ☐ Absent/CPR-time: _____
Skin:
☐ Warm/dry   ☒ Pale/cool
☐ Diaphoretic   ☐ Cyanotic

External hemorrhage:
Location: _Ⓡ hand_
Intervention: _See progress note_

TRAUMA FLOW SHEET

GLASGOW COMA SCALE (GCS)				REVISED TRAUMA SCORE		
EYES OPENING	Spontaneously	④		**A: SPONT. RESP.**	10-24	④
	To Speech	3			25-35	3
	To Pain	2			> 35	2
	None	1			< 10	1
					0	0
VERBAL	Adult		Infant/child		**B: SYSTOLIC BP**	> 90	④
	Oriented	⑤	Coos/babbles	5		70-89	3
	Confused	4	Irritable/cries, consolable	4		50-69	2
	Inappropriate	3	Cries to pain	3		< 50	1
	Incomprehensible	2	Moans to pain	2		0	0
	None	1	None	1			
MOTOR	Obeys commands	⑥	Spontaneous movements	6	**C: CONVERT GCS**	13-15	④
	Localizes	5	Withdraws to touch	5		9-12	3
	Withdraws	4	Withdraws to pain	4		6-8	2
	Flexion	3	Flexion	3		4-5	1
	Extension	2	Extension	2		3-0	0
	None	1	None	1			

Revised trauma score:
A + B + C = *12*

Secondary survey

HEAD

	Yes	No
Ear/nose bleeding	☐	☒

Blood glucose level: _____ *98* _____

	Yes	No
Battles sign	☐	☒
Facial asymmetry	☐	☒

Wounds/deformities
  Scalp: _____ *N/A* _____
  Face: _____ *N/A* _____

NECK

	Yes	No
Trachea deviated	☐	☒
Subcutaneous emphysema	☐	☒
Jugular vein distention	☐	☒

Wounds/deformities: _____ *N/A* _____

(continued)

TRAUMA FLOW SHEET

CHEST

	Yes	No
Asymmetrical movement	☐	☒
Crepitus/subcutaneous air	☐	☒

Heart sounds:
☒ Clear   ☐ Muffled

Wounds/contusions: _____N/A_____

ABDOMEN

	Yes	No
Tender	☐	☒
Rigid	☐	☒
Distended	☐	☒
Obese	☐	☒

Wounds/contusions: _____N/A_____

PELVIS/GU

Pelvis:
☒ Stable   ☐ Unstable

Blood at meatus:
☐ Yes   ☒ No

EXTREMITIES

	Pulses			Movement		Wounds/deformities
R. arm	☒ Pres	☐ Abs	☐ Dec	☒ Yes	☐ No	*Puncture wound*
L. arm	☒ Pres	☐ Abs	☐ Dec	☒ Yes	☐ No	N/A
R. leg	☒ Pres	☐ Abs	☐ Dec	☒ Yes	☐ No	N/A
L. leg	☒ Pres	☐ Abs	☐ Dec	☒ Yes	☐ No	N/A

POSTERIOR SURVEY:

Wounds/deformities: _____N/A_____

Rectal tone: ☐ Present   ☐ Absent   ☒ Deferred

TRAUMA FLOW SHEET   Trauma alert   ☐ PTA   **TRAUMA TEAM**
                         called:_____   ☐ ED

	Name		Arrival time
Trauma surgeon			
ED MD	*Jacob Smiling, MD*		*1430*
Other			
Primary RN	*Frances Baldwin, RN*		*1420*
Secondary RN			

Time	1420	1435								
BP	100/60	102/68								
Pulse	106	103								
Resp (S=Spont.)	20 S	22 S								
Temp	98.8	/								
Cardiac rhythm	NSR	NSR								
Pulse oximeter	98%	99%								
Pupils	R B / L B	R B / L B	R / L	R / L	R / L	R / L	R / L	R / L	R / L	R / L
LOC	1	1								

LOC

1 - Alert/oriented   3 - Responds to verbal   5 - Unresponsive
2 - Disoriented   4 - Responds to pain   6 - Chemically paralyzed

Pupil reaction key:

Pupil size in mm:

S - Sluggish   B - Brisk   N - Nonreactive

1 2 3 4 5 6 7 8

FLUIDS   Fluid warmer used: ☐ Yes   ☐ No

Time	Solution	Amount	Location	Rate/hr	Cath size	Additive	Amount infused	Initials
1500	NSS	1000 ml	@ arm	75/hr	18G	—		FB

MEDICATIONS

Time	1510	Tetanus	0.5 cc		I.M.		Lot #: 426718	Expires: 12/07

Time	Medication	Dose	Route	Site			Initials
1515	Toradol	30 mg	I.V.	@ arm			FB
1530	Rocephin	250 mg	I.V.	@ arm			FB

(continued)

TRAUMA FLOW SHEET

BLOOD ADMINISTRATION

Time	Unit number	Blood type	Total infused

INTAKE		OUTPUT	
Oral __250__ cc NG _____ cc		Urine __550__ cc Feces _____ cc	
IV/IVPB __600__ cc Other _____ cc		NG/emesis _____ cc Other _____ cc	

TREATMENTS AND PROCEDURES

Intubated by: _____ / _____ / _____
Size   Inserted by   Time

NG tube: _____ / _____ / _____
Size   Inserted by   Time

Chest ☐ Left _____ / _____ / _____
tube: Size   Inserted by   Time

     ☐ Right _____ / _____ / _____
Size   Inserted by   Time

Drainage: _____ / _____
Amount   Time

Foley catheter: _____ / _____ / _____ / _____
Size   Inserted by   Time   Color

Dip: ☐ Pos. ☒ Neg.

Peritoneal lavage: _____ / _____   Grossly positive? ☐ Yes ☐ No
Performed by   Timer

     Warm blankets ☐

Thoracotomy: _____ / _____   Warm fluids ☐
Performed by   Timer

Central line: _____ / _____ / _____ / _____
Size   Inserted by   Time   Location

MAJOR INJURIES

Puncture wound to ® hand from dog bite.

TRAUMA FLOW SHEET

Time	Progress Notes
1420	22-year-old white male with dog bite arrived to ED via private vehicle. Alert and oriented X3. Puncture wound to dorsal aspect of ⓡ hand. Moderate bleeding. ———————— Frances Baldwin, RN
1440	Wound irrigated c̄ NS and betadine. ———————— F. Baldwin, RN
1500	I.V. placed ⓛ arm with 18G catheter. 1000 ml NSS hung and infusing @ 75 ml/hr. 0.5 ml tetanus shot given I.M. ———— F. Baldwin, RN
1515	30 mg Toradol given I.V. push. ———————— F. Baldwin, RN
1530	250 mg Rocephin in 100 ml NSS given IVPB. ———————— F. Baldwin, RN

Police agency: _Georgetown sheriff_ ☒ Notified: _1520_ ☐ Arrived: _____

Time transfer initiated: _____ Time accepted: _____

FAMILY
☒ Present ☐ Not present but notified ☐ Unable to contact

PATIENT DISPOSITION:
Admitted to: _____ Expired: _____

Report called: _____/_____
　　　　　　　Time　　　　　Person

Transported by: _____
　　　　　　　　　　　Name

SIGNATURES:　　　　　　　　　　　　　　**INITIALS**
Frances Baldwin, RN　　　　　　　　　　　FB

UNDERSTANDING RAPE

Rape inflicts varying degrees of physical and psychological trauma. Rape-trauma syndrome typically occurs during the period after the rape or attempted rape. It refers to the victim's short- and long-term reactions and to the methods she uses to cope with the trauma.

In most cases, the rapist is a man and the victim is a woman. However, rape does occur between persons of the same gender, especially in prisons, schools, hospitals, and other institutions. Children are also commonly the victims of rape; most of the time these cases involve manual, oral, or genital contact with the child's genitalia. Commonly, the rapist is a member of the child's family. In rare instances, a woman sexually abuses a man or a child.

The prognosis is good if the rape victim receives physical and emotional support and counseling to help her deal with her feelings. The victim who articulates her feelings can cope with fears, interact with others, and return to normal routines faster than the victim who doesn't.

ment their names and badge numbers.

- Document any statements the patient makes about the attack and her state of mind during your assessment.
- Document any interventions and their outcomes. Also document interventions the patient refused such as taking the morning-after pill.
- Document patient teaching you provided the patient. If you provided the patient with names and phone numbers for a rape crisis counselor or a victim's rights advocate, document this as well.

1/10/07	2250	Admitted to ED accompanied by police officers John Hanson (badge #1234) and Teresa Collins (badge #5678). Pt. states, "I was attacked in the supermarket parking lot. I think it was about 9 p.m. He pulled me into the bushes and raped me. When he ran away, I called 911 from my cell phone." Pt. trembling and crying but able to walk into ED on her own. Placed in private room. Police officers waited in waiting room. Denies being pregnant, drug allergies, and recent illnesses including venereal disease. LMP 1/5/07. States she didn't wash or douche before coming to the hospital. Chain of evidence maintained for all specimens collected (see flow sheet). After obtaining written consent and explaining procedure, Dr. J. Smith examined pt. Pt. has reddened areas on face and anterior neck and blood on lips. Bruising noted on inner aspects of both thighs; some vaginal bleeding noted. See dr.'s note for details of pelvic exam. Specimens for venereal disease, blood, and vaginal smears collected and labeled. Evidence from fingernail scraping and pubic hair combing collected and labeled. Photographs of injuries taken. Stayed with pt. throughout exam, holding her hand and offering reassurance and comfort. Pt. cooperated with exam but was often teary. After explaining the need for prophylactic antibiotics to pt., she consented and ceftriaxone 250 mg I.M. was administered in Ⓛ dorsogluteal muscle. ——— Susan Rose, RN

1/10/07 continued	2250	Declined morning-after pill. Consented to blood screening for HIV and hepatitis. Blood samples drawn, labeled, and sent to lab. Pt. understands need for f/u tests for HIV, hepatitis, and venereal disease. States she will f/u with family dr. ———— ———— Susan Rose, RN
1/10/07	2330	June Jones, MSW, spoke with pt. at length. Gave pt. information on rape crisis center and victim's rights advocate. Pt. states, "I'll call them. Ms. Jones told me they can help me deal with this." Pt. phoned brother and sister-in-law who will come to hospital and take pt. to their home for the night. Police officers interviewed pt. with her permission regarding the details of the event. At pt.'s request Ms. Jones and myself remained with pt. ———— ———— Susan Rose, RN
1/10/07	2350	Pt.'s brother, John Muncy, and his wife, Carol Muncy, arrived to take pt. to their house. Pt. will make appt. tomorrow to f/u with own doctor next week or sooner, if needed. Pt. has names and phone numbers for rape crisis counselor, victim's rights advocate, Ms. Jones, ED, and police dept. ———— ———— Susan Rose, RN

Reportable situations

Reportable situations, which are occurrences that must be reported to the appropriate agency, vary by state. When encountering a reportable situation:

● Verify to which state agencies you need to report the situation, as there may be more than one.

● Notify the agencies of the situation, and document this notification in the patient's ED record. (See *Reportable situations in the ED,* page 247.)

Patient refusal of emergency treatment

A competent adult has the right to refuse emergency treatment. His family can't overrule the decision, and the physician isn't allowed to give the expressly refused treatment, even if the patient becomes unconscious. In most cases, the health care personnel who are responsible for the patient can remain free from legal jeopardy as long as they fully inform the patient about his medical condition and the likely consequences of refusing treatment. (See *Refusal of treatment and the courts,* page 247.) When caring for a patient who refuses emergency treatment, follow these guidelines:

● Document that the patient refuses treatment and understands the risks he consequently incurs.

● Notify the nursing supervisor and the patient's physician, and document this notification.

● Try to explain the patient's choice to his family. Emphasize that the decision is his as long as he's competent, and document your conversation.

| 1/23/07 | 1300 | Brought to ED by ambulance with chest pain, radiating to Ⓛ arm. Sitting up in bed, not in acute distress. Skin pale, RR 28, occasionally rubbing Ⓛ arm. Refusing physical exam, blood work, and ECG. States "I didn't want to come to the hospital. My coworkers called an ambulance without telling me. ———— Melissa Worthing, RN |

1/23/07	1300	I'm fine, my arm's just
continued		sore from raking leaves.
		I'm leaving." Explained
		to pt. that chest and
		arm pain may be symp-
		toms of a heart attack
		and explained the risks
		of leaving without
		treatment, including
		death. Pt. stated, "I
		told you, I'm not having
		a heart attack. I want
		to leave." Notified Mary
		Colwell, RN, nursing
		supervisor, and Dr. S.
		Lowell. Dr. S. Lowell
		explained the need for
		diagnostic tests to r/o
		MI and the risks in-
		volved in not having
		treatment. Still refus-
		ing treatment but did
		agree to sign refusal of
		treatment release form.
		Explained signs and
		symptoms of MI to pt.
		Encouraged pt. to seek
		treatment and call 911
		if symptoms persist. Pt.
		discharged with ED # to
		call with questions. ───
		─ Melissa Worthing, RN

Admission to the facility

When patients are admitted to a unit in the facility, it's important to document certain essential information:
- Document the time that the patient was admitted and the time the admitting physician was notified.
- After giving the report to the receiving nurse, document where the patient is going, the name of the nurse taking the report, mode of transfer to the unit, the condition of the patient upon transfer, and the name and time of any medications given as well as the type, solution, and rate of I.V. infusions.

Transfer to another facility

At times it becomes necessary to transfer ED patients to other facilities. You need to be particularly aware of documentation requirements for patients being transferred in order to demonstrate compliance with the Emergency Medical Treatment and Active Labor Act (EMTALA), which was designed to prevent inappropriate transfers of patients seeking emergency care or those who are in active labor. However, it usually applies to any patient seeking medical care anywhere on facility property. (See *Meeting EMTALA requirements,* page 248.)

If your patient is going to be transferred, be sure to document:
- a physician's signature certifying that the transfer is medically necessary
- the name of the receiving physician (this may be the ED physician at the receiving facility)
- that the receiving hospital has agreed to accept the patient
- that medical records are being sent with the patient
- the patient's or a relative's signature
- consent to release copies of the patient's medical record, signed by the patient or a family member
- that the patient was transferred with qualified personnel and appropriate equipment.

Discharge instructions

There's more to discharging a patient than making sure he safely leaves the facility. One of your responsibilities is to make sure that proper documentation has been filled out prior to his release. When discharging a patient, follow these documentation guidelines:

REPORTABLE SITUATIONS IN THE ED

This chart gives examples of reportable situations in the emergency department (ED) and the agencies to which they should be reported.

REPORTABLE SITUATION	AGENCY
Altercations and assaults	■ Law enforcement
Animal bites	■ Animal control
Child abuse	■ Child protective services
Communicable diseases	■ Varies by state
Deaths	■ Coroner ■ Local organ procurement (in most states)
Elder abuse	■ Adult protective services
Homicide	■ Coroner ■ Law enforcement
Motor vehicle accidents	■ Law enforcement
Suicide	■ Coroner ■ Law enforcement

● Document the patient's condition at the time of discharge or transfer to another facility.

● Document discharge instructions that you gave to the patient and his family as well as evidence of their understanding.

● If your facility uses preprinted discharge instructions, make sure that they're individualized for your patient. Include instructions for follow-up with other health care providers if needed.

● Obtain the signature of the patient or family member, and sign the discharge instructions yourself, as they become a part of the medical record.

In court

REFUSAL OF TREATMENT AND THE COURTS

The courts recognize a competent adult's right to refuse medical treatment, even when that refusal will clearly result in his death. However, the courts also recognize several circumstances that justify overruling a patient's refusal of treatment. These include:
■ when refusing treatment endangers the life of another
■ when a parent's decision threatens the child's life
■ when, despite refusing treatment, the patient makes statements that indicate he wants to live.

If none of the above grounds exist, then you have an ethical duty to defend your patient's right to refuse treatment.

Patient safety *To comply with JCAHO's Patient Safety Goals, use appropriate "hands off" communication procedures according to your facility's policy.*

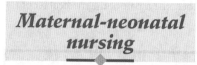

Maternal-neonatal nursing

Maternal-neonatal nursing takes place in a variety of settings, which means that as a maternal-neonatal nurse, you need to be competent to give care in multiple settings. You may care for the mother and the neonate from delivery to discharge, or you may care for high-risk, antepartum women. No matter the care you give, you must be prepared to document the care of women and infants in multifunctional settings. (See *Standards for maternal-neonatal nursing*.)

Documentation in maternal-neonatal nursing is especially sensitive and critical for two reasons that don't exist in other areas of nursing documentation:

- You're often caring for two patients at once, whose best interests may be in conflict.
- In the case of a pregnancy, labor, or birth injury, the parents or the child have until the child reaches the age of majority plus 18 months to sue.

Careful documentation of observations and interventions assures your patient quality care and provides you with the best legal protection available.

LABOR AND DELIVERY

Many institutions have a checklist or form for physical assessment of the mother on admission and another checklist or form for ongoing assessment during labor. Prior to the mother's arrival, follow these guidelines:

- If necessary, familiarize yourself with the specific procedures or protocols of your practice setting, your state's nurse practice act, and applicable national standards.
- If possible, review the prenatal record (the foundation for care and documentation during her stay) for the following information (or obtain it once the woman arrives if there's no existing record):
  - gravidity (number of pregnancies), parity (number of live births), and abortions (spontaneous or therapeutic)

– estimated due date
– weeks' gestation and the frequency of visits for prenatal care
– medical, surgical, psychiatric, and obstetric history
– laboratory results
– ultrasound or other diagnostic procedures
– allergies
– medications, including prenatal vitamins
– use of alcohol, tobacco, and illicit drugs
– complimentary therapies or supplements.

Obtain more comprehensive information from the patient upon her admission. (See *Initial assessment on admission to labor and delivery,* page 250.)

Medications

The four most common medications used in labor are antibiotics, magnesium sulfate, oxytocin, and pain relievers. When a patient receives any of these medications (or any other medications depending on the patient's preexisting health condition), document:

● medication's administration, timing, and dose
● patient's response.

Where to document

In labor and delivery, document your actions:

● on the chart, which usually contains one or more flow sheets
● in the nurses' notes
● on the delivery record
● on the monitor tracing or computerized chart and monitoring record.

Carefully transcribe appropriate information from the prenatal record to these documents. Evaluate and document fetal heart rate (FHR) and contractions according to established nursing standards as well as your facility's policy. (See *Frequency of documentation,* page 250.)

INITIAL ASSESSMENT ON ADMISSION TO LABOR AND DELIVERY

For your initial assessment of the patient on admission to labor and delivery, follow these guidelines:

■ Evaluate and document the patient's reason for coming to the labor and delivery unit. This will determine the speed of the assessment and prioritize what needs to be done as well as facilitate correct documentation. For a woman in early labor or one who's being admitted for a pregnancy-related problem, there will be plenty of time to ask questions and document as you go along. If the woman is in active labor, especially if birth is imminent, ask the most important questions, do the examination quickly, and finish the paperwork later. You're never expected to sacrifice patient care in order to do paperwork.

■ Ask the patient if she has a birth plan or what her birth plans and desires are, including positions for labor, support people, and use of medications.

■ If the patient is in labor—or if she thinks she's in labor—ask her to describe the onset of contractions, the timing and strength of contractions, and her pain level.

■ Ask the patient if there's anything else you should know in order to provide her with the best possible care.

Question the patient about:
■ gravidity, parity, and weeks' gestation
■ symptoms of gestational hypertension, diabetes, or other medical problems such as asthma
■ status of membranes.

If it's available, verify this information with the prenatal record, and enter it into the hospital record (typically on an admission flow sheet, labor flow sheet, and delivery record).

Finish your assessment with a physical examination, including:
■ baseline vital signs, understanding that there may be circumstances existing that have already changed the patient's normal vital signs (such as labor, pain, infection, gestational hypertension, or diabetes)
■ a vaginal examination, including the documentation of dilation, effacement, presenting part, and station.

FREQUENCY OF DOCUMENTATION

This chart shows documentation intervals for the patient in labor that meet Association for Women's Health, Obstetric, and Neonatal Nurses standards.

In addition to the guidelines below, the fetal heart rate (FHR) should be assessed before initiation of labor-enhancing procedures (artificial rupture of amniotic membranes), ambulation, and administration of medications or anesthesia. FHR should also be assessed after rupture of membranes, administration of medications and epidural, expulsion of an enema, catheterization, evidence of an abnormal uterine pattern, vaginal examination, ambulation, and after an increase or a decrease of a medication.

STAGE OF LABOR	LOW–RISK PATIENT	HIGH–RISK PATIENT	PITOCIN-INDUCED OR AUGMENTED LABOR
Latent	Every 60 minutes	Every 30 minutes	At a minimum, before every dose increase
Active	Every 30 minutes	Every 15 minutes	At a minimum, before every dose increase
Second stage	Every 15 minutes	Every 5 minutes	At a minimum, before every dose increase

Documenting fetal well-being

Determine whether there have been fetal problems identified during the pregnancy by reviewing the prenatal record and by asking the patient. Then apply fetal monitoring. (See *Understanding fetal monitoring*.) When documenting fetal monitoring, follow these guidelines:

● Use the fetal monitor strip to document when numerous events are occurring.

● **Alert** *When using the fetal monitor strip to document, be sure to write legibly, don't obscure any part of the tracing with writing, and don't draw attention to problems (for example, by circling an FHR deceleration). Also, transfer the documentation of significant events on the monitor strip to the patient's chart as soon as you're able.*

● When there are changes in the patient's condition or the condition of the fetus that require notification of a practitioner or midwife who isn't present on the unit, document complete information including the exact time the physician or midwife was notified, what information was given, and the response.

● If you administer medication, document the time of administration and the patient's response.

● **Patient safety** *To comply with JCAHO's Patient Safety Goals, use appropriate "hands off" communication procedures according to your facility's policy whenever you transfer care of your patient to another caregiver.*

POSTPARTUM CARE

In general, the guidelines for assessment frequency are determined by facility policy. However, be sure to keep these guidelines in mind.

● Perform and document assessments more frequently than required

> ### UNDERSTANDING FETAL MONITORING
>
> Fetal monitoring, which can be done internally or externally, assesses fetal response to uterine contractions by providing an electrocardiogram of the fetal heart rate (FHR). It precisely measures intrauterine pressure, tracks labor progress, and allows evaluation of short- and long-term FHR variability.

if any of the assessment parameters are found to be abnormal.

● Document pertinent patient teaching you provide.

NEONATAL DOCUMENTATION

Neonatal assessment includes initial and ongoing assessment as well as a thorough physical examination, all of which must be carefully documented. Special areas of neonatal documentation include Apgar scoring and the initial physical assessment.

Apgar scoring

● Provides a way to evaluate the neonate's cardiopulmonary and neurologic status

● Requires assessments at 1 and 5 minutes after birth and then every 5 minutes until the neonate stabilizes (see *Apgar scoring,* page 252)

Neonatal assessment

● Requires a thorough visual and physical examination of the neonate

● Helps identify the existence of congenital anomalies or other abnormalities (see *General guidelines for neonatal assessment,* pages 252 and 253)

Apgar scoring

This chart shows the scoring parameters for an Apgar assessment. A score of 8 to 10 indicates that the neonate is in no apparent distress; a score less than 8 indicates that resuscitative measures may be needed.

Sign	0	1	2
Heart rate	Absent	Less than 100 beats/minute	Greater than 100 beats/minute
Respiratory effort	Absent	Slow, irregular	Good crying
Muscle tone	Flaccid	Some flexion of extremities	Active motion
Reflex irritability	None	Grimace	Vigorous cry
Color	Pale, blue	Body pink, blue extremities	Completely pink

General guidelines for neonatal assessment

When performing the initial neonatal assessment, these guidelines will help you make sure that your examination and documentation are complete.

INTEGUMENTARY SYSTEM
- Assess the general appearance. Is there cyanosis or duskiness?
- Assess skin temperature.
- Assess the quality of skin turgor.
- Observe for anomalies, such as birthmarks, forceps marks, or Mongolian spots.
- Observe for the presence of erythema toxicum, lanugo, milia, petechia, or vernix, and note location and degree if present.
- Check for lacerations or abrasions. Note location and degree if present.

HEAD
- Assess the anterior and posterior fontanels. Are they sunken, soft, tense, or bulging? What's their size?
- Measure the head circumference.
- Assess the scalp. Look for the presence of bruising, caput, cephalhematoma, lacerations, and scalp electrode placement markings.
- Assess the sutures. Are they overlapping, separated (indicate in centimeters), fused, or soft?

- Assess the ears. Observe their form and positioning, and check their degree of recoil. Also check for the presence of vernix, tags, or pits.
- Assess the eyes. Are the lids fused? Is there periorbital edema? If the eyes are open, assess for pupil reaction, red reflex, and scleral hemorrhages. If there's conjunctivitis, describe drainage.
- Assess the face. Observe its general appearance for color, eye spacing, and symmetry. Look for the presence of birthmarks, edema, forceps marks, malformations, paralysis, and skin tags.
- Assess the nose. Is each nasal passage patent? Observe for nasal flaring.
- Assess the mouth and lips. Observe chin size and the integrity of the lips. (Cleft lip present?) Open the mouth and look for the presence of teeth. Observe the mucous membranes for color, moisture, and the presence of lesions. Assess the suck reflex, and follow the roof of the mouth with your finger to assess for cleft palate.
- Assess the neck. Is it supple with normal range of motion? Is the trachea aligned? Is there webbing, crepitus, or palpable glands or masses? Assess each clavicle for fracture.

General guidelines for neonatal assessment (continued)

Cardiovascular system
- Assess heart rate and rhythm. Are they regular? Are heart sounds muffled or distant?
- Assess for murmurs. If present, describe location and intensity.
- Assess peripheral pulses (brachial and femoral, bilaterally). Are they equal and regular, or bounding, weak, or thready?
- Assess the location of the point of maximal impulse (normally located at the 5th intercostal space).
- Assess capillary refill time (normally less than 3 seconds).
- Assess for edema. Note location and whether it's pitting or nonpitting.

Respiratory system
- Assess rate and rhythm of respirations. Is the pattern regular? Are there periods of apnea? Are they shallow or rapid? Does the chest expand symmetrically?
- Assess breath sounds. Are they equal, clear, and audible in all lobes? Listen for crackles, rhonchi, or wheezes.
- Assess for the presence of grunting or retracting.
- Measure the chest's circumference.
- Assess the shape of the chest as well as the placement and number of nipples. Assess breast development.

Gastrointestinal system
- Assess the umbilical cord. Note its appearance and the number of vessels.
- Observe the abdomen for general appearance. Is it round, distended, flat, or scaphoid? Is ascites present? Auscultate for bowel sounds.
- Gently palpate the abdomen. Note masses, organomegaly, or tenderness.
- Measure abdominal circumference.
- Record the first passage of meconium.
- Assess the anus for patency.

Genitourinary system
Male
- Assess the penis. Is gender obvious or is it questionable? Note the placement of the urethral meatus. (Is there epispadias or hypospadias?)
- Assess the scrotum for edema, masses, the amount of rugae, and for herniation.
- Assess the testes. Are both descended or are they still in the inguinal canal?

Female
- Assess for masses or herniation.
- Assess the clitoris and labia for size. Is gender obvious or is it questionable?
- Assess the vagina for discharge. If present, describe it.

General
- Record the first void.

Neuromuscular system
- Assess general activity. Is the neonate active, lethargic, or paralyzed? Is he jittery, tremulous, or having seizures?
- Assess the spine for limited range of motion.
- Assess the sucking, rooting, grasping, Moro, and Babinski reflexes.
- Assess tone. Is he hypotonic or hypertonic?

Extremities
- Assess for range of motion.
- Assess hips for clicks, and check gluteal fold and thigh length symmetry.
- Assess the number of digits and check for webbing, extra digits, clubbing, or cyanosis.
- Assess the soles of the feet for normal creases.
- Check the palms for Simian creases.
- Observe for gross abnormalities.

Psychosocial
- Assess the mother's status: Is she single, married, divorced, separated, widowed? Are there siblings?
- Determine the primary caregiver: mother, father, grandparent?
- Note if breast- or bottle-feeding.

THE IMPORTANCE OF PEDIATRIC NURSING DOCUMENTATION

We live in a litigious society, in which courts give children special consideration when it comes to lawsuits. For nurses working with the pediatric population, liability from malpractice may extend for years. The time requirement or statute of limitations is suspended until the age of majority (age 18), when the adult statute of limitations period begins. Therefore, a nurse can theoretically be held liable for care given 20 years prior to a child who was 2 years old at the time in question, because after the suit is filed, it may be another 2 to 3 years before the case is actually brought to court. After that length of time, the chart is typically all that one has to recall the patient and the care that was given.

Keeping this in mind, a good rule of thumb to follow is to document so thoroughly, completely, and accurately that another person, reviewing your work 2 years or more later, can see exactly what you saw and follow your train of thought in providing the nursing care and interventions that you performed. This includes your care of the child as well as your care and support of his family.

Pediatric nursing

If you're a nurse who works with children, you have special challenges. Helping a child achieve and maintain an optimal level of health means working with him and his family. Clear and accurate documentation is necessary because it allows information regarding the patient to be passed on to multiple members of the health care team in a way that oral communication can't, which may serve to protect you many years later. (See *The importance of pediatric nursing documentation*.)

SPECIAL ISSUES IN PEDIATRIC NURSING DOCUMENTATION

Special aspects for the documentation of nursing care for children include growth and development, psychological considerations, and child abuse and neglect.

Growth and development

Working with children requires skill and flexibility in providing care to a wide range of ages and developmental stages. (See *Bright Futures*.) Documentation tools:

● must have the capacity to include the different stages children go through
● must be developed using national standards
● should include current recommendations for physical assessment and health guidance.

Developmental screening

Multiple screening tools exist to assess a child's development. Tools assess:

● gross and fine motor skills
● personal and social behaviors
● language abilities
● other components of development.

One of the most commonly used tools is the Denver Developmental Screening Test II (DDST II). (See *Using the DDST II*.)

Growth charts

Growth is a continuous process that must be evaluated over time, and all growth parameters should be followed sequentially on the appropriate growth charts. Evaluating growth provides useful information for the early detection of abnormalities and provides reassurance to the parents and health care providers that the child is growing normally.

When documenting growth, utilize:

● most recent Centers for Disease Control and Prevention growth charts, developed by the National Center for Health Statistics and adopted by the World Health Organization for international use. These 16 revised charts (eight for boys, eight for girls) include weight-for-age, length/stature-for-age, and weight-forlength/stature percentile charts.

● body mass index.

Body mass index

● Helps to determine if a patient is overweight or underweight and allows early detection for those at risk of becoming overweight

● Calculated from a patient's weight and height measurements

● Interpretation depends on child's age

● Plotted for age on gender-specific charts because girls differ from boys in their percentage of body fat as they mature (See *Using pediatric growth grids,* pages 256 and 257.)

Psychosocial assessment

Psychosocial assessment is a vital part of the evaluation that is, unfortunately, commonly forgotten. It includes such topics as:

● behavior
● school performance
● family dynamics.

USING THE DDST II

The Denver Developmental Screening Test II (DDST II) is a screening tool that assesses the developmental level of children ages 1 month to 6 years; however, it isn't a diagnostic tool or intelligence test. It employs a series of developmental tasks to determine whether a child's development is within the normal range.

The DDST II looks at four domains: personal-social, fine motor adaptive, language, and gross motor skills. It's easy to administer, has been used by health care professionals for years, provides a good indication of where the child is developmentally, and is helpful in providing guidance to parents. If the child's development is questionable in any of the four areas (compared with normal standards), referral for an in-depth evaluation is recommended.

USING PEDIATRIC GROWTH GRIDS

Use a growth grid to correlate the child's height with her age and her weight with her height and age. You can also determine the child's body mass index (BMI), which is then plotted on another grid. There are separate charts for boys and girls. These sample forms show the growth of a girl tracked over a number of years. Note how her BMI was calculated and then plotted on the BMI grid.

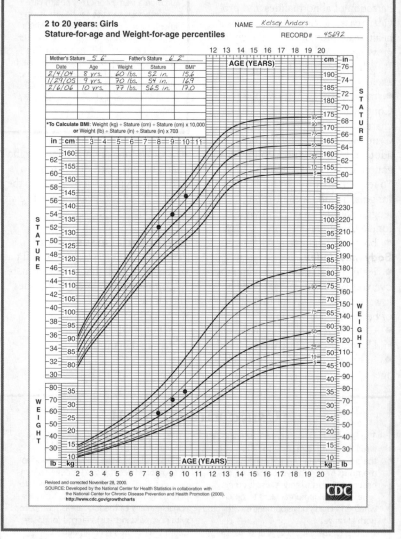

2 to 20 years: Girls
Stature-for-age and Weight-for-age percentiles

NAME *Kelsey Anders*
RECORD# *45692*

Mother's Stature *5' 6"*   Father's Stature *6' 2"*

Date	Age	Weight	Stature	BMI*
2/4/04	8 yrs.	60 lbs.	52 in.	15.6
1/29/05	9 yrs.	70 lbs.	54 in.	16.9
2/6/06	10 yrs.	77 lbs.	56.5 in.	17.0

*To Calculate BMI: Weight (kg) ÷ Stature (cm) ÷ Stature (cm) x 10,000
or Weight (lb) ÷ Stature (in) ÷ Stature (in) x 703

Revised and corrected November 28, 2000.
SOURCE: Developed by the National Center for Health Statistics in collaboration with the National Center for Chronic Disease Prevention and Health Promotion (2000).
http://www.cdc.gov/growthcharts

When performing a psychosocial assessment of a child, follow these guidelines:

- Assess and document information regarding the child's relationships with siblings and friends.

USING PEDIATRIC GROWTH GRIDS *(CONTINUED)*

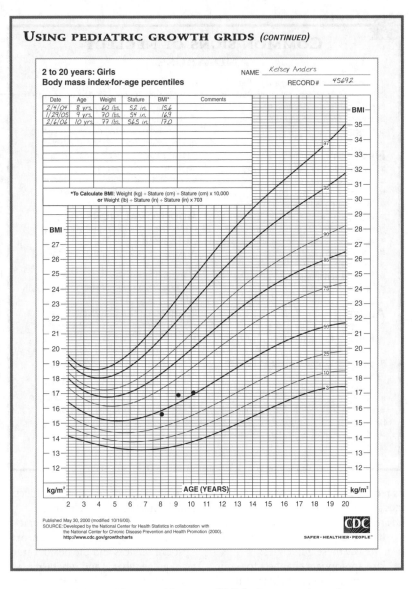

2 to 20 years: Girls
Body mass index-for-age percentiles

NAME *Kelsey Anders*

RECORD # *45692*

Date	Age	Weight	Stature	BMI*	Comments
2/4/04	8 yrs.	60 lbs.	52 in.	15.6	
1/29/05	9 yrs.	70 lbs.	54 in.	16.9	
2/6/06	10 yrs.	77 lbs.	56.5 in.	17.0	

*To Calculate BMI: Weight (kg) ÷ Stature (cm) ÷ Stature (cm) x 10,000
or Weight (lb) ÷ Stature (in) ÷ Stature (in) x 703

AGE (YEARS)

Published May 30, 2000 (modified 10/16/00).
SOURCE: Developed by the National Center for Health Statistics in collaboration with
the National Center for Chronic Disease Prevention and Health Promotion (2000).
http://www.cdc.gov/growthcharts

CDC
SAFER · HEALTHIER · PEOPLE™

- Document the child's typical behavior and reactions to stressors.
- Document how the family copes with stressful situations, such as illness and hospitalization.
- Assess current living situations, recent losses, or other ongoing or acute crises. Document your findings.

Child abuse and neglect

Child abuse (including physical, sexual, emotional, and psychological abuse) and neglect are two of the leading causes of pediatric hospital admissions. They may be suspected in any age-group, cultural setting, or environment. In most states, a nurse

COMMON SIGNS OF NEGLECT AND ABUSE

If your assessment reveals any of the following signs, consider neglect or abuse as a possible cause and document your findings. Be sure to notify the appropriate people and agencies.

NEGLECT
- Dehydration
- Failure to thrive in infants
- Failure of wounds to heal
- Inadequate clothing
- Infestations, such as scabies, lice, or maggots in a wound
- Injuries from falls
- Malnutrition
- Periodontal disease
- Poor personal hygiene
- Severe diaper rash

ABUSE
- Bleeding from body orifices
- Exposure to inappropriately harsh discipline
- Exposure to verbal abuse and belittlement
- Extreme fear or anxiety
- Genital trauma
- Head injuries or bald spots from pulling hair out
- Multiple injuries or fractures in various stages of healing
- Precocious sexual behaviors
- Pregnancy in young girls or those with physical or mental handicaps
- Recurrent injuries
- Sexually transmitted diseases in children
- Unexplained bruises, abrasions, burns, bites, damaged or missing teeth, strap or rope marks
- Verbalized accounts of being beaten, slapped, kicked, or sexually abused

ADDITIONAL SIGNS
- Abusive behavior toward younger children and pets
- Aggressive speech or behavior toward adults
- Blunted or flat affect
- Clinging behavior directed toward health care providers
- Depression or mood changes
- Lack of appropriate peer relationships
- Mistrust of others
- Nonspecific headaches, stomachaches, or eating and sleeping problems
- Runaway behavior
- Social withdrawal
- Sudden school difficulties, such as poor grades, truancy, or fighting with peers

is required by law to report signs of abuse. (See *Common signs of neglect and abuse*.)

If you suspect child abuse or neglect, follow these guidelines:
- Use appropriate channels for your facility and report suspicions to the appropriate administrator and agency.
- Document suspicions on the appropriate forms or in your nurse's notes.
- Document cultural practices the family follows. Some, such as coin rubbing in some Vietnamese families, may be mistaken for child abuse. However, regardless of cultural practices, remember that the department of social services and the health care team judge what is and what isn't abuse. (See *Your role in reporting abuse*.)
- When assessing the family, interview the child alone and try to interview his caregivers separately to identify inconsistencies with histories.

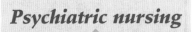

In court

YOUR ROLE IN REPORTING ABUSE

As a nurse, you play a crucial role in recognizing and reporting incidents of suspected child abuse. While caring for patients, you can readily note evidence of apparent abuse. When you do, you must pass the information along to the appropriate authorities. In many states, failure to report actual or suspected abuse constitutes a crime.

If you've ever hesitated to file an abuse report because you fear repercussions, remember that the Child Abuse Prevention and Treatment Act protects you against liability. If your report is bona fide (that is, if you file it in good faith), the law protects you from a suit filed by an alleged abuser.

1/8/07	1700	Circular burns 2 cm in
		diameter noted on lower
		® and Ⓛ scapulae in
		various stages of healing
		while auscultating breath
		sounds. Pt. states these
		injuries occurred while
		playing with cigarettes he
		found at his babysitter's
		home. When parents were
		questioned separately as
		to the cause of injuries
		on child's back, mother
		stated the child told
		her he fell off a swing
		and received a rope
		burn. Father stated he
		had no idea of the child's
		injuries. Parents stated
		the child is being watched
		after school until they
		get home by the teenager
		next door, Sally Johnson.
		Parents stated that their
		son doesn't like being
		watched by her anymore,
		but they don't know why.
		Parents state they're
		looking into alternative
		care suggestions. Dr. W.
		Gordon notified of in-
		juries and examined pt.
		at 1645. Social service
		department and nursing
		supervisor, Nancy Taylor,
		RN, notified at 1650. —
		—— Joanne M. Allen, RN

In court An injunction can be obtained to separate an abuser and the abused so the patient can be safe until the circumstances can be investigated.

Psychiatric nursing

In 1973, The American Nurses Association Coalition of Psychiatric Nursing Organizations issued standards to improve the quality of care provided by psychiatric and mental health nurses. These standards, last revised in 2000, apply to generalists and specialists working in any setting in which psychiatric and mental health nursing is practiced. (See *Coalition of Psychiatric Nursing Organizations standards,* page 261.)

SPECIAL DOCUMENTATION CONSIDERATIONS

Psychiatric nurses face a number of issues requiring special documentation. These include seclusion and restraints, substance abuse, and extrapyramidal adverse effects of therapeutic medications.

1/21/07	2000	Approached by pt. at
		1930, crying and saying
		loudly, "I can't stand it,
		they will get me." Repeat-
		ed this statement several
		times. Unable to say who
		"they" were. Pt. asked to
		sit in a seclusion room
		saying, "It's quiet and
		safe there. That's what
		I do at the psych. hospi-
		tal." Called Dr. J. Wright
		at 1935 and told him of
		pt. request. Verbal order
		given for seclusion as
		requested by pt. Dr. J.
		Wright will be in to
		evaluate pt. at 2030. Pt.
		placed in empty pt. room
		on unit in close proximity
		to nurse's station. Told
		her that because seclusion
		was voluntary she was
		free to leave seclusion
		when she felt ready. Rita
		Summers, CNA, assigned
		to continuously observe
		pt. P 82, BP 132/82, RR
		18, oral T 98.7° F. Family
		notified of pt.'s request
		for seclusion, that pt. is
		free to leave seclusion
		on her own, will be con-
		tinuously observed by
		CNA and assessed fre-
		quently by RN and that
		doctor will be by at 2030. Family stated
		they were comfortable
		with this decision.
		———— Donna Blau, RN

Restraints are defined as any method of physically restricting a person's freedom of movement, physical activity, or normal access to his body. You'll usually accomplish restraint through the application of cloth or leather wrist and ankle restraints. These can cause numerous problems, including limited mobility, skin break-down, impaired circulation, incontinence, psychological distress, and strangulation.

1/8/07	1700	Extremely agitated, cursing,
		and swinging fists and
		kicking feet at nurse and
		staff. Attempted to calm
		patient through non-
		threatening verbal com-
		munication. No I.V. access
		available. Ativan 2 mg I.M.
		given per Dr. S. Miller's
		order. After evaluation,
		Dr. S. Miller ordered 4-
		point restraints applied to
		prevent harm to patient
		and staff. Pt. informed
		that restraints would be
		removed when he could
		remain calm and refrain
		from hitting or kicking.
		Doesn't want his family to
		be notified of restraint
		application. See restraint
		monitoring sheet for fre-
		quent assessments and
		intervention notations. ——
		————Carol Sacks, RN

Seclusion and restraints

When a patient becomes dangerously out of control, you may have to employ seclusion or restraints. During seclusion, a patient is separated from others in a safe, secure, and contained environment, such as a locked room (with close nursing supervision). Secluding the patient protects him, other patients, and staff members from imminent harm.

In court *The use of seclusion and restraints poses a very sensitive legal issue and should be limited to emergencies in which the patient is at risk for harming himself or others.*

Precise documentation that covers your use of seclusion and restraints is a legal necessity. Follow your facility's policy as well as the standards set forth by the Joint Commission on Accreditation of Healthcare Organi-

COALITION OF PSYCHIATRIC NURSING ORGANIZATIONS STANDARDS

Psychiatric nursing documentation should encompass all of the standards of care as designated by the Coalition of Psychiatric Nursing Organizations. These standards are summarized below.

STANDARD I—ASSESSMENT

In this step, you gather subjective and objective information to develop a care plan, which determines the best possible care for the patient. You compile this data from information obtained during the interview, by observing the client, consulting with other members of the health care team, reviewing past medical and psychiatric records, and analyzing the results of the physical and mental examination.

STANDARD II—DIAGNOSIS

During this step, the psychiatric mental health nurse analyzes the assessment data to determine the nursing diagnoses and potential problem statements. These diagnoses and problem statements must be prioritized according to the needs of the patient and conform to accepted classifications systems, such as the North American Nursing Diagnosis Association-International (NANDA-I) Nursing Diagnosis Classification and the *Diagnostic and Statistical Manual of Mental Disorders,* 4th edition, Text Revision.

STANDARD III—OUTCOME IDENTIFICATION

Expected outcomes must be measurable and designate a specific time frame. They're patient-oriented, therapeutically sound, realistic, attainable, and cost effective. Additionally, they're derived from the diagnosis.

STANDARD IV—PLANNING

A care plan is best tailored to the patient when it involves collaboration between the patient, family, and all members of the interdisciplinary health care team. It's used to guide therapeutic interventions, document progress, and achieve the expected outcomes. It should include an educational program related to the patient's health problems, treatment regimen, and self-care activities. Its format must allow for modification, interdisciplinary access, and retrieval of data.

STANDARD V—IMPLEMENTATION

A number of interventions are used to maintain or restore mental and physical health. They must be safe, timely, appropriate, ethical, and performed according to the psychiatric–mental health nurse's level of education, practice, and certification. Interventions must be evaluated and modified based on continued assessment of the clients' response.

Subcategories of Standard V include counseling, milieu therapy, promotion of self-care activities, psychobiological interventions, health teaching, case management, health promotion and maintenance, and advanced practice interventions.

STANDARD VI—EVALUATION

Needed revisions to the care plan based on the ongoing assessment are documented.

---

zations when documenting the use of seclusion or restraints. Make sure to document:

- patient behaviors leading up to the use of seclusion or restraints
- actions taken to control the behavior before the use of seclusion or restraints

- time the patient's behavior became uncontrollable
- time the patient was placed in seclusion or restraints
- physical assessment of the patient immediately after he's placed in seclusion or restraints

- your assessment of and assistance to the patient every 15 minutes, including:
  - signs of injury associated with the application of seclusion or restraints
  - nutrition and hydration
  - circulation and range of motion
  - vital signs
  - physical and psychological status and comfort
  - readiness for discontinuation of seclusion or restraints
- medications that were given, their effectiveness, and the time of their administration
- notification of family members if the patient consented to have them informed of his care
- information given to the patient regarding conditions necessary for his release from seclusion or restraints.

Objective documentation should show evidence of proper procedures or facts on which decisions were made. In court, it can only be assumed that only those things documented were done.

Substance abuse

Patients addicted to substances may have multiple legal problems, recurrent social and interpersonal problems, and repeated absences or poor performances at work or school. When caring for a patient whom you suspect has substance abuse issues, follow these guidelines:

- Use the CAGE questionnaire if you suspect alcohol abuse. (See *Using the CAGE questionnaire*.)
- Document your findings objectively, making sure to look to the patient's family, friends, coworkers, and medical records for reliable assessment; it's common for patients with substance abuse issues to use defense mechanisms when discussing their disease.
- If your patient is at risk for substance withdrawal or shows signs of withdrawal, document that you notified the physician, the time and date of this notification, and any teaching and nursing care you provided the patient.

1/2/07	1000	Admitted to Chemical
		Dependency Unit for
		withdrawal from ethanol.
		Has a 30-year history
		of alcohol dependence
		and states, "I can't keep
		this up anymore. I
		need to get off the
		booze." Reports drinking
		a fifth of vodka per day
		for the last 2 months
		and that her last drink
		was today shortly before
		admission. Her blood
		alcohol level is 0.15%.
		She reports having gone
		through the withdrawal
		process 4 times before
		but has never completed
		rehabilitation. Reports
		the following symptoms
		during previous with-
		drawals: anxiety, nausea,
		vomiting, irritability, and
		tremulousness. Currently
		demonstrates no mani-
		festations of ethanol
		withdrawal. Dr. T. Jones
		notified of pt.'s admis-
		sion and blood alcohol
		level results. Lorazepam
		2 mg P.O. given at
		0930. Pt. instructed
		regarding s/s of ethanol
		withdrawal and associ-
		ated nursing care. She
		expressed full under-
		standing of the infor-
		mation. Will reinforce
		teaching when blood
		tests reveal no alcohol
		in blood.
		—— Brian Winters, RN

Extrapyramidal adverse effects

Nurses frequently administer antipsychotic medications to patients in psychiatric settings. Many antipsychotic medications are capable of causing profound motor effects known as *extrapyramidal adverse effects.* One of the most common extrapyramidal adverse effects is tardive dyskinesia (TD). (See *Assessing for tardive dyskinesia.*)

　　It's your responsibility to know the adverse effects of the medications the patient is receiving and to recognize and report any adverse reactions that may occur. Be sure to document:
● assessment of the patient using the Abnormal Involuntary Movement Scale tool
● notification of the physician if TD is suspected, and the time and date of this notification
● teaching provided to the patient and his family members regarding the signs and symptoms of TD and any other adverse effects that may occur due to antipsychotic medication therapy.

DOCUMENTATION IN AMBULATORY CARE

Ambulatory care has evolved greatly and includes many aspects of health care that were once unique to hospital inpatient settings, such as the performance of invasive procedures and emergency services. Today, such procedures and services are commonplace in ambulatory, outpatient, and community health care settings, which makes the necessity for accurate, complete documentation even more important. Whether your ambulatory care facility is small and independent or large and part of an integrated health care system, superior documentation remains a core component of effective and efficient patient care.

Functions of documentation in ambulatory care

The three major functions of nursing documentation in ambulatory care are:

- *Communication*—recording and exchange of information to facilitate and manage patient care
- *Regulation*—fulfilling the mandates of various accrediting bodies, governmental controls, and programmatic guidelines that allow ambulatory care facilities to operate and receive payment for their services
- *Litigation*—addressing the need for nurses and other health care providers to support their practices against possible legal challenges.

COMMUNICATION

The first function of nursing documentation in ambulatory care, as in other professional practice settings, is to communicate about patient care. Accurate, complete, timely, legible, and accessible documentation provides the most important link between understanding a patient's previous health care encounters and planning his current care. It's so important because:

- the need to coordinate patient care increases dramatically as health care

systems spread out geographically and add services.

- the number of physicians and other health care providers involved in each patient's care creates new challenges to health care communication and coordination.
- the expansion of non-physician, non-nurse personnel in the staffing of ambulatory care facilities has also increased the complexity of the communication function.

REGULATION

The second function of documentation is to meet regulatory and accreditation requirements. Health care facilities need reimbursement to survive financially. Most ambulatory care facilities, like the vast majority of other health care organizations, rely heavily on payments from:

- federal, state, and local governments
- third-party payers (insurance companies)
- various capitated or managed health plans, such as health maintenance organizations and preferred provider organizations.

LITIGATION

The third function of documentation in ambulatory care nursing is to provide legal proof of the nature, timing, and quality of care that the patient received. In fact, much of the documentation that's done in ambulatory care, as in other health care settings, revolves around avoidance of litigation and defense against litigation. When developing documentation systems for your facility, be sure to consider:

- your facility's past legal problems in the design, implementation, and evaluation of documentation systems to prevent recurrence
- issues surrounding confidentiality of and access to documentation and its maintenance.

Documentation of ambulatory care services

As indicated at the beginning of this chapter, there are multiple types of ambulatory care visits. Each type of visit requires specific documentation. In this section, you're given recommendations for the documentation of clinic and office, procedure and surgical, and chemotherapy visits; short stay and clinical decision unit assessments; and telephone encounters.

CLINIC AND OFFICE VISITS

In a clinic or professional office, each patient visit is typically documented with a narrative note from the physician, nurse practitioner, physician's assistant, or nurse who provides the care. The note should reflect:

- reason for the visit (history, chief concern, or presenting complaint)
- patient's current condition (assessment)
- what was discussed or done with the patient (interventions)
- care plan, including recommendations for follow-up.

The note should also include this routine information:

- allergies
- medications currently being taken and rationale
- medication history
- vital signs
- immunization records
- current laboratory and other tests and rationale
- any specific patient monitoring information such as diabetic management
- the name and phone number of the patient's designated "patient advocate" or specified person holding a Medical Power of Attorney for Health Care.

Patient teaching

If you provide patient teaching, make sure that you document:
- what was taught
- learning deficits that you observed (and what you did to accommodate them)
- patient's response or level of understanding
- if family members or others were included in the health teaching.

JCAHO survey

If the Joint Commission on Accreditation of Healthcare Organizations (JCAHO) or another accreditation entity surveys your ambulatory care facility, make sure that you include a summary list in the patient's record by his third clinic visit. This summary should list the types of encounters the patient has had at the facility, such as:
- well visits
- sick visits due to otitis media
- visits for immunizations.

PROCEDURE AND SURGICAL VISITS

When a patient undergoes a procedure in an ambulatory care facility, the health care provider who performs the procedure documents:
- patient consent
- procedure description
- recommended follow-up.
  Your nursing documentation should include:
- preprocedure assessment (including vital signs)
- nursing care provided before, during, and after the procedure
- postprocedure assessment (including vital signs and condition of procedure site)
- postprocedure instructions for follow-up
- patient and family teaching.

Procedure visits with conscious sedation

Some procedures, such as cardiac catheterization and endoscopy, require the patient to receive conscious sedation, which minimally lowers the patient's level of consciousness (LOC) and provides pain control while retaining the patient's protective reflexes, a patent airway, and continuous vital signs.

Preprocedure

When a patient is scheduled to receive conscious sedation, complete and document a nursing assessment before the procedure. In the assessment, be sure to include:
- patient identification and verification of patient identification
- verification of documented consent

- verification that surgical site has been identified and verified
- chief complaint
- diagnosis
- planned procedure
- ambulation status
- emotional and mental status
- neurological status
- fasting status
- pain status
- color
- drug or food allergies or allergies to other substances
- medications
- review of laboratory or other testing completed prior to the procedure
- verification and condition of procedure site
- level of sedation to be provided.

Before the start of the conscious sedation, document all care provided, including:
- vital signs and oxygen saturation
- I.V. lines started
- medications administered
- test results outside of the normal range
- communications with other health care providers regarding assessment findings (especially those that lie outside of the normal range).

Operative phase

During the operative phase—when conscious sedation is administered—document:
- patient identification and verification of patient identification
- vital signs (including pulse oximetry)
- medications administered
- patient positioning
- verification that correct surgical site is marked

- all other nursing interventions
- ongoing assessment
- patient's response to interventions.

(See *Outpatient procedure record,* pages 268 and 269.)

Postprocedure

After the procedure, verify patient identification and perform an assessment of the patient upon his arrival in the recovery area. In this assessment, document the patient's:
- vital signs and oxygen saturation
- respiratory status
- cardiovascular status
- LOC
- color and skin condition
- range of extremity movement
- pain level
- condition of the procedure site and verification of correct surgical site as marked preprocedure.

Also be sure to document:
- that drains and dressings are present
- drug allergies or adverse responses
- fluid intake and output
- communications with the health care provider who performed the procedure
- all nursing care provided and the patient's responses to your interventions.

Discharge

Use a discharge summary checklist to document the patient's readiness for discharge. This summary should include such physical and mental information as:
- vital signs (including pulse oximetry)
- level of motor control
- absence or control of nausea
- voiding status

OUTPATIENT PROCEDURE RECORD

Here is an example of an outpatient procedure record. Note how the preoperative, intra-operative, and discharge assessment all go on the same form.

Clinical Ambulatory Services
Outpatient Procedure Record

Date: _1/19/07_

Medical record number: _021839_

Name: _Cynthia Sanders_

Pre-operative assessment: Nurse: _Julie Haas, RN_

Physician: _Dr. Pat McTigue_

Condition on arrival: _"Anxious to have procedure completed."_

Consent signed: ☐ NA ☒ Yes NPO since: _1/18/07 2400_

Date/time

Allergies: _Sulfa drugs_

Pregnant: ☐ NA ☒ No ☐ Yes Trimester: _____

Dentures removed: ☒ NA ☐ No ☐ Yes

Disposition of dentures: _____

Pre-op procedure prep completed by patient: ☐ NA ☐ No ☒ Yes

Patient belongings: ☒ With patient ☐ Given to family

BP: _120/68_ Temp: _98.7°F_ P: _68_ R: _18_

Skin warmth, color, dryness: _Warm, pink, dry_

Pre-op medications: _None_

Time: _____ Route: _____

Time: _____ Route: _____

Time: _____ Route: _____

Anesthesia used: _Midazolam 1.5 mg_

Time: _1045_ Route: _I.V._

Morphine 5 mg

Time: _1045_ Route: _I.V._

I.V. access: Solution: _NSS_ Needle type: _20G_ Site: _®_ AC

Time: _1040_ Rate: _10 ml/hr_

Solution: _____ Needle type: _____ Site: _____

Time: _____ Rate: _____

Intra-operative assessment: Procedure performed: _Upper endoscopy_

If intra- and postoperative vital signs are not applicable, check here ☐

Intra-operative

TIME	TEMP	BP	P	R	O₂ SAT	O₂ RATE	LEVEL OF CONSCIOUSNESS	SKIN	MEDICATIONS TREATMENTS	NURSE'S SIGNATURE
1047	98.3	118/70	67	18	98	2 L/min	Sleeping	Warm		J. Haas RN
1050		122/72	70	20	97	2 L/min	Sleeping	Warm	Biopsy taken	J. Haas RN
1052		120/68	70	22	98	2 L/min	Sleeping	Warm	Procedure completed	J. Haas RN

Post-operative

TIME	TEMP	BP	P	R	O₂ SAT	O₂ RATE	LEVEL OF CONSCIOUSNESS	SKIN	MEDICATIONS TREATMENTS	NURSE'S SIGNATURE
1055	98.6	124/66	68	20	99	2 L/min	Easily aroused	Warm		J. Haas RN
1100		126/74	70	22	99	O₂ d/c'd	Awake	Warm	IV d/c'd	J. Haas RN
1110		128/74	72	20	99		Awake	Warm		J. Haas RN
1125		126/72	70	20	99		Awake	Warm	PO liquids tolerated	J. Haas RN

Nursing notes/interventions/monitoring equipment

Patient attached to C/R monitor, blood pressure monitor, and pulse ox. VSS. Anesth. Dr. Klein insert-
ed 20G IV in R AC, pt. tolerated well. NSS hung and infusing at 10 ml/hr. Morphine and midazolam
administered via IV, pt. sleeping but easily aroused. Upper endoscopy performed by Dr. McTigue. VSS
throughout procedure. Pt. easily aroused after procedure. O₂ and IV d/c'd and discharge instruc-
tions reviewed and written for patient and husband. Pt. verbalized understanding. Pt. discharged to
home with husband. ——————————————————————— J. Haas, RN

Specimens: ☐ NA ☒ Yes _Gastric biopsy_ Solution _Buffered formalin_ Disposition: _Outside lab_

Discharge assessment: Condition at discharge: _Alert, VSS_

Discharged to: ☒ Home ☐ IPD room: _____ ☐ Emergency room

☐ Other: _____

Discharged per: ☒ Ambulatory ☐ Wheelchair ☐ Stretcher

Accompanied by: ☒ Self ☐ Family member ☐ Other: _____

Nurse's signature/title _Julie Haas, RN_

- comfort level
- condition of dressings or appliances
- alertness and ability to understand directions
- discharge instructions and patient and family's level of understanding of instructions
- follow-up care. (See *Documenting follow-up care,* page 270.)

CHEMOTHERAPY VISITS

Many ambulatory care facilities now perform chemotherapy, and a growing number of patients are taking advantage of this new role. It's your job to document their care effectively. (See *Oncology flow sheet,* pages 272 and 273.) When documenting a patient's chemotherapy visit, follow these guidelines:

DOCUMENTING FOLLOW-UP CARE

When a patient who receives conscious sedation is discharged home, be sure to document that he has been given adequate information for obtaining emergency or needed care, including where he can receive that care. Because conscious sedation temporarily impairs memory and cognition, also document that you gave follow-up instructions to a responsible family member who will be escorting the patient home so that he can instruct the patient after the sedation wears off. Provide these instructions in writing with your facility's phone number, so the patient or family member can call with questions, and be sure you document the name of the person to whom you give the instructions, as well as his relationship to the patient.

Before discharge, document your review of all prescriptions, the evaluation by the health care provider who performed the procedure, the disposition and return of all personal patient property, and the patient's response to all instructions.

In addition to discharge paperwork, it's also your responsibility to place and docu-ment a follow-up phone call to the patient 72 hours after the conscious sedation. During this phone call, you'll collect important information, including level of pain, presence of nausea and vomiting, oral intake, sleep comfort or disturbances, bleeding or discharges, voiding, and activity patterns. Also be sure to address and document patient and family questions at this time. If the patient was referred to another health care provider at the time of discharge, assess and document the patient's referral status.

If the patient or a family member can't be reached after a predetermined number of attempts, a message should be left for the patient, and the failure to reach the patient should be documented. Many patients who have procedures or ambulatory surgery are back to work or out of the home the day after surgery. All calls and call attempts must be documented fully. When using voicemail or message recording devices to facilitate patient contact, use due caution. Make sure that the message doesn't violate patient confidentiality in any way.

- At every visit, document the patient's:
  - weight
  - infection symptoms
  - new lesions, if present
  - hydration and antiemetic regimen
  - specific chemotherapeutic agent and dose given
  - up-to-date laboratory results
  - other significant comments.
- Fully document changes in treatment and teaching.
- If the patient is in a research study or on a clinical trial protocol, include documentation that's specific to the study.

- When a patient is new to chemotherapy, document that you taught the patient about self-care measures and when to call for assistance.
- Provide written instructions for home care and written information about the specific chemotherapeutic drug that has been prescribed.

SHORT STAY AND CLINICAL DECISION UNITS

Clinical decision units offer the opportunity for patients to receive care or be observed for up to 23 hours in an ambulatory care facility. When working in a clinical decision unit,

follow these documentation guidelines:

- Assess every patient upon admission, and document your findings. (See *Short stay nurses' admission assessment form,* page 274.)
- Document the reason for the patient's admission, which could be for surgery, infusion therapy, medical monitoring, or some other reason.
- If your facility develops patient care protocols for each patient type, follow your facility's guidelines, and fill out all the appropriate documentation.
- On discharge, give written discharge instructions, and have the patient or caregiver sign them. Be sure to document your actions.

TELEPHONE ENCOUNTERS

Telephone encounters are common in ambulatory care. They may initiate a visit, require advice from you or another health care provider, or initiate a prescription renewal or a follow-up visit. In order to prevent confusion, your facility should develop a format for documenting these encounters to prevent the omission of significant information, while also providing a way to accurately organize the information you obtain. When documenting telephone encounters, include:

- date and time of the call
- who called (the patient or the patient's caregiver)
- name of the patient and the patient's primary health care provider
- patient's chief complaint
- reported temperature
- pregnancy status (if applicable)
- allergies

- chronic diseases
- current medications
- your assessment of the situation and the advice you gave.

Also follow these documentation guidelines:

- If a patient calls asking for a prescription to be refilled, document the name of the patient's pharmacy and its telephone number as well as the medication's:
  - name
  - strength
  - dosage
  - quantity
  - refill amount.
- Keep the telephone encounter form in the patient's record. (See *Telephone encounter form,* page 275.)
- Documentation that in any way identifies a patient by name, address, telephone number, or clinical condition must be either filed as part of the official record or securely destroyed by shredding. All paper, including paper with informal "scratch" documentation made during phone encounters, should be secured to ensure patient confidentiality.

ONCOLOGY FLOW SHEET

Oncology flow sheets, such as this example, can be used for chemotherapy administration in the ambulatory care setting.

Oncology Flow Sheet   Name _____

				1/28/07					
DATE				1/28/07					
DAY ON STUDY									
TREATMENT	1	Anzemet I.V.	‡	100 mg					
	2	Decadron I.V.	‡	10 mg					
	3	Adriamycin I.V.	‡	100 mg					
	4	Cytoxan I.V.	‡	1000 mg					
	5	Antibiotics	(✓)						
	6	Transfusions amount							
	7								
	8	X R T (	)						
MARROW	9	Cellularity	(N-I-D)						
	10	Tumor cells	%						
	11								
	12								
LAB	13	Hgb	gm	12.5					
	14	Hct	Vol %						
	15	Reticulocytes	%						
	16	Platelets mm^3	(10^3)	350,000					
	17	WBC mm^3	(10^3)	4.5					
	18	Neutrophils	%	60%					
	19	Lymphocytes	%						
	20	Monocytes	%						
	21	Eosinophils	%						
	22	ANC		2.7					
	23	BUN	mg%						
	24								
	25								
	26								
	27								
	28								
	29								
	30								
	31								
	32								
PHYSICAL	33	Temp							
	34	Weight (kg) (lb)		150 lb					
	35	Hemorrhage	•						
	36	Infection	•						
	37								
	38								
	39								
MEASURABLE LESIONS	40								
	41								
	42								
	43								
	44								
	45								
	46	New lesions	(✓)						
SYMPTOMS	47	Performance status							
	48		•						
	49		•						
	50		•						
	51		•						
TOXICITY	52		•						
	53		•						
	54		•						
	55		•						
	56		•						
RESP	57	Objective	†						
	58	Subjective	†						

Form used courtesy of the Henry Ford Health System, West Bloomfield, Michigan

Date 1/28/07

Medical record number B698437

Pt. No. _____ Reg. Date _____

Study _____ Rx. No. _____

Disease Category _____

Progress notes and remarks:
(Signature/Title/Date each)

1/28/07 @ 1330
Pt. and family viewed video "So Many Questions." Reviewed medication
names, adverse effects, and management with pt. and family. All questions answered. Weight 150 lb, Height 65", BSA 2.0 ────────
I.V. started with 22G angiocatheter, ⊕ blood return. 500cc NSS
hung and infusing. I.V. patent. Pt. premedicated with Anzemet and
Decadron, followed by Adriamycin and Cytoxan — each infused via I.V.
without incident. I.V. d/c'd. Patient will see doctor prior to next
treatment, to have weekly CBC, and will call with any questions or
problems. ──────────────────────────── Ana Cumming, RN

‡ Record amount of drug administered in manner specified in protocol
• Describe under remarks and rate severity: 0 = none; 1 = mild; 2 = moderate; 3 = severe; 4 = fatal
† Rate response as: C (Complete), P (Partial), M (Mixed), N (No change), or I (Increasing disease)

SHORT STAY NURSES' ADMISSION ASSESSMENT FORM

Short stay, observation, or clinical decision units have their own admission assessment forms for nurses. Here's an example.

Short Stay/CDU Nurses' Admission Assessment Form

Date: _1/25/07_

Name: _Susanna Jackson_

Medical record number: _018263_

Patient type: ☐ DEM ☐ MED ☒ SURG ☐ OTHER _____

Arrival time: _1130_　　Arrived: ☐ Walking ☒ Wheelchair ☐ Other _____

Patient identified: ☒ Name ☒ Bracelet Age: _41_ Height: _5′ 6″_ Weight: _135 lb_

Emotional status: ☒ Calm ☐ Apprehensive ☐ Combative ☐ Crying

Neurological: ☒ Oriented ☒ Awake ☐ Easily aroused ☐ Confused ☐ Lethargic
　　　　　　☐ Asleep ☐ Unresponsive

Color: ☒ Pink ☐ Pale ☐ Cyanotic ☐ Jaundiced

Skin: ☒ Warm ☐ Cool ☒ Dry ☐ Moist

Diagnosis: _Cholecystitis, S/P laparoscopic cholecystectomy_

Consents correct and signed: ☒ Yes ☐ No Explain: _____

Nursing care considerations: _Monitor vital signs, wound checks for_
bleeding, pain management, nausea management.

Personal items:

Dentures/Partials	Glasses/Contacts	Hearing aids
☐ Retained	☐ Retained	☐ Retained
☐ Removed	☐ Removed	☐ Removed
☒ None	☒ None	☒ None

Drug allergies/sensitivities: _Penicillin: rash_ ☐ NKDA

Current medications: _Prochlorperazine 5 mg IV every 4° prn_
nausea and vomiting; morphine 5 mg IV every 4° prn pain.

Pertinent medical history:

☐ Diabetes ☐ Pulmonary disease ☐ Arthritis ☐ Cardiovascular disease
☒ Hypertension ☐ Psychiatric disease ☐ Seizure disorder ☐ Stroke
☐ Kidney disease ☐ Substance abuse ☐ Migraine headache ☐ No significant history
☐ Other_____

Initial vital signs: BP _138/80_ P _76_ R _20_ T _98.4°F_ Spo₂ _98_ %
　　　　　　☐ RA ☒ O₂ _2_ L/min

Signature/Title: _Karen Sands, RN_ Date: _1/25/07_ Time: _1200_

Form used courtesy of the Henry Ford Health System, West Bloomfield, Michigan

TELEPHONE ENCOUNTER FORM

Some ambulatory care facilities have developed forms to be used for telephone encounters, which become part of the medical record. The bottom section of the sample form here can be used for patients requiring prescription refills.

Telephone Encounter Form

MRN: _0193802_
Patient's name: _Joseph DiLorenzo_
DOB: _4/18/1935_

Date of call: 1/14/07	Time of call: 1045	Site: Twin City Health Clinic		

Caller:
Emily DiLorenzo, patient's wife   Telephone number: Provider: Insurance:
_(843)555-3547_   Dr. McManus   Medicare

Chief complaint:
States her husband has been complaining of muscle weakness, and he has been nauseous since yesterday, has vomited twice today.

Temperature: Pregnant: Allergies:
98.9°F orally   ☒ N ☐ Y   ☐ N ☒ Y   _penicillin: rash_

Chronic diseases:
Hypertension, heart failure

Current medications:
_Digoxin 0.5 mg PO daily   Furosemide 40 mg PO b.i.d.
Enalapril 2.5 mg PO b.i.d._

Assessment/Advice:
Pt's wife stated symptoms started yesterday. Took Maalox yesterday for nausea but didn't help. Stated pt. had cardiology appointment on 1/11/07 and that the doses of his "heart" medicines were increased. Reports no signs or symptoms of infection. Told to bring pt. to clinic today for evaluation and digoxin level.

Lauren Wilson, RN   _1/14/07_

Signature   Title   Date

Pharmacy name: Telephone number:

Medications:	Strength:	Dosage:	Quantity:	Refill:

Provider's signature: _____
                      Signature   Title   Date

Called by: _____
          Signature   Title   Date

Form used courtesy of the Henry Ford Health System, West Bloomfield, Michigan

9

DOCUMENTATION IN LONG-TERM CARE

Long-term care facilities provide continuing care for chronically ill or disabled patients. (Patients who reside in nursing homes are referred to as *residents.*) Their focus of care is to attain or maintain the highest level of functioning possible; however, their role is slowly changing. Today, many long-term care facilities find that they're admitting more patients who require short-term skilled nursing services and who may eventually be discharged back into the community.

Maintaining accurate, complete documentation in long-term care is vital for these reasons:

- Documentation of assessment findings, therapeutic interventions, and patient outcomes helps maintain communication among the many disciplines involved in caring for patients in a long-term care facility.
- State and federal agencies compile data gathered from medical record documentation into databases, where the data is compared with similar data from other long-term care facilities. Media outlets then publish the results of these comparisons for consumer information.

- State and federal agencies strictly regulate long-term care facilities, necessitating high standards of accurate and complete documentation. These agencies utilize documentation entered on the Minimum Data Set (MDS) form to focus the survey process on specific patients, to pinpoint reviews that statistically indicate areas of concern, and trigger care planning for skilled nursing needs.
- The health care facility may use documentation to defend itself and its personnel in court.
- Documentation is now directly related to reimbursement, and good documentation ensures certification, licensure, and accreditation. Without accurate and complete documentation, such programs as Medicare and Medicaid may deny payment and put the facility and practitioner under fraud and abuse scrutiny.

Although some forms and requirements of documentation in long-term care share many similarities with documentation in other practice settings, long-term care documentation differs in two important ways:

- The MDS form has become a central focus for documentation concerns in long-term care facilities. (See "Minimum Data Set," page 279.)
- Documentation of intermediate care patients who stay for weeks or months in a long-term care facility may not be required as often as in the acute care setting, but specific parameters must be followed.

Levels of care

Long-term care facilities usually offer two levels of care, skilled and intermediate, but they can specialize in one or the other. They each come with their own specialized documentation needs:
- If you're working in a skilled care facility or nursing unit, where patient care involves specialized nursing skills, make sure you know how to document:
  - I.V. therapy
  - medications
  - parenteral nutrition
  - respiratory care
  - wound management
  - mechanical ventilation
  - physical, occupational, or speech therapy.
- If you're working in an intermediate care facility or nursing unit, where patient care may mean managing chronic illness, your documentation will cover less complex nursing practices such as assistance with activities of daily living (ADLs).

Patients at both levels may need short- or long-term care and may move from one level to another according to their progress or decline. Living arrangements, geography, networks, and other factors help determine the patient's length of stay.

Regulations and regulatory agencies

Many government programs, laws, and agencies regulate documentation in long-term care facilities, including:
- programs such as Medicare and Medicaid
- laws such as the Omnibus Budget Reconciliation Act (OBRA) of 1987
- government agencies such as the Centers for Medicare & Medicaid Services (CMS) (formerly the Health Care Financing Administration)
- accrediting agencies such as the Joint Commission on Accreditation of Healthcare Organizations (JCAHO).

MEDICARE
Medicare is a federal health insurance program for:
- people age 65 or older
- people younger than age 65 with disabilities
- people with end-stage renal disease.

Medicare has two parts:
- Part A covers care provided as a hospital inpatient, hospice care, home health care, and care received in skilled nursing facilities.
- Part B helps pay for physician's services, outpatient hospital care, and some other medically necessary services that Part A doesn't cover, such as physical and occupational therapy.

In order for a facility to receive payment for Part A care, a nurse—usually a registered nurse assessment coordinator (RNAC)—must assure that specific criteria are met prior to admission and that skilled services are provided, assessed, and documented daily.

MEDICAID

Medicaid is a jointly funded federal and state health insurance program for low-income and needy people. It covers:

- children
- people who are eligible to receive federally assisted income maintenance payments
- elderly, blind, or disabled people.

Most patients in long-term care facilities are enrolled in Medicaid and receive either skilled or intermediate care.

- For skilled care, Medicaid requires daily documentation of all aspects of patient care.
- For intermediate care, Medicaid requires daily documentation of medications, treatments, and restorative nursing and ADL care provided.

OBRA

In 1987, Congress enacted OBRA, which imposed dozens of new requirements on long-term care facilities and home health care agencies to protect the rights of patients receiving long-term care. This law requires that a comprehensive assessment, or a *Resident Assessment Instrument* (RAI), be performed within 14 days of a patient's admission to a long-term care facility. This assessment consists of:

- *MDS:* provides key information required for patient assessment
- *Triggers:* conditions documented on the MDS that indicate patients who may be at risk for developing specific functional problems and require further evaluation using Resident Assessment Protocols (RAPs)
- *RAPs:* provide a problem-oriented approach for analyzing conditions triggered on the MDS.

Information from the MDS and RAPs then form the basis for developing an individualized care plan, which, under OBRA, must be developed within 7 days of completion of the RAI.

CMS

The role of CMS, a branch of the Department of Health and Human Services, is to ensure compliance by health care facilities with federal Medicare and Medicaid standards. As part of the Nursing Home Initiative to promote quality care in nursing homes, the CMS:

- publicizes statistical information gleaned from the MDS
- compares nursing homes against one another in such categories as pressure ulcers, pain, and ADL assistance.

Nursing homes that perform poorly may be denied Medicare and Medicaid reimbursement, which is why your documentation using the MDS needs to be accurate and complete.

JCAHO

JCAHO accredits long-term care facilities using standards developed in conjunction with health care experts. Accreditation by JCAHO is volun-

tary. Standard performance is documented in:

- assessments
- progress notes
- care plans
- discharge plans.

Standardized and required documents

Some forms are commonly used in multiple health care settings; others are specific to long-term care. Forms discussed in this section include the MDS, RAPs, care plans, the Preadmission Screening and Annual Resident Review (PASARR), the initial nursing assessment form, other assessment forms, nursing summaries, and discharge and transfer forms.

MINIMUM DATA SET

Mandated by OBRA, the MDS is a federal regulatory form that must be filled out for every patient admitted to a long-term care facility. (See *Understanding the Minimum Data Set.* Also see *Minimum Data Set form,* pages 280 to 288.) The requirements for completion of the MDS vary with the type of admission.

- For intermediate care patients, complete the MDS at these times:
  - admission assessment—required by day 14
  - quarterly review assessment—performed every 90 days
  - annual assessment
  - significant change in status assessment.
- For skilled care Medicare Part A patients under the prospective payment system, Medicare mandates a more frequent schedule of assessments. This schedule accompanies the OBRA schedule and requires completion at these times:
  - 5-day assessment
  - 14-day assessment
  - 30-day assessment
  - 60-day assessment
  - 90-day assessment
  - readmission or return assessment
  - at the completion of skilled rehabilitation services, called an *Other Medicare Required Assessment.*

The RNAC is responsible for monitoring and coordinating these stringent assessment schedules.

Helpful hints for completing the MDS

- Data documented on the MDS requires information from specific

---

UNDERSTANDING THE MINIMUM DATA SET

Initially designed to be a primary source document for standard assessments, the Minimum Data Set (MDS) has evolved into a tool for determining resource utilization groups or payment categories. In this capacity, surveyors and auditors require that information documented on the MDS be obtained from information documented elsewhere in the medical record. Each facility may have different types of methods or forms for documenting this information, but an electronic medical record where daily notes are automatically documented on the MDS is the most efficient process.

MINIMUM DATA SET FORM

Numeric Identifier_____

MINIMUM DATA SET (MDS) — *VERSION 2.0*
FOR NURSING HOME RESIDENT ASSESSMENT AND CARE SCREENING

BASIC ASSESSMENT TRACKING FORM

SECTION AA. IDENTIFICATION INFORMATION

1. **RESIDENT NAME** — Mary P. Klein
   a. (First)   b. (Middle Initial)   c. (Last)   d. (Jr/Sr)

2. **GENDER**   1. Male   2. Female — 2

3. **BIRTHDATE** — 11 - 05 - 1933
   Month   Day   Year

4. **RACE/ETHNICITY**
   1. American Indian/Alaskan Native
   2. Asian/Pacific Islander
   3. Black, not of Hispanic origin
   4. Hispanic
   5. White, not of Hispanic origin — 5

5. **SOCIAL SECURITY AND MEDICARE NUMBERS**
   a. Social Security Number — 050-50-5000
   b. Medicare number (or comparable railroad insurance number)

6. **FACILITY PROVIDER NO.**
   a. State No.
   b. Federal No.

7. **MEDICAID NO.** ["+" if pending, "N" if not a Medicaid recipient]

8. **REASONS FOR ASSESSMENT** [Note—Other codes do not apply to this form]
   a. Primary reason for assessment
      1. Admission assessment (required by day 14)
      2. Annual assessment
      3. Significant change in status assessment
      4. Significant correction of prior full assessment
      5. Quarterly review assessment
      10. Significant correction of prior quarterly assessment
      0. NONE OF ABOVE — 1

   b. Codes for assessments required for Medicare PPS or the State
      1. Medicare 5 day assessment
      2. Medicare 30 day assessment
      3. Medicare 60 day assessment
      4. Medicare 90 day assessment
      5. Medicare readmission/return assessment
      6. Other state required assessment
      7. Medicare 14 day assessment
      8. Other Medicare required assessment — 1

9. **Signatures of Persons who Completed a Portion of the Accompanying Assessment or Tracking Form**

I certify that the accompanying information accurately reflects resident assessment or tracking information for this resident and that I collected or coordinated collection of this information on the dates specified. To the best of my knowledge, this information was collected in accordance with applicable Medicare and Medicaid requirements. I understand that this information is used as a basis for ensuring that residents receive appropriate and quality care, and as a basis for payment from federal funds. I further understand that payment of such federal funds and continued participation in the government-funded health care programs is conditioned on the accuracy and truthfulness of this information, and that I may be personally subject to or may subject my organization to substantial criminal, civil, and/or administrative penalties for submitting false information. I also certify that I am authorized to submit this information by this facility on its behalf.

Signature and Title	Sections	Date
a. Sue Rayne, MSW	B, F	1/8/07
b. Sandra Landry, RN	C, D, E, G, H, I, J, L	1/8/07
c. D.T. Arnold, Activities	N	1/8/07
d. Mary Jo Pope, RD	K	1/8/07
e. Jane Gold, PT	G3, G4, P1b, T	1/8/07
f. Janie K. Kauffman, RN	M, O, P, Q	1/8/07
g.		
h.		
i.		
j.		
k.		
l.		

GENERAL INSTRUCTIONS

Complete this information for submission with all full and quarterly assessments (Admission, Annual, Significant Change, State or Medicare required assessments, or Quarterly Reviews, etc.)

Ⓚ = Key items for computerized resident tracking

☐ = When box blank, must enter number or letter   a. = When letter in box, check if condition applies

MDS 2.0 September, 2000

---

time periods. For example, section G, Physical functioning and structural problems, has a look-back period of 7 days, where section E, Mood and behavior patterns, has a look-back period of 30 days. All look-back periods are determined by the assessment reference date that's documented in section A3 of the MDS; the RNAC is responsible for determining this date.

● Make sure the scores documented within the MDS are consistent between sections. For example:

– If you document aphasia in section I, Disease diagnoses, the symptoms should correspond to the coding in

Resident: *Mary P. Klein*   Numeric Identifier: _____

MINIMUM DATA SET (MDS) — *VERSION 2.0*
FOR NURSING HOME RESIDENT ASSESSMENT AND CARE SCREENING

BACKGROUND (FACE SHEET) INFORMATION AT ADMISSION

SECTION AB. DEMOGRAPHIC INFORMATION

1.	DATE OF ENTRY	Date the stay began. Note — Does not include readmission if record was closed at time of temporary discharge to hospital. In such cases, use prior admission date

`0 1 - 0 2 - 2 0 0 7`
Month   Day   Year

2. **ADMITTED FROM (AT ENTRY)**   1. Private home/apt. with no home health services   2. Private home/apt. with home health services   3. Board and care/assisted living/group home   4. Nursing home   5. Acute care hospital   6. Psychiatric hospital, MR/DD facility   7. Rehabilitation hospital   8. Other   — **5**

3. **LIVED ALONE (PRIOR TO ENTRY)**   0. No   1. Yes   2. In other facility — **0**

4. **ZIP CODE OF PRIOR PRIMARY RESIDENCE** — `1 8 9 0 1`

5. **RESIDENTIAL HISTORY 5 YEARS PRIOR TO ENTRY**   *(Check all settings resident lived in during 5 years prior to date of entry given in item AB1 above)*

Prior stay at this nursing home	a.
Stay in other nursing home	b.
Other residential facility—board and care home, assisted living, group home	c.
MH/psychiatric setting	d.
MR/DD setting	e.
NONE OF ABOVE	f. ✓

6. **LIFETIME OCCUPATION(S)** [Put "/" between two occupations] — *Teacher*

7. **EDUCATION (Highest Level Completed)**   1. No schooling   2. 8th grade/less   3. 9-11 grades   4. High school   5. Technical or trade school   6. Some college   7. Bachelor's degree   8. Graduate degree — **8**

8. **LANGUAGE**   *(Code for correct response)*   a. Primary Language   0. English   1. Spanish   2. French   3. Other — **0**   b. If other, specify

9. **MENTAL HEALTH HISTORY**   Does resident's RECORD indicate any history of mental retardation, mental illness, or developmental disability problem?   0. No   1. Yes — **0**

10. **CONDITIONS RELATED TO MR/DD STATUS**   *(Check all conditions that are related to MR/DD status that were manifested before age 22, and are likely to continue indefinitely)*

Not applicable—no MR/DD (Skip to AB11)	a. ✓
MR/DD with organic condition	
Down's syndrome	b.
Autism	c.
Epilepsy	d.
Other organic condition related to MR/DD	e.
MR/DD with no organic condition	f.

11. **DATE BACKGROUND INFORMATION COMPLETED** — `0 1 - 0 3 - 2 0 0 7`
Month   Day   Year

SECTION AC. CUSTOMARY ROUTINE

1. **CUSTOMARY ROUTINE**   *(Check all that apply. If all information UNKNOWN, check last box only)*

(In year prior to DATE OF ENTRY to this nursing home, or year last in community if now being admitted from another nursing home)

CYCLE OF DAILY EVENTS

Stays up late at night (e.g., after 9 pm)	a. ✓
Naps regularly during day (at least 1 hour)	b.
Goes out 1+ days a week	c.
Stays busy with hobbies, reading, or fixed daily routine	d. ✓
Spends most of time alone or watching TV	e.
Moves independently indoors (with appliances, if used)	f.
Use of tobacco products at least daily	g.
NONE OF ABOVE	h.
EATING PATTERNS	
Distinct food preferences	i.
Eats between meals all or most days	j. ✓
Use of alcoholic beverage(s) at least weekly	k.
NONE OF ABOVE	l.
ADL PATTERNS	
In bedclothes much of day	m.
Wakens to toilet all or most nights	n. ✓
Has irregular bowel movement pattern	o.
Showers for bathing	p.
Bathing in PM	q. ✓
NONE OF ABOVE	r.
INVOLVEMENT PATTERNS	
Daily contact with relatives/close friends	s.
Usually attends church, temple, synagogue (etc.)	t. ✓
Finds strength in faith	u.
Daily animal companion/presence	v.
Involved in group activities	w. ✓
NONE OF ABOVE	x.
UNKNOWN—Resident/family unable to provide information	

SECTION AD. FACE SHEET SIGNATURES

SIGNATURES OF PERSONS COMPLETING FACE SHEET:

Sue Rayne, MSW

	Date
a. Signature of RN Assessment Coordinator — *Marie Smith, RNAC*	*1/4/07*

I certify that the accompanying information accurately reflects resident assessment or tracking information for this resident and that I collected or coordinated collection of this information on the dates specified. To the best of my knowledge, this information was collected in accordance with applicable Medicare and Medicaid requirements. I understand that this information is used as a basis for ensuring that residents receive appropriate and quality care, and as a basis for payment from federal funds. I further understand that payment of such federal funds and continued participation in the government-funded health care programs is conditioned on the accuracy and truthfulness of this information, and that I may be personally subject to or may subject my organization to substantial criminal, civil, and/or administrative penalties for submitting false information. I also certify that I am authorized to submit this information by this facility on its behalf.

Signature and Title	Sections	Date
b.		
c.		
d.		
e.		
f.		
g.		

☐ = When box blank, must enter number or letter   ☐ a. = When letter in box, check if condition applies

MDS 2.0 September, 2000

(continued)

section C, Communication/Hearing patterns. You should also mark and grade sections C4, Making self understood, and C6, Ability to understand others, appropriately.
– If you document the performance of physical therapy, occupational therapy, or speech therapy in Section P, Special treatments and procedures, be sure to document that either the patient or the direct care staff believe that the patient is capable of increased independence.
– Ensure that the diagnosis listed in section I, Disease diagnoses, accu-

MINIMUM DATA SET FORM *(CONTINUED)*

Resident *Mary P. Klein* Numeric Identifier ____

MINIMUM DATA SET (MDS) — *VERSION 2.0*
FOR NURSING HOME RESIDENT ASSESSMENT AND CARE SCREENING
FULL ASSESSMENT FORM
(Status in last 7 days, unless other time frame indicated)

SECTION A. IDENTIFICATION AND BACKGROUND INFORMATION

No.	Item	Content	Entry
1.	RESIDENT NAME	*Mary* a. (First) / *P.* b. (Middle Initial) / *Klein* c. (Last) / d. (Jr/Sr)	
2.	ROOM NUMBER	B215	
3.	ASSESSMENT REFERENCE DATE	a. *Last day of MDS observation period* 01-07-2007 (Month, Day, Year) b. Original (0) or corrected copy of form (enter number of correction)	
4a.	DATE OF REENTRY	**Date of reentry from most recent temporary discharge to a hospital in last 90 days (or since last assessment or admission if less than 90 days)** __-__-____ (Month, Day, Year)	
5.	MARITAL STATUS	1. Never married 2. Married 3. Widowed 4. Separated 5. Divorced	2
6.	MEDICAL RECORD NO.	121105	
7.	CURRENT PAYMENT SOURCES FOR N.H. STAY	(*Billing Office to indicate; **check all that apply in last 30 days***) a. Medicaid per diem b. Medicare per diem X c. Medicare ancillary part A d. Medicare ancillary part B e. CHAMPUS per diem f. VA per diem g. Self or family pays for full per diem X h. Medicaid resident liability or Medicare co-payment i. Private insurance per diem (including co-payment) j. Other per diem	
8.	REASONS FOR ASSESSMENT [***Note—If this is a discharge or reentry assessment, only a limited subset of MDS items need be completed***]	a. Primary reason for assessment 1. Admission assessment (required by day 14) 2. Annual assessment 3. Significant change in status assessment 4. Significant correction of prior full assessment 5. Quarterly review assessment 6. Discharged—return not anticipated 7. Discharged—return anticipated 8. Discharged prior to completing initial assessment 9. Reentry 10. Significant correction of prior quarterly assessment 0. *NONE OF ABOVE*	1
		b. ***Codes for assessments required for Medicare PPS or the State*** *1. Medicare 5 day assessment* *2. Medicare 30 day assessment* *3. Medicare 60 day assessment* *4. Medicare 90 day assessment* *5. Medicare readmission/return assessment* *6. Other state required assessment* *7. Medicare 14 day assessment* *8. Other Medicare required assessment*	1
9.	RESPONSIBILITY/ LEGAL GUARDIAN	(***Check all that apply***) a. Legal guardian b. Other legal oversight c. Durable power of attorney/health care d. Durable power attorney/financial e. Family member responsible f. Patient responsible for self X g. *NONE OF ABOVE*	
10.	ADVANCED DIRECTIVES	(*For those items with supporting **documentation** in the medical record, **check all that apply***) a. Living will X b. Do not resuscitate c. Do not hospitalize d. Organ donation e. Autopsy request f. Feeding restrictions g. Medication restrictions h. Other treatment restrictions i. *NONE OF ABOVE*	

SECTION B. COGNITIVE PATTERNS

No.	Item	Content	Entry
1.	COMATOSE	(*Persistent vegetative state/no discernible consciousness*) 0. No 1. Yes (**If yes, skip to Section G**)	0
2.	MEMORY	(*Recall of what was learned or known*) a. Short-term memory OK—seems/appears to recall after 5 minutes 0. Memory OK 1. Memory problem	1
		b. Long-term memory OK—seems/appears to recall long past 0. Memory OK 1. Memory problem	0
3.	MEMORY/ RECALL ABILITY	(***Check all that resident was normally able to recall during last 7 days***) a. Current season X b. Location of own room c. Staff names/faces d. That he/she is in a nursing home X e. *NONE OF ABOVE* are recalled	
4.	COGNITIVE SKILLS FOR DAILY DECISION-MAKING	(*Made decisions regarding tasks of daily life*) 0. *INDEPENDENT*—decisions consistent/reasonable 1. *MODIFIED INDEPENDENCE*—some difficulty in new situations only 2. *MODERATELY IMPAIRED*—decisions poor; cues/supervision required 3. *SEVERELY IMPAIRED*—never/rarely made decisions	2
5.	INDICATORS OF DELIRIUM—PERIODIC DISORDERED THINKING/ AWARENESS	(*Code for behavior in the last 7 days.*) [***Note: Accurate assessment requires conversations with staff and family who have direct knowledge of resident's behavior over this time***]. 0. Behavior not present 1. Behavior present, not of recent onset 2. Behavior present, over last 7 days appears different from resident's usual functioning (e.g., new onset or worsening)	
		a. EASILY DISTRACTED—(e.g., difficulty paying attention; gets sidetracked)	1
		b. PERIODS OF ALTERED PERCEPTION OR AWARENESS OF SURROUNDINGS—(e.g., moves lips or talks to someone not present; believes he/she is somewhere else; confuses night and day)	0
		c. EPISODES OF DISORGANIZED SPEECH—(e.g., speech is incoherent, nonsensical, irrelevant, or rambling from subject to subject; loses train of thought)	0
		d. PERIODS OF RESTLESSNESS—(e.g., fidgeting or picking at skin, clothing, napkins, etc; frequent position changes; repetitive physical movements or calling out)	0
		e. PERIODS OF LETHARGY—(e.g., sluggishness; staring into space; difficult to arouse; little body movement)	0
		f. MENTAL FUNCTION VARIES OVER THE COURSE OF THE DAY—(e.g., sometimes better, sometimes worse; behaviors sometimes present, sometimes not)	1
6.	CHANGE IN COGNITIVE STATUS	Resident's cognitive status, skills, or abilities have changed as compared to status of **90 days ago** (or since last assessment if less than 90 days) 0. No change 1. Improved 2. Deteriorated	0

SECTION C. COMMUNICATION/HEARING PATTERNS

No.	Item	Content	Entry
1.	HEARING	(*With hearing appliance, if used*) 0. *HEARS ADEQUATELY*—normal talk, TV, phone 1. *MINIMAL DIFFICULTY* when not in quiet setting 2. *HEARS IN SPECIAL SITUATIONS ONLY*—speaker has to adjust tonal quality and speak distinctly 3. *HIGHLY IMPAIRED*/absence of useful hearing	1
2.	COMMUNICATION DEVICES/ TECHNIQUES	(***Check all that apply** during last 7 days*) a. Hearing aid, present and used X b. Hearing aid, present and not used regularly c. Other receptive comm. techniques used (e.g., lip reading) d. *NONE OF ABOVE*	
3.	MODES OF EXPRESSION	(***Check all used** by resident to make needs known*) a. Speech X b. Writing messages to express or clarify needs c. American sign language or Braille d. Signs/gestures/sounds e. Communication board f. Other g. *NONE OF ABOVE*	
4.	MAKING SELF UNDERSTOOD	(*Expressing information content—however able*) 0. *UNDERSTOOD* 1. *USUALLY UNDERSTOOD*—difficulty finding words or finishing thoughts 2. *SOMETIMES UNDERSTOOD*—ability is limited to making concrete requests 3. *RARELY/NEVER UNDERSTOOD*	2
5.	SPEECH CLARITY	(*Code for speech in the last 7 days*) 0. *CLEAR SPEECH*—distinct, intelligible words 1. *UNCLEAR SPEECH*—slurred, mumbled words 2. *NO SPEECH*—absence of spoken words	1
6.	ABILITY TO UNDERSTAND OTHERS	(*Understanding verbal information content—however able*) 0. *UNDERSTANDS* 1. *USUALLY UNDERSTANDS*—may miss some part/intent of message 2. *SOMETIMES UNDERSTANDS*—responds adequately to simple, direct communication 3. *RARELY/NEVER UNDERSTANDS*	2
7.	CHANGE IN COMMUNICATION/ HEARING	Resident's ability to express, understand, or hear information has changed as compared to status of **90 days ago** (or since last assessment if less than 90 days) 0. No change 1. Improved 2. Deteriorated	2

[ ] = When box blank, must enter number or letter [a.] = When letter in box, check if condition applies

MDS 2.0 September, 2000

rately reflects the reason for rehabilitation services.

- Pay particular attention to accurately scoring the late-loss ADLs (bed mobility, transfer, eating, toilet use) in Section G, Physical functioning and structural problems. These scores impact directly on all resource utilization groups (RUG) payment categories. Many facilities have developed specific ADL forms that capture daily information on function, including a patient's self-performance code and a code documenting the amount of ADL support provided by the staff.

Resident **Mary P. Klein**   Numeric Identifier _____

SECTION D. VISION PATTERNS

1.	VISION	(Ability to see in adequate light and with glasses if used) 0. *ADEQUATE*—sees fine detail, including regular print in newspapers/books 1. *IMPAIRED*—sees large print, but not regular print in newspapers/books 2. *MODERATELY IMPAIRED*—limited vision; not able to see newspaper headlines, but can identify objects 3. *HIGHLY IMPAIRED*—object identification in question, but eyes appear to follow objects 4. *SEVERELY IMPAIRED*—no vision or sees only light, colors, or shapes; eyes do not appear to follow objects	1
2.	VISUAL LIMITATIONS/ DIFFICULTIES	Side vision problems—decreased peripheral vision (e.g., leaves food on one side of tray, difficulty traveling, bumps into people and objects, misjudges placement of chair when seating self) Experiences any of following: sees halos or rings around lights; sees flashes of light; sees "curtains" over eyes NONE OF ABOVE	a. ☐ b. ☐ c. X
3.	VISUAL APPLIANCES	Glasses; contact lenses; magnifying glass 0. No 1. Yes	1

SECTION E. MOOD AND BEHAVIOR PATTERNS

1.	INDICATORS OF DEPRES- SION, ANXIETY, SAD MOOD	(Code for indicators observed in last 30 days, irrespective of the assumed cause) 0. Indicator not exhibited in last 30 days 1. Indicator of this type exhibited up to five days a week 2. Indicator of this type exhibited daily or almost daily (6, 7 days a week)	

VERBAL EXPRESSIONS OF DISTRESS

a. Resident made negative statements—e.g., "Nothing matters; Would rather be dead; What's the use; Regrets having lived so long; Let me die"	0	
b. Repetitive questions—e.g., "Where do I go; What do I do?"	0	
c. Repetitive verbalizations—e.g., calling out for help, ("God help me")	0	
d. Persistent anger with self or others—e.g., easily annoyed, anger at placement in nursing home; anger at care received	0	
e. Self deprecation—e.g., "I am nothing; I am of no use to anyone"	0	
f. Expressions of what appear to be unrealistic fears—e.g., fear of being abandoned, left alone, being with others	0	
g. Recurrent statements that something terrible is about to happen—e.g., believes he or she is about to die, have a heart attack	0	

h. Repetitive health complaints—e.g., persistently seeks medical attention, obsessive concern with body functions	0
i. Repetitive anxious complaints/concerns (non-health related) e.g., persistently seeks attention/ reassurance regarding schedules, meals, laundry, clothing, relationship issues	0

SLEEP-CYCLE ISSUES

j. Unpleasant mood in morning	0
k. Insomnia/change in usual sleep pattern	0

SAD, APATHETIC, ANXIOUS APPEARANCE

l. Sad, pained, worried facial expressions—e.g., furrowed brows	1
m. Crying, tearfulness	0
n. Repetitive physical movements—e.g., pacing, hand wringing, restlessness, fidgeting, picking	0

LOSS OF INTEREST

o. Withdrawal from activities of interest—e.g., no interest in long standing activities or being with family/friends	0
p. Reduced social interaction	0

2.	MOOD PERSIS- TENCE	One or more indicators of depressed, sad or anxious mood were not easily altered by attempts to "cheer up", console, or reassure the resident over last 7 days 0. No mood 1. Indicators present, 2. Indicators present, indicators easily altered not easily altered	2
3.	CHANGE IN MOOD	Resident's mood status has changed as compared to status of 90 days ago (or since last assessment if less than 90 days) 0. No change 1. Improved 2. Deteriorated	0
4.	BEHAVIORAL SYMPTOMS	(A) Behavioral symptom *frequency* in last 7 days 0. Behavior not exhibited in last 7 days 1. Behavior of this type occurred 1 to 3 days in last 7 days 2. Behavior of this type occurred 4 to 6 days, but less than daily 3. Behavior of this type occurred daily (B) Behavioral symptom *alterability* in last 7 days 0. Behavior not present OR behavior was easily altered 1. Behavior was not easily altered	(A) (B)
		a. WANDERING (moved with no rational purpose, seemingly oblivious to needs or safety)	0 0
		b. VERBALLY ABUSIVE BEHAVIORAL SYMPTOMS (others were threatened, screamed at, cursed at)	0 0
		c. PHYSICALLY ABUSIVE BEHAVIORAL SYMPTOMS (others were hit, shoved, scratched, sexually abused)	0 0
		d. SOCIALLY INAPPROPRIATE/DISRUPTIVE BEHAVIORAL SYMPTOMS (made disruptive sounds, noisiness, screaming, self-abusive acts, sexual behavior or disrobing in public, smeared/threw food/feces, hoarding, rummaged through others' belongings)	1 1
		e. RESISTS CARE (resisted taking medications/ injections, ADL assistance, or eating)	0 0

SECTION F. PSYCHOSOCIAL WELL-BEING

1.	SENSE OF INITIATIVE/ INVOLVE- MENT	At ease interacting with others	a. X
		At ease doing planned or structured activities	b. X
		At ease doing self-initiated activities	c. X
		Establishes own goals	d. ☐
		Pursues involvement in life of facility (e.g., makes/keeps friends; involved in group activities; responds positively to new activities; assists at religious services)	e. ☐
		Accepts invitations into most group activities	f. ☐
		NONE OF ABOVE	g. ☐
2.	UNSETTLED RELATION- SHIPS	Covert/open conflict with or repeated criticism of staff	a. ☐
		Unhappy with roommate	b. ☐
		Unhappy with residents other than roommate	c. ☐
		Openly expresses conflict/anger with family/friends	d. ☐
		Absence of personal contact with family/friends	e. ☐
		Recent loss of close family member/friend	f. ☐
		Does not adjust easily to change in routines	g. X
3.	PAST ROLES	Strong identification with past roles and life status	a. ☐
		Expresses sadness/anger/empty feeling over lost roles/status	b. ☐
		Resident perceives that daily routine (customary routine, activities) is very different from prior pattern in the community	c. X
		NONE OF ABOVE	d. ☐

SECTION G. PHYSICAL FUNCTIONING AND STRUCTURAL PROBLEMS

1.	(A) ADL SELF-PERFORMANCE—(Code for resident's PERFORMANCE OVER ALL SHIFTS during last 7 days—Not including setup)	

0. *INDEPENDENT*—No help or oversight —OR— Help/oversight provided only 1 or 2 times during last 7 days
1. *SUPERVISION*—Oversight, encouragement or cueing provided 3 or more times during last 7 days —OR— Supervision (3 or more times) plus physical assistance provided only 1 or 2 times during last 7 days
2. *LIMITED ASSISTANCE*—Resident highly involved in activity; received physical help in guided maneuvering of limbs or other nonweight bearing assistance 3 or more times —OR—More help provided only 1 or 2 times during last 7 days
3. *EXTENSIVE ASSISTANCE*—While resident performed part of activity, over last 7-day period, help of following type(s) provided 3 or more times:
— Weight-bearing support
— Full staff performance during part (but not all) of last 7 days
4. *TOTAL DEPENDENCE*—Full staff performance of activity during entire 7 days
8. *ACTIVITY DID NOT OCCUR* during entire 7 days

(B) ADL SUPPORT PROVIDED—(Code for MOST SUPPORT PROVIDED OVER ALL SHIFTS during last 7 days; code regardless of resident's self-performance classification)
0. No setup or physical help from staff
1. Setup help only
2. One person physical assist
3. Two+ persons physical assist
8. ADL activity itself did not occur during entire 7 days

			(A) SELF-PERF	(B) SUPPORT
a.	BED MOBILITY	How resident moves to and from lying position, turns side to side, and positions body while in bed	3	3
b.	TRANSFER	How resident moves between surfaces—to/from: bed, chair, wheelchair, standing position (EXCLUDE to/from bath/toilet)	3	2
c.	WALK IN ROOM	How resident walks between locations in his/her room	2	2
d.	WALK IN CORRIDOR	How resident walks in corridor on unit	2	3
e.	LOCOMO- TION ON UNIT	How resident moves between locations in his/her room and adjacent corridor on same floor. If in wheelchair, self-sufficiency once in chair	2	2
f.	LOCOMO- TION OFF UNIT	How resident moves to and returns from off unit locations (e.g., areas set aside for dining, activities, or treatments). If facility has only one floor, how resident moves to and from distant areas on the floor. If in wheelchair, self-sufficiency once in chair	2	2
g.	DRESSING	How resident puts on, fastens, and takes off all items of street clothing, including donning/removing prosthesis	3	2
h.	EATING	How resident eats and drinks (regardless of skill). Includes intake of nourishment by other means (e.g., tube feeding, total parenteral nutrition)	1	1
i.	TOILET USE	How resident uses the toilet room (or commode, bedpan, urinal); transfer on/off toilet, cleanses, changes pad, manages ostomy or catheter, adjusts clothes	3	2
j.	PERSONAL HYGIENE	How resident maintains personal hygiene, including combing hair, brushing teeth, shaving, applying makeup, washing/drying face, hands, and perineum (EXCLUDE baths and showers)	3	2

5.	CHANGE IN BEHAVIORAL SYMPTOMS	Resident's behavior status has changed as compared to status of 90 days ago (or since last assessment if less than 90 days) 0. No change 1. Improved 2. Deteriorated	0

MDS 2.0 September, 2000

(continued)

RESIDENT ASSESSMENT PROTOCOLS

Another federally mandated form, the RAP summary lists identified problems and documents the existence of a corresponding care plan. For example, if the patient has a stage II pressure ulcer documented in the MDS, the RAP summary should indicate the need for a care plan to treat the pressure ulcer. (See *Resident assessment protocol summary,* page 289.)

CARE PLANS

Each patient in a long-term care facility must have a documented interdis-

MINIMUM DATA SET FORM *(CONTINUED)*

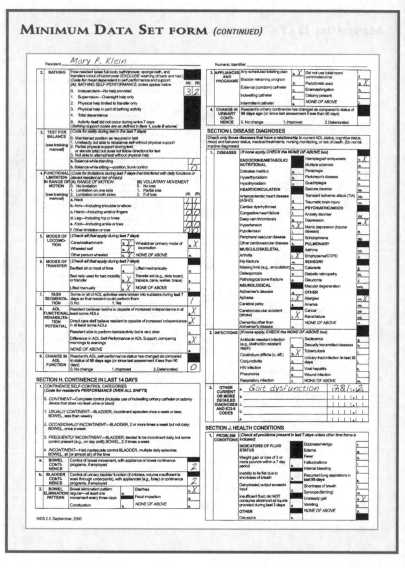

ciplinary care plan. The care plan must include:

- a problem list (to include items identified on the RAP summary)
- a measurable goal for each problem identified
- approaches that will be used to attain those goals.

When using a care plan, follow these guidelines:

- make sure that an interdisciplinary care plan is completed within 7 days of the completion of the MDS. Your health care team may utilize an interim care plan (which should be in place within 24 hours of admission)

Resident: *Mary P. Klein*

Numeric Identifier _____

SECTION M. SKIN CONDITION

				Number at Stage
2	PAIN SYMPTOMS	(Code the highest level of pain present in the last 7 days)		
		a. FREQUENCY with which resident complains or shows evidence of pain 0. No pain (skip to J4) 1. Pain less than daily 2. Pain daily	**b. INTENSITY** of pain 1. Mild pain 2. Moderate pain 3. Times when pain is horrible or excruciating	0
3	PAIN SITE	(If pain present, check all sites that apply in last 7 days)		
		Back pain	a. X Incisional pain	f.
		Bone pain	b. Joint pain (other than hip)	g.
		Chest pain while doing usual activities	c. Soft tissue pain (e.g., lesion, muscle)	h.
		Headache	d. Stomach pain	i.
		Hip pain	e. Other	j.
4	ACCIDENTS	(Check all that apply)		
		Fell in past 30 days	a. X Hip fracture in last 180 days	c.
		Fell in past 31–180 days	b. Other fracture in last 180 days	d.
			NONE OF ABOVE	e.
5	STABILITY OF CONDITIONS	Conditions/diseases make resident's cognitive, ADL, mood or behavior patterns unstable—(fluctuating, precarious, or deteriorating)		a.
		Resident experiencing an acute episode or a flare-up of a recurrent or chronic problem		b.
		End-stage disease, 6 or fewer months to live		c.
		NONE OF ABOVE		d. X

SECTION K. ORAL/NUTRITIONAL STATUS

1	ORAL PROBLEMS	Chewing problem — a.
		Swallowing problem — b.
		Mouth pain — c.
		NONE OF ABOVE — d.
2	HEIGHT AND WEIGHT	Record (a.) height in inches and (b.) weight in pounds. Base weight on most recent measure in last 30 days; measure weight consistently in accord with standard facility practice—e.g., in a.m. after voiding, before meal, with shoes off, and in nightclothes a. HT (in.) 66 b. WT (lb.) 170
3	WEIGHT CHANGE	a. Weight loss—5% or more in last 30 days; or 10% or more in last 180 days 0. No 1. Yes — 0
		b. Weight gain—5% or more in last 30 days; or 10% or more in last 180 days 0. No 1. Yes — 0
4	NUTRITIONAL PROBLEMS	Complains about the taste of many foods — a. Leaves 25% or more of food uneaten at most meals — c.
		Regular or repetitive complaints of hunger — b. NONE OF ABOVE — d. X
5	NUTRITIONAL APPROACHES	(Check all that apply in last 7 days)
		Parenteral/IV — a. Dietary supplement between meals — f.
		Feeding tube — b.
		Mechanically altered diet — c. Plate guard, stabilized built-up utensil, etc. — g.
		Syringe (oral feeding) — d. On a planned weight change program — h.
		Therapeutic diet — e. NONE OF ABOVE — i.
6	PARENTERAL OR ENTERAL INTAKE	(Skip to Section L if neither 5a nor 5b is checked)
		a. Code the proportion of total calories the resident received through parenteral or tube feedings in the last 7 days 0. None 3. 51% to 75% 1. 1% to 25% 4. 76% to 100% 2. 26% to 50%
		b. Code the average fluid intake per day by IV or tube in last 7 days 0. None 3. 1001 to 1500 cc/day 1. 1 to 500 cc/day 4. 1501 to 2000 cc/day 2. 501 to 1000 cc/day 5. 2001 or more cc/day

SECTION L. ORAL/DENTAL STATUS

1	ORAL STATUS AND DISEASE PREVENTION	Debris (soft, easily movable substances) present in mouth prior to going to bed at night — a.
		Has dentures or removable bridge — b.
		Some/all natural teeth lost—does not have or does not use dentures (or partial plates) — c.
		Broken, loose, or carious teeth — d.
		Inflamed gums (gingiva); swollen or bleeding gums; oral abscesses; ulcers or rashes — e.
		Daily cleaning of teeth/dentures or daily mouth care—by resident or staff — f. X
		NONE OF ABOVE — g.

SECTION M. SKIN CONDITION

			Number at Stage
1	ULCERS (Due to any cause)	(Record the number of ulcers at each ulcer stage—regardless of cause. If none present at a stage, record "0" (zero). Code all that apply during last 7 days. Code 9 = 9 or more.) [Requires full body exam.]	
		a. Stage 1. A persistent area of skin redness (without a break in the skin) that does not disappear when pressure is relieved.	1
		b. Stage 2. A partial thickness loss of skin layers that presents clinically as an abrasion, blister, or shallow crater.	0
		c. Stage 3. A full thickness of skin is lost, exposing the subcutaneous tissues - presents as a deep crater with or without undermining adjacent tissue.	0
		d. Stage 4. A full thickness of skin and subcutaneous tissue is lost, exposing muscle or bone.	0
2	TYPE OF ULCER	(For each type of ulcer, code for the highest stage in the last 7 days using scale in item M1—i.e., 0=none; stages 1, 2, 3, 4)	
		a. Pressure ulcer—any lesion caused by pressure resulting in damage of underlying tissue	1
		b. Stasis ulcer—open lesion caused by poor circulation in the lower extremities	0
3	HISTORY OF RESOLVED ULCERS	Resident had an ulcer that was resolved or cured in LAST 90 DAYS 0. No 1. Yes	0
4	OTHER SKIN PROBLEMS OR LESIONS PRESENT	(Check all that apply during last 7 days)	
		Abrasions, bruises	a. X
		Burns (second or third degree)	b.
		Open lesions other than ulcers, rashes, cuts (e.g., cancer lesions)	c.
		Rashes—e.g., intertrigo, eczema, drug rash, heat rash, herpes zoster	d.
		Skin desensitized to pain or pressure	e.
		Skin tears or cuts (other than surgery)	f.
		Surgical wounds	g.
		NONE OF ABOVE	h.
5	SKIN TREATMENTS	(Check all that apply during last 7 days)	
		Pressure relieving device(s) for chair	a. X
		Pressure relieving device(s) for bed	b. X
		Turning/repositioning program	c.
		Nutrition or hydration intervention to manage skin problems	d. X
		Ulcer care	e.
		Surgical wound care	f.
		Application of dressings (with or without topical medications) other than to feet	g.
		Application of ointments/medications (other than to feet)	h.
		Other preventative or protective skin care (other than to feet)	i. X
		NONE OF ABOVE	j.
6	FOOT PROBLEMS AND CARE	(Check all that apply during last 7 days)	
		Resident has one or more foot problems—e.g., corns, callouses, bunions, hammer toes, overlapping toes, pain, structural problems	a.
		Infection of the foot—e.g., cellulitis, purulent drainage	b.
		Open lesions on the foot	c.
		Nails/calluses trimmed during last 90 days	d. X
		Received preventative or protective foot care (e.g., used special shoes, inserts, pads, toe separators)	e.
		Application of dressings (with or without topical medications)	f.
		NONE OF ABOVE	g.

SECTION N. ACTIVITY PURSUIT PATTERNS

1	TIME AWAKE	(Check appropriate time periods over last 7 days) Resident awake all or most of time (i.e., naps no more than one hour per time period) in the:
		Morning — a. X Evening — c.
		Afternoon — b. NONE OF ABOVE — d.
		(If resident is comatose, skip to Section O)
2	AVERAGE TIME INVOLVED IN ACTIVITIES	(When awake and not receiving treatments or ADL care) 0. Most—more than 2/3 of time 2. Little—less than 1/3 of time 1. Some—from 1/3 to 2/3 of time 3. None — 2
3	PREFERRED ACTIVITY SETTINGS	(Check all settings in which activities are preferred)
		Own room — a. Outside facility — d.
		Day/activity room — b. X
		Inside NH/off unit — c. NONE OF ABOVE — e.
4	GENERAL ACTIVITY PREFERENCES (adapted to resident's current abilities)	(Check all PREFERENCES whether or not activity is currently available to resident)
		Cards/other games — a. Trips/shopping — f.
		Crafts/arts — b. Walking/wheeling outdoors — g.
		Exercise/sports — c. Watching TV — h. X
		Music — d. X Gardening or plants — i.
		Reading/writing — e. X Talking or conversing — j.
		Spiritual/religious activities — f. X Helping others — k.
			NONE OF ABOVE — l.

MDS 2.0 September, 2000

(continued)

until there's an interdisciplinary care conference regarding the patient.

• Make sure that a documented review of the plan is completed every 3 months, when a patient's condition changes, or when unplanned events such as a fall occur.

PASARR

Federal statues require the completion of the PASARR form on or prior to admission to a long-term care facility. Filling out the form is usually the responsibility of a social worker or the admissions director. It screens for:

• mental illness

Resident __Mary P. Klein__   Numeric Identifier _____

5.	PREFERS CHANGE IN DAILY ROUTINE	Code for resident preferences in daily routines 0. No change 1. Slight change 2. Major change	
		a. Type of activities in which resident is currently involved	
		b. Extent of resident involvement in activities	

SECTION O. MEDICATIONS

1.	NUMBER OF MEDICA- TIONS	(Record the number of different medications used in the last 7 days; enter "0" if none used)	07
2.	NEW MEDICA- TIONS	(Resident currently receiving medications that were initiated during the last 90 days) 0. No 1. Yes	0
3.	INJECTIONS	(Record the number of DAYS injections of any type received during the last 7 days; enter "0" if none used)	0
4.	DAYS RECEIVED THE FOLLOWING MEDICATION	(Record the number of DAYS during last 7 days; enter "0" if not used. Note—enter "1" for long-acting meds used less than weekly)	
		a. Antipsychotic	0
		b. Antianxiety	3
		c. Antidepressant	7
		d. Hypnotic	0
		e. Diuretic	0

SECTION P. SPECIAL TREATMENTS AND PROCEDURES

1.	SPECIAL TREAT- MENTS, PROCE- DURES, AND PROGRAMS	a. SPECIAL CARE—Check treatments or programs received during the last 14 days	

TREATMENTS

TREATMENTS		PROGRAMS	
Chemotherapy	a.	Ventilator or respirator	l.
Dialysis	b.	Alcohol/drug treatment program	m.
IV medication	c.	Alzheimer's/dementia special care unit	n.
Intake/output	d.	Hospice care	o.
Monitoring acute medical condition	e.	Pediatric unit	p.
Oxostomy care	f.	Respite care	q.
Oxygen therapy	g.	Training in skills required to return to the community (e.g., taking medications, house work, shopping, transportation, ADLs)	r.
Radiation	h.		
Suctioning	i.		
Tracheostomy care	j.		
Transfusions	k.	NONE OF ABOVE	X

b. THERAPIES - Record the number of days and total minutes each of the following therapies was administered (for at least 15 minutes a day) in the last 7 calendar days (Enter 0 if none or less than 15 min. daily) [Note—count only post admission therapies]		DAYS	MIN
(A) = # of days administered for 15 minutes or more		(A)	(B)
(B) = total # of minutes provided in last 7 days			
a. Speech - language pathology and audiology services		3	105
b. Occupational therapy		0	
c. Physical therapy		4	120
d. Respiratory therapy		0	
e. Psychological therapy (by any licensed mental health professional)		1	30

2.	INTERVEN- TION PROGRAMS FOR MOOD, BEHAVIOR, COGNITIVE LOSS	(Check all interventions or strategies used in last 7 days—no matter where received)	
		Special behavior symptom evaluation program	X
		Evaluation by a licensed mental health specialist in last 90 days	X
		Group therapy	c.
		Resident-specific deliberate changes in the environment to address mood/behavior patterns—e.g., providing bureau in which to rummage	d.
		Reorientation—e.g., cueing	e.
		NONE OF ABOVE	f.

3.	NURSING REHABILITA- TION/ RESTOR- ATIVE CARE	Record the NUMBER OF DAYS each of the following rehabilitation or restorative techniques or practices was provided to the resident for more than or equal to 15 minutes per day in the last 7 days (Enter 0 if none or less than 15 min. daily)	
		a. Range of motion (passive)	0
		b. Range of motion (active)	0
		c. Splint or brace assistance	0
		TRAINING AND SKILL PRACTICE IN:	
		d. Bed mobility	0
		e. Transfer	0
		f. Walking	0
		g. Dressing or grooming	5
		h. Eating or swallowing	0
		i. Amputation/prosthesis care	0
		j. Communication	0
		k. Other	0

4.	DEVICES AND RESTRAINTS	(Use the following codes for last 7 days:) 0. Not used 1. Used less than daily 2. Used daily	
		Bed rails	
		a. — Full bed rails on all open sides of bed	0
		b. — Other types of side rails used (e.g., half rail, one side)	0
		c. Trunk restraint	0
		d. Limb restraint	0
		e. Chair prevents rising	0
5.	HOSPITAL STAY(S)	Record number of times resident was admitted to hospital with an overnight stay in last 90 days (or since last assessment if less than 90 days). (Enter 0 if no hospital admissions)	01
6.	EMERGENCY ROOM (ER) VISIT(S)	Record number of times resident visited ER without an overnight stay in last 90 days (or since last assessment if less than 90 days). (Enter 0 if no ER visits)	01
7.	PHYSICIAN VISITS	In the LAST 14 DAYS (or since admission if less than 14 days in facility) how many days has the physician (or authorized assistant or practitioner) examined the resident? (Enter 0 if none)	02
8.	PHYSICIAN ORDERS	In the LAST 14 DAYS (or since admission if less than 14 days in facility) how many days has the physician (or authorized assistant or practitioner) changed the resident's orders? Do not include order renewals without change. (Enter 0 if none)	02
9.	ABNORMAL LAB VALUES	Has the resident had any abnormal lab values during the last 90 days (or since admission)? 0.No 1.Yes	1

SECTION Q. DISCHARGE POTENTIAL AND OVERALL STATUS

1.	DISCHARGE POTENTIAL	a. Resident expresses/indicates preference to return to the community 0. No 1. Yes	1
		b. Resident has a support person who is positive towards discharge 0. No 1. Yes	1
		c. Stay projected to be of a short duration— discharge projected within 90 days (do not include expected discharge due to death) 0. No 1. Within 30 days 2. Within 31-90 days 3. Discharge status uncertain	2
2.	OVERALL CHANGE IN CARE NEEDS	Resident's overall self sufficiency has changed significantly as compared to status of 90 days ago (or since last assessment if less than 90 days) 0. No change 1. Improved—receives fewer supports, needs less restrictive level of care 2. Deteriorated—receives more support	0

SECTION R. ASSESSMENT INFORMATION

1.	PARTICIPA- TION IN ASSESS- MENT	a. Resident: 0. No 1. Yes	1
		b. Family: 0. No 1. Yes 2. No family	1
		c. Significant other: 0. No 1. Yes 2. None	
2.	SIGNATURE OF PERSON COORDINATING THE ASSESSMENT:		
		Marie Smith, RNAC	
		a. Signature of RN Assessment Coordinator (sign on above line)	
		b. Date RN Assessment Coordinator signed as complete	01-10-2007
			Month Day Year

MDS 2.0 September, 2000

- mental retardation
- other conditions that may affect ADL functioning.

INITIAL NURSING ASSESSMENT

The initial nursing assessment must be performed and documented for all patients admitted to a long-term care facility. Many facilities have forms that cue staff on obtaining and documenting complete assessment information. However, in general, if you utilize the topic categories of the MDS, you'll perform a comprehensive assessment.

Minimum Data Set form (continued)

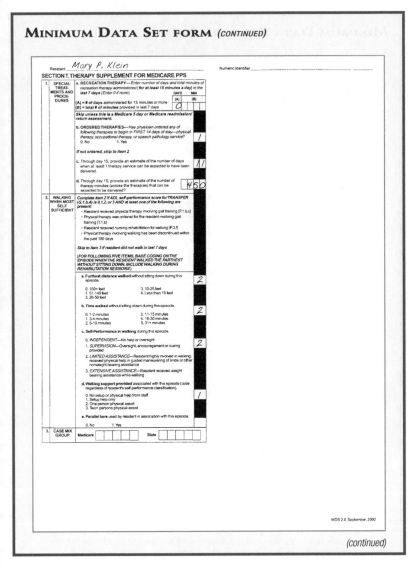

Among the areas that you'll assess are:
- cognitive function
- communication and hearing patterns (document the presence of a hearing aid)
- continence
- disease processes, including system assessments, vital signs, height, and weight
- health conditions
- mood and behavior
- oral, dental, diet, and nutritional status (be sure to note if dentures are present)

(continued)

MINIMUM DATA SET FORM *(CONTINUED)*

SECTION V. RESIDENT ASSESSMENT PROTOCOL SUMMARY   Numeric Identifier _____

Resident's Name: *Mary P. Klein*   Medical Record No.: _____

1. Check if RAP is triggered.
2. For each triggered RAP, use the RAP guidelines to identify areas needing further assessment. Document relevant assessment information regarding the resident's status.

   - Describe:
     — Nature of the condition (may include presence or lack of objective data and subjective complaints).
     — Complications and risk factors that affect your decision to proceed to care planning.
     — Factors that must be considered in developing individualized care plan interventions.
     — Need for referrals/further evaluation by appropriate health professionals.

   - Documentation should support your decision-making regarding whether to proceed with a care plan for a triggered RAP and the type(s) of care plan interventions that are appropriate for a particular resident.

   - Documentation may appear anywhere in the clinical record (e.g., progress notes, consults, flowsheets, etc.).

3. Indicate under the <u>Location of RAP Assessment Documentation</u> column where information related to the RAP assessment can be found.
4. For each triggered RAP, indicate whether a new care plan, care plan revision, or continuation of current care plan is necessary to address the problem(s) identified in your assessment. The Care Planning Decision column must be completed within 7 days of completing the RAI (MDS and RAPs).

A. RAP PROBLEM AREA	(a) Check if triggered	Location and Date of RAP Assessment Documentation	(b) Care Planning Decision—check if addressed in care plan
1. DELIRIUM			
2. COGNITIVE LOSS			
3. VISUAL FUNCTION			
4. COMMUNICATION	X	1/5/07 Progress notes	X
5. ADL FUNCTIONAL/ REHABILITATION POTENTIAL	X	1/6/07 Progress notes	X
6. URINARY INCONTINENCE AND INDWELLING CATHETER			
7. PSYCHOSOCIAL WELL-BEING			
8. MOOD STATE	X	1/6/07 Progress notes	X
9. BEHAVIORAL SYMPTOMS	X	1/6/07 Progress notes	X
10. ACTIVITIES	X	1/5/07 Progress notes	X
11. FALLS	X	1/6/07 Progress notes	X
12. NUTRITIONAL STATUS			
13. FEEDING TUBES			
14. DEHYDRATION/FLUID MAINTENANCE			
15. DENTAL CARE			
16. PRESSURE ULCERS			
17. PSYCHOTROPIC DRUG USE			
18. PHYSICAL RESTRAINTS			

B. *Marie Smith, RNAC*   2. 0|1 – 1|1 – 2|0|0|7   Month Day Year
1. Signature of RN Coordinator for RAP Assessment Process

Jamie K. Kauffman, RN   4. 0|1 – 1|1 – 2|0|0|7   Month Day Year
3. Signature of Person Completing Care Planning Decision

MDS 2.0 September, 2000

Source: Centers for Medicare and Medicaid Services. Baltimore. Available at: *www.cms.hhs.gov/quality/mds20*. Last accessed September 21, 2006.

- physical functioning and structural problems
- psychosocial well-being
- skin conditions
- vision.

Other assessment forms

In addition to the initial nursing assessment, you'll commonly use other forms to collect patient information. Certain risk assessment forms can help to quantify a patient's risk for falls and skin breakdown. (See *Fall*

RESIDENT ASSESSMENT PROTOCOL SUMMARY

After recording the certification data on the MDS form, analyze it to identify the patient's primary problems and care needs. Then fill in the Resident Assessment Protocol (RAP) Summary, shown here. The completed form verifies that you've written a care plan.

Resident's name: *Leo Mancuso* | Medical record no.: *0839-2547*

Signature of RN assessment coordinator: *M. Burns, RN, BSN*

RESIDENT ASSESSMENT PROTOCOL SUMMARY

1. For each RAP area triggered, show whether you are proceeding with care plan intervention.

2. Document problems, complications, and risk factors; the need for referral to appropriate health care professional; and the reason for deciding to proceed or not proceed to care planning. Documentation may appear anywhere the facility routinely keeps such information, such as problem sheets or progress notes.

3. Identify the location of this information.

RAP problem area	Care planning decision		Location of information
	Proceed	Do not proceed	
Delirium	☐	☑	*N/A See neuro note 1/2/07*
Cognitive loss and dementia	☑	☐	*Care plan #1*
Visual function	☑	☐	*Care plan #3*
Communication	☑	☐	*Care plan #3*
ADL function and rehabilitation potential	☑	☐	*Care plan #3*
Urinary incontinence and indwelling catheter	☑	☐	*Care plan #4*
Psychosocial well-being	☑	☐	*Care plan #21*
Mood state	☑	☐	*Care plan #2*
Behavior problem	☑	☐	*Care plan #5*
Activities	☑	☐	*Care plan #7*
Falls	☑	☐	*Care plan #6*
Nutritional status	☑	☐	*Care plan #1*
Feeding tubes	☑	☐	*N/A See dietary note 1/2/07*
Dehydration and fluid maintenance	☐	☑	*Care plan #6*
Dental care	☑	☐	*Care plan #3*
Pressure ulcers	☑	☐	*Care plan #9*
Psychotropic drug use	☐	☑	*N/A See neuro note 1/2/07*
Physical restraints	☑	☐	*Care plan #7*

---

assessment and action plan, pages 290 and 291. Also see *Braden scale for predicting pressure sore risk,* pages 292 to 295.)

DISCHARGE AND TRANSFER FORMS

When the facility discharges a patient to home or another institution, document:

- reason for discharge
- patient's destination

- mode of transportation
- disposition of personal property
- person or staff member accompanying him.

If the patient is transferred home:

- review medication and treatments with the patient or responsible caregiver, and document their understanding
- document all other patient teaching.

(Text continues on page 294.)

FALL ASSESSMENT AND ACTION PLAN

This standardized assessment tool can help you evaluate your patient's risk for falls and plan preventive measures if needed.

Patient's name: _Kevin Lawson_
Does the patient have problems with:

ISSUE	ASSESSMENT	ACTION
Comfort • Pain	≥ 3 ___ Yes ✓ No	___ Notify physician of pain level. ___ Offer thermal modalities 4x/day while awake. ___ Tailor pain medication schedule to wake-up time/therapy schedule/HS. ___ Reposition as needed.
Elimination • Incontinence	✓ Yes ___ No	✓ Time void q2 hours while awake and q4 hours at night as needed. ___ Initiate bowel program. ✓ Restrict fluids after 1900 hours unless contraindicated. ✓ Place commode at bedside on dominant side. ✓ Orient to call bell and location of bathroom/bathroom safety.
Tubings • I.V.s • Chest tubes • Urinary catheter	✓ Yes ___ No ___ Yes ✓ No ___ Yes ✓ No	✓ Position tube and pole for safety. ✓ Verbal reminder to patient. ___ Use leg bag during waking hours.
Mobility • Unsteady gait; poor balance	___ Yes ✓ No	___ Physical assistance required at all times. ___ Consult physical therapy if appropriate.
• Transfer	≥ min assist ___ Yes ✓ No	___ Ensure at least one bottom side rail is down on dominant side. ___ Ensure top two side rails are up to help with transfers. ___ Ensure appropriate number of staff available for transfer. ___ Place sign "CALL AND WAIT FOR ASSISTANCE" in bathroom.
• Limited endurance	✓ Yes ___ No	✓ Schedule rest periods in daily activity schedule.
• Orthostatic hypotension	✓ Yes ___ No	✓ Instruct in gradual position change.

ISSUE	ASSESSMENT	ACTION
Mental status • Cognitive deficit present	✓ Yes ___ No	✓ 24-hour usage of bed/chair alarm. ✓ Time void q2 hours while awake and q4 hours at night as needed. ✓ Implement appropriate seating device. ✓ Track and document behavioral patterns. ✓ Provide appropriate diversional activities. ✓ Orient to environment. ✓ Check medication list.
Communication barrier • Non-English speaking	___ Yes ✓ No	___ Arrange for interpreter. ___ Ask for help from family if appropriate.
• Unable to make needs known	___ Yes ✓ No	___ Use picture/communication board.
• Hearing deficit	✓ Yes ___ No	___ Ensure hearing aid is present and functional. ___ Use amplification devices.
• Visual deficit	___ Yes ✓ No	___ Clear pathways and ensure ambulation aids are close to patient. ___ Orient to environment.
Medications • Cardiovascular	✓ Yes ___ No	✓ If cardiovascular meds used and symptoms or dizziness present, check orthostatic blood pressure and heart rate. Call physician if needed.
• Psychoactive/sleep	___ Yes ✓ No	___ If psychoactive/sleep meds used and symptoms or dizziness present, notify physician of adverse effects, and check orthostatic blood pressure.
• Diuretics	___ Yes ✓ No	___ If diuretics used, time void q2 hours while awake and q4 hours at night as needed.
• Anesthetic (1st 24hr. post-op)	___ Yes ✓ No	___ If 1st 24 hr. post-op, physical assistance provided at all times.
• Anticoagulants	___ Yes ✓ No	___ If anticoagulants used, implement Anticoagulant Therapy Protocol.

Above action plan reviewed and implemented:

DATE _1/9/07_ TIME _0800_ NAME _J. Kuka, RN_
DATE _1/9/07_ TIME _1600_ NAME _H. Cane, RN_
DATE _1/10/07_ TIME _2400_ NAME _P. Seria, RN_

Adapted with permission from Abington Memorial Hospital Department of Nursing, Abington, Pa.

BRADEN SCALE FOR PREDICTING PRESSURE SORE RISK

The Braden scale, shown here, is the most reliable of several existing instruments for assessing the older patient's risk of developing pressure sores. The lower the score, the greater the risk.

Patient's name ___Kevin Lawson___

SENSORY PERCEPTION Ability to respond meaningfully to pressure-related discomfort	**1. Completely limited:** Unresponsive (does not moan, flinch, or grasp) to painful stimuli because of diminished level of consciousness or sedation OR Limited ability to feel pain over most of body surface	**2. Very limited:** Responds only to painful stimuli; cannot communicate discomfort except by moaning or restlessness OR Has a sensory impairment that limits the ability to feel pain or discomfort over half of body
MOISTURE Degree to which skin is exposed to moisture	**1. Constantly moist:** Skin is kept moist almost constantly by perspiration, urine, and so forth; dampness is detected every time patient is moved or turned	**2. Very moist:** Skin is often but not always moist; linen must be changed at least once per shift
ACTIVITY Degree of physical activity	**1. Bedfast:** Confined to bed	**2. Chairfast:** Ability to walk severely limited or nonexistent; cannot bear own weight and must be assisted into chair or wheelchair
MOBILITY Ability to change and control body position	**1. Completely immobile:** Does not make even slight changes in body or extremity position without assistance	**2. Very limited:** Makes occasional slight changes in body or extremity position but unable to make frequent or significant changes independently
NUTRITION Usual food intake pattern	**1. Very poor:** Never eats a complete meal; rarely eats more than one-third of any food offered; eats two servings or less of protein (meat or dairy products) per day; takes fluids poorly; does not take a liquid dietary supplement OR Is NPO or maintained on clear liquids or I.V. fluids for more than 5 days	**2. Probably inadequate:** Rarely eats a complete meal and generally eats only about half of any food offered; protein intake includes only three servings of meat or dairy products per day; occasionally will take a dietary supplement OR Receives less than optimum amount of liquid diet or tube feeding

Evaluator's name _Joan Norris, RN_   Date of assessment _1/18/07_

3. Slightly limited: Responds to verbal commands but cannot always communicate discomfort or need to be turned OR Has some sensory impairment that limits ability to feel pain or discomfort in one or two extremities	**4. No impairment:** Responds to verbal commands; has no sensory deficit that would limit ability to feel or voice pain or discomfort	3
3. Occasionally moist: Skin is occasionally moist, requiring an extra linen change approximately once per day	**4. Rarely moist:** Skin is usually dry; linen requires changing only at routine intervals	3
3. Walks occasionally: Walks occasionally during day, but for very short distances, with or without assistance; spends majority of each shift in bed or chair	**4. Walks frequently:** Walks outside the room at least twice per day and inside room at least once every 2 hours during waking hours	4
3. Slightly limited: Makes frequent though slight changes in body or extremity position independently	**4. No limitations:** Makes major and frequent changes in position without assistance	4
3. Adequate: Eats more than half of most meals; eats four servings of protein (meat, dairy products) each day; occasionally will refuse a meal, but will usually take a supplement if offered OR Is on a tube feeding or total parenteral nutrition regimen that probably meets most nutritional needs	**4. Excellent:** Eats most of every meal and never refuses a meal; usually eats four or more servings of meat and dairy products; occasionally eats between meals; does not require supplementation	4

(continued)

If a patient is transferred to the hospital, document all equipment and devices sent with the patient, such as a walker, dentures, or hearing aids. (If these items are lost while in the hospital, this documentation may save the long-term care facility the expense of replacing the items.) (See *Transfer and personal belongings form,* pages 296 to 298.)

DOCUMENTATION GUIDELINES

In a long-term care facility, consider these points when updating your records:

● When writing nursing summaries, be sure to address all specific patient problems documented in the care plan.

● When writing progress notes, confirm that the patient's progress is being evaluated and reevaluated continually in relation to the goals or outcomes defined in the care plan. If the patient's goals aren't met, this failure also needs to be addressed. Additional actions should be described and documented.

● Document transfers and discharges according to your facility's protocol.

● Document, as part of the transfer information, the medication the patient has been receiving or has been prescribed.

● Document changes in the patient's condition, and report them to the physician and the family as soon as possible, but within 24 hours.

● Document follow-up interventions or other measures implemented in response to a reported change in the patient's condition.

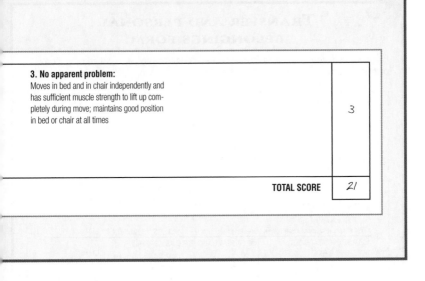

3. No apparent problem:
Moves in bed and in chair independently and has sufficient muscle strength to lift up completely during move; maintains good position in bed or chair at all times

3

TOTAL SCORE 21

- Document visits from the patient's family or friends and phone calls to the patient.
- If an incident occurs, such as a fall or a treatment error, fill out an incident report, and write follow-up notes for at least 48 hours after the incident (or follow your facility's policy).
- Keep detailed documentation on each shift per your facility's policy.
- Keep reimbursement issues in mind when documenting. For a facility to qualify for payment, its records must clearly reflect the level of care given to the patient.
- Make sure that your documentation accurately reflects all skilled services that the patient receives.
- Always document a physician's verbal and telephone orders, and make sure that the physician counter-signs these orders within the time frames specified by state regulations and your facility's policy.
- Document physician visits to the patient.

TRANSFER AND PERSONAL BELONGINGS FORM

Patients in long-term care facilities may be admitted to the hospital, discharged to home, or transferred to other facilities. The forms here are used during this process.

1. PATIENT'S LAST NAME	FIRST NAME	MI
Clark	Robert	T

2. SEX	3. SOCIAL SECURITY NUMBER
Male	144-44-4444

4. PATIENT'S ADDRESS (Street, City, State, Zip Code)
1 Wise Street, Springhouse, PA 19411

5. DATE OF BIRTH	6. RELIGION
2-8-35	unknown

7. DATE OF THIS TRANSFER	8. FACILITY NAME AND ADDRESS TRANSFERRING TO
1/29/01	Seniors Care Facility, 22 Elderly Way, Phila., PA

9. PHYSICIAN IN CHARGE AT TIME OF TRANSFER
Dr. Nicholas
Will this physician care for patient after admission to new facility? ❏ YES ☒ NO

10. DATES OF STAY AT FACILITY TRANSFERRING FROM	11. PAYMENT SOURCE FOR CHARGES TO PATIENT		
	A. ☒ SELF OR FAMILY	C. ❏ BLUE CROSS BLUE SHIELD	E. ❏ PUBLIC AGENCY (Give name)
ADMISSION DISCHARGE	B. ❏ PRIVATE INSURANCE	D. ❏ EMPLOYER OR UNION	F. ❏ OTHER (Explain)
12/14/06 1/29/01			

12-A. NAME AND ADDRESS OF FACILITY TRANSFERRING FROM

Community Hospital   3000 Medical Way, Phila., PA

12-B. NAMES AND ADDRESSES OF ALL HOSPITALS AND EXTENDED CARE FACILITIES FROM WHICH PATIENT WAS DISCHARGED IN PAST 60 DAYS.

13. CLINIC APPOINTMENT DATE TIME	CLINIC APPOINTMENT CARD ATTACHED	14. DATE OF LAST PHYSICAL EXAMINATION
		1/26/01

15. RELATIVE OR GUARDIAN: Name   Address   Phone number
Katherine Clark 1 Wise Street, Springhouse, PA 19411 1-215-999-9000

16. DIAGNOSES AT TIME OF TRANSFER	EMPLOYMENT RELATED:
(a) Primary Stroke	❏ YES
(b) Secondary Type 1 diabetes	☒ NO

VITALS AT TIME OF TRANSFER	ADVANCE DIRECTIVES ☒ YES ❏ NO
	❏ COPY ATTACHED
T 98⁶ P 68 R 20 B/P 140/82	CODE STATUS Full code

CHECK ALL THAT APPLY	☑ Speech	**Activity Tolerance**	**Potential for Rehabilitation**
Disabilities	❏ Hearing	**Limitations**	❏ Good
❏ Amputation	☑ Vision	❏ None	❏ Fair
☑ Paralysis ① side	❏ Sensation	☑ Moderate	☑ Poor
❏ Contracture	**Incontinence**	❏ Severe	IMPORTANT MEDICAL INFORMATION
❏ Pressure Ulcer	☑ Bladder	**Patient knows diagnosis?**	(State allergies if any)
Impairments	☑ Bowel	☑ Yes	PCN
❏ Mental	☑ Saliva	❏ No	

TRANSFER AND PERSONAL BELONGINGS
FORM (CONTINUED)

DIET, DRUGS, AND OTHER THERAPY at time of discharge

-Mechanical soft diet (2,000 cal)
-Megace 4 tabs Q6h
-Lasix 40 mg P.O. b.i.d.
-Aspirin 81 mg P.O. q.d.
-Humulin 70/30 20 units daily in a.m. & h.s.

(Physician, please sign below)

_____

SUGGESTIONS FOR ACTIVE CARE

BED
Position in good body alignment and change
position every __2__ hrs.
Avoid __flat supine__ position
Prone position __2__ time/day as tolerated.

WEIGHT BEARING
☐ Full
☑ Partial
☐ None
on_____leg

EXERCISES
Range of motion __3__ times/day.
to __(L)__ extremities _____ by
☐ patient ☐ nurse ☐ family
Stand __3__ min. __2__ times/day.

SITTING
__4__ hr __3__ times/day

LOCOMOTION
Walk____unable____times/day.

SOCIAL ACTIVITIES
Encourage (☑ group ☐ individual) activities (☑ within ☐ outside) home.
Transportation: ☑ Ambulance ☐ Car ☐ Car for handicapped ☐ Bus

Signature of Physician or Nurse __John Brown, RN__   Date____1 / 29 / 01____

Any articles of clothing or other belongings left at the hospital will be held for 30 days after discharge. Items remaining after this period will be disposed of by the hospital.

COMMENTS

Date: 1/29/01		
Initials: RC		
VALUABLES DESCRIBE		
Wallet:	✔	1 brown leather wallet
Money (Amount): $25.00	✔	1-$20 bill 5 $ 1 bills
Watch:		
Jewelry:		
Glasses/Contacts: Glasses	✔	Wire rim — gold
Hearing Aids:		
Dentures:	✔	
Partial		
Complete	✔	Container labeled
Keys		

(continued)

TRANSFER AND PERSONAL BELONGINGS
FORM (CONTINUED)

Any articles of clothing or other belongings left at the hospital will be held for 30 days after discharge. Items remaining after this period will be disposed of by the hospital.

ARTICLE	DESCRIBE		COMMENTS
Ambulatory Aids:			
Cane, Walker, Etc.			
Bedclothes		✔	1 pair plaid pajamas
Belt			
Dress			
Outer Wear			
Pants			
Pocketbook			
Shirt			
Shoes			
Sweater			
Undergarments			
Other			

All belongings were sent home with patient's family: YES   (NO)

Patient's Signature _____ *Bob Park* _____

Witnessed by Hospital Personnel _____ *Mary Jones, RN* _____

10

DOCUMENTATION IN HOME HEALTH CARE

Federal, state, and local laws and agencies regulate home health care agencies. These regulatory standard bearers require home health care agencies to provide accurate, complete documentation and a high standard of care. If a home health care agency fails to meet these regulatory standards, it jeopardizes its licensure, accreditation, and reimbursement.

Home health care growth

Recent trends have contributed to the growth of the home health care industry, including:
- the development of a prospective payment system for home health care agencies, which was implemented in October 2000 and requires Medicare to pay home health care agencies a predetermined base payment that's adjusted for the health care needs of the patient
- improved utilization review, which has caused a decrease in the average length of a patient's hospitalization, resulting in patients who are typically

sicker and more reliant on home health care after discharge
- greater patient diversity, including expanded services to new populations representing all age groups and a variety of medical conditions, has led to the emergence of home health care subspecialties, such as home infusion agencies and high-tech, cancer-related home health care (see *Hospice care services,* pages 300 and 301)
- more affordable support services, which has increased the availability of home health care and may eventually make the home health care industry the primary supplier of health care in the United States.

Standardized and required documents

In the home health care setting, the nurse is more responsible for ensuring reimbursement payments than in any other health care setting. Your agency's success or failure virtually depends on your documentation skills because home health care agencies are paid prospectively, meaning

HOSPICE CARE SERVICES

Many home health care agencies provide hospice care services. Hospice programs provide palliative care to the terminally ill in both homes and hospitals.

MEDICARE COVERAGE

Since 1983, patients who have met specific admission criteria can qualify for the hospice Medicare benefit instead of the traditional Medicare benefit, allowing greater freedom to choose the hospice alternative for terminal care. The patient receives noncurative medical and support services not otherwise covered by Medicare.

Medicare coverage for hospice care is available if:

■ The patient is eligible for Medicare Part A, which covers skilled nursing home and hospital care. People eligible for Medicare are those age 65 or older, long-term disabled patients, and people with end-stage renal disease.

■ The patient's physician and the hospice medical director certify that the patient is terminally ill with a life expectancy of 6 months or less.

■ The patient receives care from a Medicare-approved hospice program.

A Medicare-approved hospice will usually provide care in the patient's home. The hospice team and the patient's physician establish a care plan for medical and support services for the management of a terminal illness.

A patient without coverage for hospice benefits may be eligible for free or reduced-cost care through local programs or foundations. Alternatively, a patient may pay privately for hospice services.

UNDERSTANDING AND ACCEPTANCE OF TREATMENT

With hospice care, the patient and primary caregiver must complete documentation indicating their understanding of hospice care. The patient and caregiver must sign an informed consent form that outlines everyone's responsibilities. They must also sign a form indicating their understanding and acceptance of the role of the primary caregiver. The form here is an example of this type of document.

---

they receive two payments of a preset amount of money based on the documentation of the initial nursing assessment. If the patient's care requires more than the preset reimbursement level, the agency is responsible for covering the difference in cost, which is why home health care organizations have a tightly structured documentation system.

As a home health care nurse:
● you're bound by all the controls imposed by the professional standards and nurse practice acts that govern nurses in all other settings.
● you'll need to become familiar with your agency's requirements because every home health care agency has its own standards, requirements, and forms to be used when documenting a patient's care.

● you'll find that all agencies and payers require certain types of documentation, even if they use different forms to report the information.
● you'll need to ensure certain types of documentation, including:
– referral for home health care
– Medicare and Medicaid forms
– assessment, including the Outcome and Assessment Information Set (OASIS)-B1
– nursing care plan
– medical update
– progress notes
– nursing summaries

– patient or caregiver teaching
– recertification
– discharge summary.

REFERRAL FORMS

Before you begin caring for a patient in his home, your agency will verify that the patient qualified for home health care by evaluating these criteria:

- *clinical criteria*—skilled care needed, appropriately prescribed therapy that can be done in the home, caregiver available to assist patient
- *technical criteria (patient or caregiver)*—senses intact, ability to learn and follow procedures, ability to recognize complications and initiate emergency medical procedures
- *environmental criteria*—access to a telephone, electricity, and water; clean living environment
- *financial criteria*—verification of insurance coverage, full knowledge of copayment or out-of-pocket expenses, agreement to comply with the conditions of participation.

The referral form is used to make sure that the agency can provide services the patient needs before it agrees to take the new case. (See *Using a referral form for home care,* pages 302 to 304.)

(Text continues on page 304.)

USING A REFERRAL FORM
FOR HOME CARE

Also called an intake form, a referral form is used to document a new patient's needs when you begin your evaluation. Use the sample here as a guide.

Date of referral: _1/17/07_   Branch: _North_   Chart #: _97-413_ H ✓
Info taken by: _Beth Isham, RN_   Admit date: _1/18/07_
Patient's name: _Geraldine Rush_
Address: _66 Newton St._
City: _Burlington_   State: _VT_ Zip: _05402_
Phone: _(802) 123-4567_   Date of birth: _4/3/39_
Primary caregiver name & phone number: _husband (Dennis)_ _(802) 123-4567_
Insurance name: _Medicare_   Ins. #: _123-45-6789_
Is this a managed care policy (HMO)? _no_
Primary Dx: (Code _162.5_) _lung cancer_   Date: _12/11/00_
               (Code _877_) _pressure ulcer (coccyx)_   Date: _3/13/02_
               (Code _714.0_) _rheumatoid arthritis_   Date: _1990s_
Procedures: (Code _86.28_) _ulcer care_   Date: _3/14/04_
Referral source: _J. Silva, hospital SW_   Phone: _765-2813_
Doctor name & phone #: _Frank Crabbe_   Phone: _765-4321_
Doctor address: _9073 Parkway Drive, Burlington_
Hospital: _University Hospital_   Admit: _1/1/07_ Discharge: _1/16/07_
Functional limitations: _Pain management, nonambulatory, poor fine motor skills 2°_
rheumatoid arthritis
ORDERS/SERVICES: (specify amount, frequency, and duration)
(SN:) _SN visits 3x/week & p.r.n. x 2 months_
(AL:) _CNA visits daily 5 days/week x 2 months_
(PT, OT,)ST: _PT & OT evaluations and visits 2-3 x/week & p.r.n. x 2 months_
(MSW:) _MSW evaluation & weekly visits x 2 months_
Spiritual coordinator: _Rev. Carlson, St. Paul's Lutheran Church_
Counselor: _JoAnne Knowton, MSW_
Volunteer: _Rosalie Marshall (niece) will provide care on weekends_
Other services provided: _shopping, laundry, meal prep_
Goals: _wound care, pain management, terminal care @ home_
Equipment: _Needs commode, hospital bed, bedpan, Hoyer lift, side rail w/c_
Company & phone number: _Scott Medical Equipment 765-9931_
Safety measures: _side rails up X 4_
Nutritional req _diet as tolerated_
FUNCTIONAL LIMITATIONS: (Circle applicable)

1. Amputation	5. Paralysis	9. Legally blind
2. Bowel/Bladder	⑥ Endurance	10. Dyspnea with
3. Contracture	⑦ Ambulation	minimal exer
4. Hearing	8. Speech	⑪ Other _RA_

USING A REFERRAL FORM FOR HOME CARE *(CONTINUED)*

ACTIVITIES PERMITTED: (Circle applicable)

1. Complete bed rest
2. Bed rest BRP
3. Up as tolerated
4. Transfer bed/chair *(circled)*

6. Partial wgt bearing
7. Independent at home
8. Crutches
9. Cane

10. Wheelchair *(circled)*
11. Walker
12. No restriction
13. Other -specify _____

Accessibility to bath: Y - N *(N circled)*   Shower   Y - N *(N circled)*   Bathroom   Y - N *(N circled)*   Exit   Y *(circled)* - N

Mental status (Circle): Oriented Comatose Forgetful (Depressed) Disoriented Lethargic Agitated

Other _____

Allergies: _none known_

- Hospice appropriate meds
- Med company: _Walker Pharmacy_

MEDICATIONS:

morphine sulfate liq. 20 mg/ml 40 mg P.O. every 6h p.r.n. pain

Compazine 10 mg P.O. every 4-6h p.r.n. n/v

Colace   200 mg P.O. daily p.r.n. constipation

Benadryl 25 - 50 mg P.O. @ bedtie p.r.n. sleeplessness

Living will   Yes _✓_   No _____   Obtained _____

Family to mail to office _____

Guardian, POA, or responsible person: _husband_

Address & phone number: _same_

Other family members: _____

ETOH: _0_   Drug use: _0_

Smoker: _2 ppd x 40 years; quit 2 yrs ago_

History: _Other than problems associated with arthritis, was in general good health until_
12/04, Dx: lung CA - husband cared for @ home until 1/1/05.

Social history (place of birth, education, jobs, retirement, etc.): _Born & raised in Toronto,_
became U.S. citizen when married in 1951. 2 yrs. college - majored in music. Retired
church organist.

ADMISSION NOTES: VS: T _98.4° P.O._   AP _86_   RR _18_   BP _140/72_

Lungs: _decreased breath sounds LLL_

Extremities: _cool to touch; pedal pulses present_

Wgt: _118_   Recent wgt (loss)/gain of _40 lb over 6 months_

Admission narrative: _Visit made to pt/husband in hospital before discharge. Both have_
been told that she is failing rapidly, and would like her to return home with Hospice
services. Niece willing to help 2 days/week. Pt apprehensive; husband blames himself for the
coccygeal decubitus ulcer which developed under his care.

(continued)

Psychosocial issues: *Pt. has always cared for husband. Describes self as depressed that she is no longer able to do so; worries who will care for him after she dies.*

Environmental concerns: *need smoke detectors*

Are there any cultural or spiritual customs or beliefs of which we should be aware before providing Hospice services? *Pt. would like Holy Communion just before death (& weekly)*

Funeral home: *not yet chosen*   Contact made: Yes _____ No *X*

DIRECTIONS: *Corner Newton & Elm; duplex, white with green trim. Door on @ says 66. Bell broken — knock loudly.*

Agency representative signature: *Beth Isham, RN   Home Care Supervisor*

Date: *1/18/07*

MEDICARE AND MEDICAID FORMS

By mandate in 1985, the Centers for Medicare and Medicaid Services (CMS) required home health care agencies to standardize and update their record-keeping and documentation methods. Since the implementation of OASIS, the collection of specific data is required. For each qualified Medicare or Medicaid recipient:

● the agency must complete a Home Health Certification and Plan of Care form (Form 485) and submit it for approval every 60 days. (See *Certifying home health care needs.*)

● the agency must complete a Medical Update and Patient Information form (Form 486) to provide data needed to make coverage determinations for additional home care or whenever Medicare requests it for review. (See *Providing updated medical and patient information,* page 306.)

These forms allow Medicare reviewers, also known as *fiscal intermediaries,* to evaluate each claim in accordance with the criteria for coverage. If you work for an agency that uses these forms, remember that:

● you're responsible for completing these forms for your patients unless your agency utilizes an admission team for this purpose (Only registered nurses and therapists are authorized to complete these forms.)

● data are usually filed after completing a comprehensive nursing assessment and devising a suitable care plan

● you (or the therapist) and the attending physician must sign and date these forms.

Remember: Medicare won't provide payment unless the required forms

CERTIFYING HOME HEALTH CARE NEEDS

The Home Health Certification and Plan of Care form (also known as Form 485) is the official form required by Medicare to authorize coverage for home care. To maintain Medicare coverage, this form must be updated and resubmitted every 60 days.

Department of Health and Human Services Health Care Financing Administration			Form Approved OMB No. 0938-0357	
HOME HEALTH CERTIFICATION AND PLAN OF CARE				
1. Patient's HI Claim No. *III-III*	2. Start Of Care Date *01/08/06*	3. Certification Period From: *03/12/07* To: *05/13/07*	4. Medical Record No. *78-9101*	5. Provider No. *11-1213*

6. Patient's Name and Address
Mary Long
2218 Central Ave.
Wichita, Kansas

7. Provider's Name, Address and Telephone Number
Home Health Agency
301 Main Street
Wichita, Kansas

8. Date of Birth *06/04/29*		9. Sex ☐ M ☑ F

11. ICD-9-CM	Principal Diagnosis	Date
4-27-31	*atrial fibrillation*	*12/20/06*

12. ICD-9-CM	Surgical Procedure	Date
0000	*gastrostomy tube insertion*	*01/02/07*

13. ICD-9-CM	Other Pertinent Diagnoses	Date
4280	*heart failure*	*12/31/06*
496	*chronic airway obstruction*	*11/29/06*

10. Medications: Dose/Frequency/Route (N)ew (C)hanged
digoxin 0.125 mg P.O. daily; Lasix 20 mg P.O. daily; warfarin 5 mg P.O. daily; Capoten 12.5 mg b.i.d.; Proventil 2 puffs q.i.d. p.r.n.; MVI one P.O. daily; FeSO₄ 325 mg daily; Ex-Strength Tylenol 500 mg every 4h p.r.n.; albuterol 0.5 cc with 3 cc NSS via nebulizer b.i.d.; aspirin 325 mg P.O. qd

14. DME and Supplies
Gastrostomy tube supplies, cane

15. Safety Measures:
Prevent falls

16. Nutritional Req. *Magnacal 80 ml/hr*

17. Allergies: *NKA*

18.A. Functional Limitations

1 ☐ Amputation	5 ☐ Paralysis	9 ☐ Legally Blind
2 ☐ Bowel/Bladder (Incontinence)	6 ☑ Endurance	A ☐ Dyspnea With Minimal Exertion
3 ☐ Contracture	7 ☐ Ambulation	B ☐ Other (Specify)
4 ☐ Hearing	8 ☐ Speech	

18.B. Activities Permitted

1 ☐ Complete Bedrest	6 ☐ Partial Weight Bearing	A ☐ Wheelchair
2 ☐ Bedrest BRP	7 ☐ Independent At Home	B ☐ Walker
3 ☑ Up As Tolerated	8 ☐ Crutches	C ☐ No Restrictions
4 ☐ Transfer Bed/Chair	9 ☑ Cane	D ☐ Other (Specify)
5 ☐ Exercises Prescribed		

19. Mental Status:

1 ☑ Oriented	3 ☐ Forgetful	5 ☐ Disoriented	7 ☐ Agitated
2 ☐ Comatose	4 ☐ Depressed	6 ☐ Lethargic	8 ☐ Other

20. Prognosis: 1 ☐ Poor 2 ☐ Guarded 3 ☐ Fair 4 ☑ Good 5 ☐ Excellent

21. Orders for Discipline and Treatments (Specify Amount/Frequency/Duration)

RN: Assess heart failure, effects of digoxin, monitor complaints of arthritis pain control; monitor gastrostomy tube site, help with gastrostomy feedings and tube care. Draw blood as ordered by MD. AIDE: 2-3wk; assist with personal care and ADLs.

22. Goals/Rehabilitation Potential/Discharge Plans
Patient will demonstrate correct colostomy care within 2 weeks. Patient will verbalize 2 emotional support systems before discharge.

23. Nurse's Signature and Date of Verbal SOC Where Applicable: *N. Smith, RN 01/08/07*	25. Date HHA Received Signed POT *01/08/07*

24. Physician's Name and Address
M. Raser, MD
555 Main St.
Wichita, Kansas

26. I certify/recertify that this patient is confined to his/her home and needs intermittent skilled nursing care, physical therapy and/or speech therapy or continues to need occupational therapy. The patient is under my care, and I have authorized the services on this plan of care and will periodically review the plan.

27. Attending Physician's Signature and Date Signed
M. Raser, MD 01/8/07

28. Anyone who misrepresents, falsifies, or conceals essential information required for payment of Federal funds may be subject to fine, imprisonment, or civil penalty under applicable Federal laws.

Form HCFA-485 (C-4) (02-94) (Print Aligned)   PROVIDER

PROVIDING UPDATED MEDICAL AND PATIENT INFORMATION

To continue providing reimbursable skilled nursing care to a patient at home, Medicare requires that the home health care agency submit a Medical Update and Patient Information form (also known as Form 486) after the first 60 days of home care. A sample of this form appears here.

Department of Health and Human Services Health Care Financing Administration		Form Approved OMB No. 0938-0357	

Department of Health and Human Services
Health Care Financing Administration
Form Approved
OMB No. 0938-0357

MEDICAL UPDATE AND PATIENT INFORMATION

1. Patient's HI Claim No. 98-7850	2. SOC Date 06/08/06	3. Certification Period From: 11/08/06 To: 01/07/07	4. Medical Record No. 75-4099	5. Provider No. 98-7654

6. Patient's Name and Address James Dole, 412 Main Street, Newark, NJ	7. Provider's Name Home Health Agency

8. Medicare Covered: ☑Y ☐N	9. Date Physician Last Saw Patient: 10/24/04	10. Date Last Contacted Physician: 10/25/04

11. Is the Patient Receiving Care in an 1861 (J)(1) Skilled Nursing Facility or Equivalent? ☐Y ☑N ☐ Do Not Know	12. ☐ Certification ☑ Recertification ☐ Modified

13. Dates of Last Inpatient Stay: Admission 05/31/04	Discharge 06/05/04	14. Type of Facility: A

15. Updated information: New Orders/Treatments/Clinical Facts/Summary from Each Discipline

Discipline	Visits (this bill)	Frequency and duration	Treatment codes	Total visits projected this cert.
SN	00	2 times a week X 3 weeks	N	06
Aide	00	3 times a week X 4 weeks	A6	12

SN: A&O x 3. Skin warm, dry, pale, slight dyspnea noted with activity. Trace bilat. pedal edema, lungs clear. No complaints. Improved & increased feeling of well-being demonstrated. Peg tube patent and functioning well. Correctly demonstrates checking for residual, peg tube site care.

Aide: pt seen 3x/wk. Increased difficulty ambulating. Expressed feelings of despair and hopelessness associated with physical condition.

16. Functional Limitations (Expand From 485 and Level of ADL) Reason Homebound/Prior Functional Status *Interaction between pt and daughter who wants pt to strive to live. Pt increasingly fearful of institutional care. Pt agrees to join gastrostomy support group. CCSN to facilitate. Needs more encouragement to perform ADLs. Daughter more involved with care.*

17. Supplementary Plan of Care on File from Physician Other than Referring Physician: (If Yes, Please Specify Giving Goals/Rehab. Potential/Discharge Plan)	☐Y ☐N

18. Unusual Home/Social Environment *N/A*

19. Indicate Any Time When the Home Health Agency Made a Visit and Patient was Not Home and Reason Why if Ascertainable	20. Specify Any Known Medical and/or Non-Medical Reasons the Patient Regularly Leaves Home and Frequency of Occurrence

21. Nurse or Therapist Completing or Reviewing Form *Anita M. Haffner, RN*	Date (Mo., Day, Yr.) 1/14/07

Form HCFA-486 (C3) (02-94) (Print Aligned)   **PROVIDER**

are properly completed, signed, dated, and submitted. To meet Medicare's criteria for home health care reimbursement, the patient must meet all of these conditions:

- He must be confined to his home.

PHYSICIAN'S TELEPHONE ORDERS

Home health nurses rely heavily on the use of telephone orders. The agency must make sure that its nurses follow guidelines established by the Centers for Medicare and Medicaid Services for taking and documenting these orders. Here is an example of a form used by one agency to fulfill documentation requirements. The physician must sign the order within 48 hours.

Facility name

Suburban Home Health Agency

Address

123 Main Street, Phila. PA 19111

Last name   First name

Smith   _Kevin_

Attending physician   Admission no.

Bedricki   _147–111–471_

Date ordered	Date discontinued	ORDERS
1/18/07	1/21/07	Tylenol 650 mg P.O. every 6h p.r.n. Temp greater than 101° F

Signature of nurse receiving order   Time

  Mary Perro, RN   _1820_

Signature of physician   Date

- He must need skilled services, such as a skilled nurse or a physical, occupational, or speech therapist.
- He must need those skilled services on an intermittent basis.
- The care he needs must be reasonable and medically necessary.
- He must be under a physician's care.

In addition, home health care nurses must document a physician's telephone orders using CMS established guidelines. Some agencies develop their own forms to fulfill these requirements. (See *Physician's telephone orders.*)

Agency assessment

When a patient is referred to a home health care agency, the agency must complete and document a thorough and specific assessment using the most recently revised version of the OASIS, the OASIS-B1—unless the patient is younger than age 18 or a woman receiving maternal-child services. When performing this assessment, make sure you document the patient's:

- physical status
- nutritional status
- mental and emotional status
- home environment in relation to safety and supportive services and groups, such as family, neighbors, and community
- knowledge of his disease or current condition, prognosis, and treatment plan
- potential for complying with the treatment plan.

It's also important to comply with assessment time lines mandated by the OASIS regulations. Patient assessment must be completed:

- within 5 days of the initiation of care and at 60 days and 120 days (if needed)
- when the patient is transferred to another agency
- when there's a significant change in the patient's condition
- when the patient resumes care following an inpatient stay of 24 hours or longer.

OASIS forms

The OASIS forms were developed specifically to measure outcomes for adults who receive home health care. Using this instrument, you'll collect data to measure changes in your pa-

tient's health status over time. Typically, you'll collect OASIS data:

- when a patient starts home health care
- at the 60-day recertification point
- when the patient is discharged or transferred to another facility such as a hospital or subacute care facility. (See *Using the OASIS-B1 form.*)

Care plan

As in any health care setting, the nursing process forms the basis for developing the care plan. Some agencies use the Home Health Certification and Plan of Care form (Form 485) as the patient's official care plan. Other agencies require a separate care plan. If a patient is receiving more than one service, such as physical or occupational therapy, agencies use an interdisciplinary care plan. (See *Interdisciplinary care plan,* pages 342 and 343.)

In court *A care plan is the most direct evidence of your nursing judgment. If you outline a care plan and then deviate from it, a court may decide that you strayed from a reasonable standard of care. Be sure to update your care plan, and make sure that it fits the patient's needs.*

To document most effectively on your care plan, follow these suggestions:

- Keep a copy of the care plan in the patient's home for easy reference by him and his family.
- Make sure that the plan is comprehensive by including more than the patient's physiologic problems. Also document the home environment, the resources needed, and the attitudes of the patient, his family, and primary caregiver.

(Text continues on page 341.)

USING THE OASIS-B1 FORM

The OASIS-B1 form includes more than 80 topics, such as socioeconomic, physiologic, and functional data; service utilization information; and mental, behavioral, and emotional data.

OUTCOME AND ASSESSMENT INFORMATION SET (OASIS-B1)

START OF CARE Assessment (also used for Resumption of Care Following Inpatient Stay)	Client's Name: _____ Client Record No. _____

The Outcome and Assessment Information Set (OASIS) is the intellectual property of The Center for Health Services Research, Denver, Colorado. It is used with permission.

DEMOGRAPHIC/GENERAL INFORMATION

1. (M0010) Agency Medicare Provider Number:

   _____

2. (M0012) Agency Medicaid Provider Number:

   _____

> **Branch Identification** *(Optional, for Agency Use)*
>
> 3. (M0014) Branch State: _____
> 4. (M0016) Branch ID Number:
>
>   _____
>   Agency-assigned

5. (M0020) Patient ID Number:

   QCB/811757

6. (M0030) Start of Care Date: <u>*01*</u> / <u>*02*</u> / <u>*2007*</u>
                         month   day   year

7. (M0032) Resumption of Care Date:

   _____ / _____ / _____   ☒ NA - Not Applicable
   month   day   year

8. (M0040) Patient Name:

   Terry   *S*
   First   MI
   Elliot   *Mr.*
   Last   Suffix

   Patient Address:
   11 Second Street
   Street, Route, Apt. Number
   Hometown
   City

   (M0050) Patient State of Residence: <u>*PA*</u>

   (M0060) Patient Zip Code: <u>*10981*</u> - <u>*1234*</u>

   Phone: (<u>*881*</u>) <u>*555*</u> - <u>*2937*</u>

(continued)

---

9. (M0063) Medicare Number:

134765482 A
including suffix

☐ NA - No Medicare

10. (M0064) Social Security Number:

111 - *22* - *3333*

☐ UK - Unknown or Not Available

11. (M0065) Medicaid Number:

☒ NA - No Medicaid

12. (M0066) Birth Date: *07* / *08* / *1928*
month   day   year

13. (M0069) Gender:

☒ 1 - Male   ☐ 2 - Female

14. (M0072) Primary Referring Physician ID:

222222   (UPIN#)

☐ UK - Unknown or Not Available

Name *Dr. Kyle Stevens*

Address *10 State St.*

Hometown, PA 10981

Phone: (*881*) *555* - *6900*

FAX: (*881*) *555* - *6974*

15. (M0080) Discipline of Person Completing Assessment:

☒ 1-RN   ☐ 2-PT   ☐ 3-SLP/ST   ☐ 4-OT

16. (M0090) Date Assessment Completed:

01 /*02* / *2007*
month   day   year

17. (M0100) This Assessment is Currently Being Completed for the Following Reason:

Start/Resumption of Care

☒ 1 - Start of care — further visits planned

☐ 2 - Resumption of care (after inpatient stay)

Follow-Up

☐ 3 - Recertification (follow-up) reassessment
[Go to *M0150*]

☐ 4 - Other follow-up [Go to *M0150*]

Transfer to an Inpatient Facility

☐ 5 - Transferred to an inpatient facility — patient not
discharged from agency [Go to *M0150*]

☐ 6 - Transferred to an inpatient facility — patient
discharged from agency [Go to *M0150*]

Discharge from Agency — Not to an Inpatient Facility

☐ 7 - Death at home [Go to *M0150*]

☐ 8 - Discharge from agency [Go to *M0150*]

☐ 9 - Discharge from agency — no visits completed
after start/resumption of care assessment
[Go to *M0150*]

18. Marital status:

☐ Not Married ☒ Married ☐ Widowed
☐ Divorced ☐ Separated ☐ Unknown

19. (M0140) Race/Ethnicity (as identified by patient):
(Mark all that apply.)

☐ 1 - American Indian or Alaska Native

☐ 2 - Asian

☐ 3 - Black or African-American

☐ 4 - Hispanic or Latino

☐ 5 - Native Hawaiian or Pacific Islander

☒ 6 - White

☐ UK - Unknown

20. Emergency contact:

Name _Susan Elliot_

Address _11 Second St._

Hometown, PA 10981

Phone: (_881_) _555_ - _2937_

(continued)

21. **(M0150) Current Payment Sources for Home Care:**
(Mark all that apply.)

☐ 0 - None; no charge for current services
☒ 1 - Medicare (traditional fee-for-service)
☐ 2 - Medicare (HMO/managed care)
☐ 3 - Medicaid (traditional fee-for-service)
☐ 4 - Medicaid (HMO/managed care)
☐ 5 - Workers' compensation
☐ 6 - Title programs (e.g., Title III, V, or XX)
☐ 7 - Other government (e.g., CHAMPUS, VA, etc.)
☐ 8 - Private insurance
☐ 9 - Private HMO/managed care
☐ 10 - Self-pay
☐ 11 - Other (specify) _____
☐ UK - Unknown

22. **(M0160) Financial Factors** limiting the ability of the patient/family to meet basic health needs:
(Mark all that apply.)

☒ 0 - None
☐ 1 - Unable to afford medicine or medical supplies
☐ 2 - Unable to afford medical expenses that are not covered by insurance/Medicare (e.g., copayments)
☐ 3 - Unable to afford rent/utility bills
☐ 4 - Unable to afford food
☐ 5 - Other (specify)

PATIENT HISTORY

23. **(M0175)** From which of the following **Inpatient Facilities** was the patient discharged *during the past 14 days*?
(Mark all that apply.)

☐ 1 - Hospital
☐ 2 - Rehabilitation facility
☐ 3 - Skilled nursing facility
☐ 4 - Other nursing home
☐ 5 - Other (specify) _____
☒ NA - Patient was not discharged from an inpatient facility [If NA, go to *M0200*]

24. **(M0180) Inpatient Discharge Date** (most recent):

_____ / _____ / _____
month   day   year

☐ UK - Unknown

25. **(M0190)** List each inpatient Diagnosis and ICD code at the level of highest specificity *for only those conditions treated during an inpatient facility stay within the last 14 days* (no surgical, E-codes, or V-codes):

    Inpatient Facility Diagnosis   ICD-9-CM

    a. _____   (_____ . _____)

    b. _____   (_____ . _____)

26. **(M0200)** Medical or Treatment Regimen Change Within Past 14 Days: Has this patient experienced a change in medical or treatment regimen (e.g., medication, treatment, or service change due to new or additional diagnosis, etc.) within the last 14 days?

    ☐ 0 - No   [If No, go to *M0220*]

    ☒ 1 - Yes

27. **(M0210)** List the patient's **Medical Diagnosis** and ICD code at the level of highest specificity for those conditions requiring changed medical or treatment regimen (no surgical, E-codes, or V-codes):

    Changed Medical Regimen Diagnosis   ICD-9-CM

    a. *open wound @ ankle*   (*891* . *00*)

    b. _____   (_____ . _____)

    c. _____   (_____ . _____)

    d. _____   (_____ . _____)

28. **(M0220)** Conditions Prior to Medical or Treatment
    Regimen Change or Inpatient Stay Within Past 14 Days:
    If this patient experienced an inpatient facility discharge or change in medical or treatment regimen within the past 14 days, indicate any conditions which existed *prior to* the inpatient stay or change in medical or treatment regimen. **(Mark all that apply.)**

    ☐ 1 - Urinary incontinence

    ☐ 2 - Indwelling/suprapubic catheter

    ☐ 3 - Intractable pain

    ☐ 4 - Impaired decision-making

    ☐ 5 - Disruptive or socially inappropriate behavior

    ☐ 6 - Memory loss to the extent that supervision required

    ☒ 7 - None of the above

    ☐ NA - No inpatient facility discharge *and* no change in medical or treatment regimen in past 14 days

    ☐ UK - Unknown

(continued)

29. (M0230/M0240) Diagnoses and Severity Index: List each diagnosis and ICD-9-CM code at the level of highest specificity (no surgical codes) for which the patient is receiving home care. Rate each condition using the following severity index. **(Choose one value that represents the most severe rating appropriate for each diagnosis.)** E-codes (for M0240 only) or V-codes (for M0230 or 240) may be used. ICD-9-CM sequencing requirements must be followed if multiple coding is indicated for any diagnoses. If a V-code is reported in place of a case mix diagnosis, then M0245 Payment Diagnosis should be completed. Case mix diagnosis is a primary or first secondary diagnosis that determines the Medicare PPS case mix group.

0 - Asymptomatic, no treatment needed at this time

1 - Symptoms well controlled with current therapy

2 - Symptoms controlled with difficulty, affecting daily functioning; patient needs ongoing monitoring

3 - Symptoms poorly controlled, patient needs frequent adjustment in treatment and dose monitoring

4 - Symptoms poorly controlled, history of rehospitalizations

(M0230) Primary Diagnosis   ICD-9-CM

a. *open wound @ ankle*   (*891* . *00*)

Severity Rating ☐ 0 ☐ 1 ☒ 2 ☐ 3 ☐ 4

(M0240) Other Diagnoses   ICD-9-CM

b. *Type 2 diabetes*   (*250* . *72*)

Severity Rating ☐ 0 ☐ 1 ☒ 2 ☐ 3 ☐ 4

c. *PVD*   (*443* . *89*)

Severity Rating ☐ 0 ☐ 1 ☐ 2 ☒ 3 ☐ 4

d. _____ (___ . ___)

Severity Rating ☐ 0 ☐ 1 ☐ 2 ☐ 3 ☐ 4

e. _____ (___ . ___)

Severity Rating ☐ 0 ☐ 1 ☐ 2 ☐ 3 ☐ 4

f. _____ (___ . ___)

Severity Rating ☐ 0 ☐ 1 ☐ 2 ☐ 3 ☐ 4

(M0245) Payment diagnosis (optional): If a V-code was reported in M0230 in place of a case mix diagnosis, list the primary diagnosis and ICD-9-CM code determined in accordance with OASIS requirements in effect before October 1, 2003 — no V-codes, E-codes, or surgical codes allowed. ICD-9-CM sequencing requirements must be followed. Complete both lines (a) and (b) if the case mix diagnosis is a manifestation code or in other situations where multiple coding is indicated for the primary diagnosis; otherwise, complete line (a) only.

(M0245) Primary Diagnosis   ICD-9-CM

a. _____ (___ . ___)

(M0245) First Secondary Diagnosis   ICD-9-CM

a. _____ (___ . ___)

30. Patient/family knowledge and coping level regarding present illness:

    Patient _Knowledgeable about disease process_

    Family _Anxious to assist in care_

31. Significant past health history:

    PVD

    Type 2 diabetes

    Ⓡ BKA

32. **(M0250) Therapies** the patient receives *at home*:
    (Mark all that apply.)

    ☐ 1 - Intravenous or infusion therapy (excludes TPN)

    ☐ 2 - Parenteral nutrition (TPN or lipids)

    ☐ 3 - Enteral nutrition (nasogastric, gastrostomy, jejunostomy, or any other artificial entry into the alimentary canal)

    ☒ 4 - None of the above

33. **(M0260) Overall Prognosis:** BEST description of patient's overall prognosis for *recovery from this episode of illness.*

    ☐ 0 - Poor: little or no recovery is expected and/or further decline is imminent

    ☒ 1 - Good/Fair: partial to full recovery is expected

    ☐ UK - Unknown

34. **(M0270) Rehabilitative Prognosis:** BEST description of patient's prognosis for *functional status.*

    ☒ 0 - Guarded: minimal improvement in functional status is expected; decline is possible

    ☐ 1 - Good: marked improvement in functional status is expected

    ☐ UK - Unknown

35. **(M0280) Life Expectancy:** (Physician documentation is not required.)

    ☐ 0 - Life expectancy is greater than 6 months

    ☒ 1 - Life expectancy is 6 months or fewer

(continued)

36. Immunization/screening tests:

Immunizations:

Flu	☒ Yes ☐ No	Date	10/06
Tetanus	☒ Yes ☐ No	Date	3/03
Pneumonia	☒ Yes ☐ No	Date	10/05
Other _____		Date	_____

Screening:

Cholesterol level	☒ Yes ☐ No	Date	11/05
Mammogram	☐ Yes ☒ No	Date	
Colon cancer screen	☒ Yes ☐ No	Date	11/02
Prostate cancer screen	☒ Yes ☐ No	Date	11/02

Self-exam frequency:

Breast self-exam frequency _____

Testicular self-exam frequency _____

37. Allergies: *NKA*

38. **(M0290) High Risk Factors** characterizing this patient:
    (Mark all that apply.)

    ☒ 1 - Heavy smoking

    ☐ 2 - Obesity

    ☐ 3 - Alcohol dependency

    ☐ 4 - Drug dependency

    ☐ 5 - None of the above

    ☐ UK - Unknown

LIVING ARRANGEMENTS

39. **(M0300) Current Residence:**

    ☒ 1 - Patient's owned or rented residence (house, apartment, or mobile home owned or rented by patient/couple/significant other)

    ☐ 2 - Family member's residence

    ☐ 3 - Boarding home or rented room

    ☐ 4 - Board and care or assisted living facility

    ☐ 5 - Other (specify) _____

40. **(M0310) Structural Barriers** in the patient's environment limiting independent mobility: **(Mark all that apply.)**

☐ 0 - None

☒ 1 - Stairs inside home which *must* be used by the patient (e.g., to get to toileting, sleeping, eating areas)

☐ 2 - Stairs inside home which are used optionally (e.g., to get to laundry facilities)

☒ 3 - Stairs leading from inside house to outside

☐ 4 - Narrow or obstructed doorways

41. **(M0320) Safety Hazards** found in the patient's current place of residence: **(Mark all that apply.)**

☒ 0 - None

☐ 1 - Inadequate floor, roof, or windows

☐ 2 - Inadequate lighting

☐ 3 - Unsafe gas/electric appliance

☐ 4 - Inadequate heating

☐ 5 - Inadequate cooling

☐ 6 - Lack of fire safety devices

☐ 7 - Unsafe floor coverings

☐ 8 - Inadequate stair railings

☐ 9 - Improperly stored hazardous materials

☐ 10 - Lead-based paint

☐ 11 - Other (specify) _____

42. **(M0330) Sanitation Hazards** found in the patient's current place of residence: **(Mark all that apply.)**

☒ 0 - None

☐ 1 - No running water

☐ 2 - Contaminated water

☐ 3 - No toileting facilities

☐ 4 - Outdoor toileting facilities only

☐ 5 - Inadequate sewage disposal

☐ 6 - Inadequate/improper food storage

☐ 7 - No food refrigeration

☐ 8 - No cooking facilities

☐ 9 - Insects/rodents present

☐ 10 - No scheduled trash pickup

☐ 11 - Cluttered/soiled living area

☐ 12 - Other (specify) _____

(continued)

43. (M0340) Patient Lives With: (Mark all that apply.)

☐ 1 - Lives alone
☒ 2 - With spouse or significant other
☐ 3 - With other family member
☐ 4 - With a friend
☐ 5 - With paid help (other than home care agency staff)
☐ 6 - With other than above
Comments: _____

_____

_____

44. Others living in household:

Name _Susan_ Age _70_ Sex _F_
Relationship _wife_ Able/willing to assist ☒ Yes ☐ No
Name _____ Age_____ Sex _____
Relationship _____ Able/willing to assist ☐ Yes ☐ No
Name _____ Age_____ Sex _____
Relationship _____ Able/willing to assist ☐ Yes ☐ No
Name _____ Age_____ Sex _____
Relationship _____ Able/willing to assist ☐ Yes ☐ No
Name _____ Age_____ Sex _____
Relationship _____ Able/willing to assist ☐ Yes ☐ No
Name _____ Age_____ Sex _____
Relationship _____ Able/willing to assist ☐ Yes ☐ No

SUPPORTIVE ASSISTANCE

45. Persons/Organizations providing assistance:

_____

_____

_____

_____

46. (M0350) Assisting Person(s) Other than Home Care Agency Staff:
(Mark all that apply.)

☐ 1 - Relatives, friends, or neighbors living outside the home
☒ 2 - Person residing in the home (EXCLUDING paid help)
☐ 3 - Paid help
☐ 4 - None of the above
      [If None of the above, go to *Review of Systems*]
☐ UK - Unknown [If Unknown, go to *Review of Systems*]

47. **(M0360) Primary Caregiver** taking *lead* responsibility for providing or managing the patient's care, providing the most frequent assistance, etc. (other than home care agency staff):

☐ 0 - No one person [If No one person, go to *M0390*]

☒ 1 - Spouse or significant other

☐ 2 - Daughter or son

☐ 3 - Other family member

☐ 4 - Friend or neighbor or community or church member

☐ 5 - Paid help

☐ UK - Unknown [If Unknown, go to *M0390*]

48. **(M0370) How Often** does the patient receive assistance from the primary caregiver?

☒ 1 - Several times during day and night

☐ 2 - Several times during day

☐ 3 - Once daily

☐ 4 - Three or more times per week

☐ 5 - One to two times per week

☐ 6 - Less often than weekly

☐ UK - Unknown

49. **(M0380) Type of Primary Caregiver Assistance:**
(Mark all that apply.)

☒ 1 - ADL assistance (e.g., bathing, dressing, toileting, bowel/bladder, eating/feeding)

☒ 2 - IADL assistance (e.g., meds, meals, housekeeping, laundry, telephone, shopping, finances)

☐ 3 - Environmental support (housing, home maintenance)

☒ 4 - Psychosocial support (socialization, companionship, recreation)

☒ 5 - Advocates or facilitates patient's participation in appropriate medical care

☐ 6 - Financial agent, power of attorney, or conservator of finance

☐ 7 - Health care agent, conservator of person, or medical power of attorney

☐ UK - Unknown

Comments: _____

(continued)

REVIEW OF SYSTEMS

SENSORY STATUS

(Mark S for subjective, O for objectively assessed problem. If no problem present or if not assessed, mark NA.)

Head *NA* Dizziness

NA Headache (describe location, duration) _____

Eyes *O* Glasses *NA* Cataracts *NA* Blurred/double vision

O PERRL ___ Other (specify) _____

50. (M0390) Vision with corrective lenses if the patient usually wears them:

☒ 0 - Normal vision: sees adequately in most situations; can see medication labels, newsprint.

☐ 1 - Partially impaired: cannot see medication labels or newsprint, but *can* see obstacles in path, and the surrounding layout; can count fingers at arm's length.

☐ 2 - Severely impaired: cannot locate objects without hearing or touching them *or* patient nonresponsive.

Ears *NA* Hearing aid *NA* Tinnitus

___ Other (specify) _____

51. (M0400) Hearing and Ability to Understand Spoken Language in patient's own language (with hearing aids if the patient usually uses them):

☒ 0 - No observable impairment. Able to hear and understand complex or detailed instructions and extended or abstract conversation.

☐ 1 - With minimal difficulty, able to hear and understand most multi-step instructions and ordinary conversation. May need occasional repetition, extra time, or louder voice.

☐ 2 - Has moderate difficulty hearing and understanding simple, one-step instructions and brief conversation; needs frequent prompting or assistance.

☐ 3 - Has severe difficulty hearing and understanding simple greetings and short comments. Requires multiple repetitions, restatements, demonstrations, additional time.

☐ 4 - *Unable* to hear and understand familiar words or common expressions consistently, *or* patient nonresponsive.

Oral ___ Gum problems ___ Chewing problems

___ Dentures ___ Other (specify) _____

52. **(M0410) Speech and Oral (Verbal) Expression of Language** (in patient's own language):

☒ 0 - Expresses complex ideas, feelings, and needs clearly, completely, and easily in all situations with no observable impairment.

☐ 1 - Minimal difficulty in expressing ideas and needs (may take extra time; makes occasional errors in word choice, grammar or speech intelligibility; needs minimal prompting or assistance).

☐ 2 - Expresses simple ideas or needs with moderate difficulty (needs prompting or assistance, errors in word choice, organization, or speech intelligibility). Speaks in phrases or short sentences.

☐ 3 - Has severe difficulty expressing basic ideas or needs and requires maximal assistance or guessing by listener. Speech limited to single words or short phrases.

☐ 4 - *Unable* to express basic needs even with maximal prompting or assistance but is not comatose or unresponsive (e.g., speech is nonsensical or unintelligible).

☐ 5 - Patient nonresponsive or unable to speak.

Nose and sinus

N/A Epistaxis ____ Other (specify)_____

Neck and throat

N/A Hoarseness *N/A* Difficulty swallowing

____ Other (specify) _____

Musculoskeletal, Neurological

N/A Hx arthritis	*N/A* Joint pain	*N/A* Syncope
N/A Gout	*N/A* Weakness	*N/A* Seizure
N/A Stiffness	*S* Leg cramps	*N/A* Tenderness
N/A Swollen joints	*S* Numbness	*N/A* Deformities
N/A Unequal grasp	*O* Temp changes	*N/A* Comatose
N/A Tremor	*N/A* Aphasia/inarticulate speech	

N/A Paralysis (describe) _____

N/A Amputation (location) _____

N/A Other (specify) _____

Coordination, gait, balance (describe) *Gait steady* _____

_____

_____

_____

Comments (Prosthesis, appliances) *Uses a walker* _____

_____

_____

_____

_____

(continued)

Pain location: ____Ⓛ ankle_____

Type:

___ Acute   _X_ Recent onset   ___ Chronic

Duration:

_X_ Intermittent   ___ Constant   ___ Other _____

Intensity Scale (0-10): ___4___

Precipitating factors: _____

Control Measures:

_X_ Rest   ___ Heat/Cold   ___ Tens Unit

___ Relaxation   ___ Music Therapy   ___ Biofeedback

___ Massage   ___ Medication   ___ Other: _____

Best Response to Control Measures (0-10): ___/_____

MD contacted to discuss pain management alternatives for unrelieved pain: _____

Pain comments _____

53. (M0420) Frequency of Pain interfering with patient's activity or movement:

☐ 0 - Patient has no pain or pain does not interfere with activity or movement

☐ 1 - Less often than daily

☒ 2 - Daily, but not constantly

☐ 3 - All of the time

54. (M0430) Intractable Pain: Is the patient experiencing pain that is *not easily relieved,* occurs at least daily, and affects the patient's sleep, appetite, physical or emotional energy, concentration, personal relationships, emotions, or ability or desire to perform physical activity?

☒ 0 - No

☐ 1 - Yes

Comments (pain management) _____

_____

_____

_____

INTEGUMENTARY STATUS

_O_ Hair changes (where) _Balding_

_NA_ Pruritus _____ Other (specify)_____

Skin condition (Record type # on body area. Indicate size to right of numbered category.)

#5

Type	Size
1. Lesions	
2. Bruises	
3. Masses	
4. Scars	
5. Stasis Ulcers	_1/2" round_
6. Pressure Ulcers	
7. Incisions	
8. Other (specify)	

55. **(M0440)** Does this patient have a **Skin Lesion** or an **Open Wound**? This excludes "OSTOMIES."

☐ 0 - No [If No, go to *Cardio/respiratory status*]

☒ 1 - Yes

56. **(M0445)** Does this patient have a **Pressure Ulcer**?

☒ 0 - No [If No, go to *M0468*]

☐ 1 - Yes

(continued)

57. **(M0450)** Current Number of Pressure Ulcers at Each Stage: (Circle one response for each stage.)

Pressure Ulcer Stages

Number of Pressure Ulcers

a) Stage 1: Nonblanchable erythema of intact skin; the heralding of skin ulceration. In darker-pigmented skin, warmth, edema, hardness, or discolored skin may be indicators.   0 1 2 3 4 or more

b) Stage 2: Partial thickness skin loss involving epidermis and/or dermis. The ulcer is superficial and presents clinically as an abrasion, blister, or shallow crater.   0 1 2 3 4 or more

c) Stage 3: Full-thickness skin loss involving damage or necrosis of subcutaneous tissue which may extend down to, but not through, underlying fascia. The ulcer presents clinically as a deep crater with or without undermining of adjacent tissue.   0 1 2 3 4 or more

d) Stage 4: Full-thickness skin loss with extensive destruction, tissue necrosis, or damage to muscle, bone, or supporting structures (e.g., tendon, joint capsule, etc.)

e) In addition to the above, is there at least one pressure ulcer that cannot be observed due to the presence of eschar or a nonremovable dressing, including casts?   0 1 2 3 4 or more

- ☐ 0 - No
- ☐ 1 - Yes

58. **(M0460)** Stage of Most Problematic (Observable) Pressure Ulcer:

- ☐ 1 - Stage 1
- ☐ 2 - Stage 2
- ☐ 3 - Stage 3
- ☐ 4 - Stage 4
- ☐ NA - No observable pressure ulcer

59. **(M0464)** Status of Most Problematic (Observable) Pressure Ulcer:

- ☐ 1 - Fully granulating
- ☐ 2 - Early/partial granulation
- ☐ 3 - Not healing
- ☐ NA - No observable pressure ulcer

60. **(M0468)** Does this patient have a **Stasis Ulcer**?

- ☐ 0 - No [If No, go to *M0482*]
- ☒ 1 - Yes

61. (M0470) Current Number of Observable Stasis Ulcer(s):
   - ☐ 0 - Zero
   - ☒ 1 - One
   - ☐ 2 - Two
   - ☐ 3 - Three
   - ☐ 4 - Four or more

62. (M0474) Does this patient have at least one **Stasis Ulcer that Cannot be Observed** due to the presence of a nonremovable dressing?
   - ☒ 0 - No
   - ☐ 1 - Yes

63. (M0476) Status of Most Problematic (Observable) Stasis Ulcer:
   - ☐ 1 - Fully granulating
   - ☒ 2 - Early/partial granulation
   - ☐ 3 - Not healing
   - ☐ NA - No observable stasis ulcer

64. (M0482) Does this patient have a **Surgical Wound?**
   - ☒ 0 - No [If No, go to *Cardio/Respiratory Status*]
   - ☐ 1 - Yes

65. (M0484) Current Number of (Observable) Surgical Wounds: (If a wound is partially closed but has *more* than one opening, consider each opening as a separate wound.)
   - ☐ 0 - Zero
   - ☐ 1 - One
   - ☐ 2 - Two
   - ☐ 3 - Three
   - ☐ 4 - Four or more

66. (M0486) Does this patient have at least one **Surgical Wound that Cannot be Observed** due to the presence of a nonremovable dressing?
   - ☐ 0 - No
   - ☐ 1 - Yes

67. (M0488) Status of Most Problematic (Observable) Surgical Wound:
   - ☐ 1 - Fully granulating
   - ☐ 2 - Early/partial granulation
   - ☐ 3 - Not healing
   - ☐ NA - No observable surgical wound

(continued)

CARDIO/RESPIRATORY STATUS

Temperature _99°_   Respirations _18_

Blood pressure
  Lying _132/80_ Sitting _130/78_ Standing _130/76_

Pulse
  Apical rate _72_   Radial rate _72_
  Rhythm _Regular_   Quality _____

Cardiovascular
  _N/A_ Palpitations   _N/A_ Chest pains
  _S_ Claudication   _N/A_ Murmurs
  _S_ Fatigues easily   _O_ Edema
  _N/A_ BP problems   _N/A_ Cyanosis
  _N/A_ Dyspnea on exertion   _N/A_ Varicosities
  _N/A_ Paroxysmal nocturnal dyspnea
  _N/A_ Orthopnea (# of pillows)
  _N/A_ Cardiac problems (specify) _____
  _N/A_ Pacemaker _____
              (Date of last battery change)
  Other (specify) _____
  Comments _____
  _____
  _____
  _____

Respiratory
  History of
  _N/A_ Asthma   _N/A_ Pleurisy
  _N/A_ TB   _N/A_ Pneumonia
  _S_ Bronchitis   _N/A_ Emphysema
  Other (specify) _____
  Present condition
  _S_ Cough (describe) _Dry_____
  _O_ Breath sounds (describe) _Clear_____
  _N/A_ Sputum (character and amount) _____
  Other (specify) _____

68. **(M0490)** When is the patient dyspneic or noticeably **Short of Breath**?

  ☒ 0 - Never, patient is not short of breath

  ☐ 1 - When walking more than 20 feet, climbing stairs

  ☐ 2 - With moderate exertion (e.g., while dressing, using commode or bedpan, walking distances less than 20 feet)

  ☐ 3 - With minimal exertion (e.g., while eating, talking, or performing other ADLs) or with agitation

  ☐ 4 - At rest (during day or night)

69. (M0500) Respiratory Treatments utilized at home:
(Mark all that apply.)

☐ 1 - Oxygen (intermittent or continuous)

☐ 2 - Ventilator (continually or at night)

☐ 3 - Continuous positive airway pressure

☐ 4 - None of the above

Comments _____

_____

_____

_____

ELIMINATION STATUS

Genitourinary Tract

N/A Frequency	*N/A* Prostate disorder
N/A Pain	*N/A* Dysmenorrhea
N/A Hematuria	*N/A* Lesions
N/A Vaginal discharge/bleeding	*N/A* Hx hysterectomy
S Nocturia	*N/A* Gravida/Para
N/A Urgency	*N/A* Contraception
N/A Date last PAP _____	

Other (specify) _____

70. (M0510) Has this patient been treated for a **Urinary Tract Infection** in the past 14 days?

☒ 0 - No

☐ 1 - Yes

☐ NA - Patient on prophylactic treatment

☐ UK - Unknown

71. (M0520) Urinary Incontinence or Urinary Catheter Presence:

☒ 0 - No incontinence or catheter (includes anuria or ostomy for urinary drainage)
   [If No, go to *M0540*]

☐ 1 - Patient is incontinent

☐ 2 - Patient requires a urinary catheter (i.e., external, indwelling, intermittent, suprapubic) [Go to *M0540*]

(continued)

72. (M0530) When does Urinary Incontinence occur?

☐ 0 - Timed-voiding defers incontinence

☐ 1 - During the night only

☐ 2 - During the day and night

Comments (e.g., appliances and care, bladder programs, catheter type, frequency of irrigation and change) _____

_____

_____

_____

_____

_____

Gastrointestinal Tract

N/A Indigestion   N/A Rectal bleeding

N/A Nausea/vomiting   N/A Hemorrhoids

N/A Ulcers   N/A Gallbladder problems

N/A Pain   N/A Jaundice

N/A Diarrhea/constipation   N/A Tenderness

N/A Hernias (where) _____

Other (specify) _____

73. (M0540) Bowel Incontinence Frequency:

☒ 0 - Very rarely or never has bowel incontinence

☐ 1 - Less than once weekly

☐ 2 - One to three times weekly

☐ 3 - Four to six times weekly

☐ 4 - On a daily basis

☐ 5 - More often than once daily

☐ NA - Patient has ostomy for bowel elimination

☐ UK - Unknown

74. (M0550) Ostomy for Bowel Elimination: Does this patient have an ostomy for bowel elimination that (within the last 14 days):

a) was related to an inpatient facility stay, *or*

b) necessitated a change in medical or treatment regimen?

☒ 0 - Patient does *not* have an ostomy for bowel elimination.

☐ 1 - Patient's ostomy was *not* related to an inpatient stay and did *not* necessitate change in medical or treatment regimen.

☐ 2 - The ostomy *was* related to an inpatient stay or *did* necessitate change in medical or treatment regimen.

Comments (bowel function, stool color, bowel program, GI series, abd. girth) _____

_____

_____

Nutritional status

N/A Weight loss/gain last 3 mos. (Give amount _____)

N/A Over/under weight ____ Change in appetite

Diet _20% protein 30% fat_____

Other (specify) _____

Meals prepared by _Wife_____

Comments _____

_____

_____

_____

_____

Breasts (For both male and female)

N/A Lumps   *N*/A Tenderness

N/A Discharge   *N*/A Pain

Other (specify) _____

Comments _____

_____

_____

_____

_____

NEURO/EMOTIONAL/BEHAVIORAL STATUS

N/A Hx of previous psych. illness

Other (specify) _____

75. (M0560) Cognitive Functioning: (Patient's current level of alertness, orientation, comprehension, concentration, and immediate memory for simple commands.)

☐ 0 - Alert/oriented, able to focus and shift attention, comprehends and recalls task directions independently.

☒ 1 - Requires prompting (cueing, repetition, reminders) only under stressful or unfamiliar conditions.

☐ 2 - Requires assistance and some direction in specific situations (e.g., on all tasks involving shifting of attention), or consistently requires low stimulus environment due to distractibility.

☐ 3 - Requires considerable assistance in routine situations. Is not alert and oriented or is unable to shift attention and recall directions more than half the time.

☐ 4 - Totally dependent due to disturbances such as constant disorientation, coma, persistent vegetative state, or delirium.

(continued)

76. (M0570) When Confused (Reported or Observed):

- [X] 0 - Never
- [ ] 1 - In new or complex situations only
- [ ] 2 - On awakening or at night only
- [ ] 3 - During the day and evening, but not constantly
- [ ] 4 - Constantly
- [ ] NA - Patient nonresponsive

77. (M0580) When Anxious (Reported or Observed):

- [ ] 0 - None of the time
- [ ] 1 - Less often than daily
- [X] 2 - Daily, but not constantly
- [ ] 3 - All of the time
- [ ] NA - Patient nonresponsive

78. (M0590) Depressive Feelings Reported or Observed in Patient: (Mark all that apply.)

- [ ] 1 - Depressed mood (e.g., feeling sad, tearful)
- [ ] 2 - Sense of failure or self-reproach
- [X] 3 - Hopelessness
- [ ] 4 - Recurrent thoughts of death
- [ ] 5 - Thoughts of suicide
- [ ] 6 - None of the above feelings observed or reported

79. (M0600) Patient Behaviors (Reported or Observed): (Mark all that apply.)

- [ ] 1 - Indecisiveness, lack of concentration
- [ ] 2 - Diminished interest in most activities
- [ ] 3 - Sleep disturbances
- [ ] 4 - Recent change in appetite or weight
- [ ] 5 - Agitation
- [ ] 6 - A suicide attempt
- [X] 7 - None of the above behaviors observed or reported

80. (M0610) Behaviors Demonstrated *at Least Once a Week* (Reported or Observed): (Mark all that apply.)

- [ ] 1 - Memory deficit: failure to recognize familiar persons/places, inability to recall events of past 24 hours, significant memory loss so that supervision is required
- [ ] 2 - Impaired decision making: failure to perform usual ADLs or IADLs, inability to appropriately stop activities, jeopardizes safety through actions
- [ ] 3 - Verbal disruption: yelling, threatening, excessive profanity, sexual references, etc.

☐ 4 - Physical aggression: aggressive or combative to self and others (e.g., hits self, throws objects, punches, dangerous maneuvers with wheelchair or other objects)

☐ 5 - Disruptive, infantile, or socially inappropriate behavior (**excludes** verbal actions)

☐ 6 - Delusional, hallucinatory, or paranoid behavior

☒ 7 - None of the above behaviors demonstrated

81. **(M0620) Frequency of Behavior Problems (Reported or Observed)** (e.g., wandering episodes, self-abuse, verbal disruption, physical aggression, etc.):

☒ 0 - Never

☐ 1 - Less than once a month

☐ 2 - Once a month

☐ 3 - Several times each month

☐ 4 - Several times a week

☐ 5 - At least daily

82. **(M0630)** Is this patient receiving **Psychiatric Nursing Services** at home provided by a qualified psychiatric nurse?

☒ 0 - No

☐ 1 - Yes

Comments _____

_____

_____

_____

Endocrine and hematopoietic

_S_ Diabetes   _N/A_ Polydipsia

_N/A_ Polyuria   _N/A_ Thyroid problem

_N/A_ Excessive bleeding or bruising

_S_ Intolerance to heat and cold

Fractionals

Usual results _____

Frequency checked _____

Other (specify) _____

Comments _____

_____

(continued)

ADL/IADLs

For M0640-M0800, complete the "Current" column for all patients. For
these same items, complete the "Prior" column only at start of care and
at resumption of care; mark the level that corresponds to the patient's
condition 14 days prior to start of care date (M0030) or resumption of
care date (M0032). In all cases, record what the patient is *able to do.*

83. (M0640) **Grooming:** Ability to tend to personal hygiene needs (i.e., washing face and hands,
hair care, shaving or makeup, teeth or denture care, fingernail care).

Prior Current

☒ ☐ 0 - Able to groom self unaided, with or without the use of assistive devices or
adapted methods.

☐ ☒ 1 - Grooming utensils must be placed within reach before able to complete
grooming activities.

☐ ☐ 2 - Someone must assist the patient to groom self.

☐ ☐ 3 - Patient depends entirely upon someone else for grooming needs.

☐   UK - Unknown

84. (M0650) **Ability to Dress *Upper* Body** (with or without dressing aids) including undergarments,
pullovers, front-opening shirts and blouses, managing zippers, buttons, and snaps:

Prior Current

☒ ☐ 0 - Able to get clothes out of closets and drawers, put them on and remove them
from the upper body without assistance.

☐ ☒ 1 - Able to dress upper body without assistance if clothing is laid out or handed
to the patient.

☐ ☐ 2 - Someone must help the patient put on upper body clothing.

☐ ☐ 3 - Patient depends entirely upon another person to dress the upper body.

☐   UK - Unknown

85. (M0660) **Ability to Dress *Lower* Body** (with or without dressing aids) including undergarments, slacks, socks or nylons, shoes:

Prior Current

☒ ☐ 0 - Able to obtain, put on, and remove clothing and shoes without assistance.

☐ ☐ 1 - Able to dress lower body without assistance if clothing and shoes are laid out
or handed to the patient.

☐ ☒ 2 - Someone must help the patient put on undergarments, slacks, socks or nylons, and shoes.

☐ ☐ 3 - Patient depends entirely upon another person to dress lower body.

☐   UK - Unknown

86. (M0670) Bathing: Ability to wash entire body. *Excludes* grooming (washing face and hands only).

Prior   Current

☐ ☐ 0 - Able to bathe self in *shower or tub* independently

☒ ☐ 1 - With the use of devices, is able to bathe self in shower or tub independently.

☐ ☐ 2 - Able to bathe in shower or tub with the assistance of another person:
       (a) for intermittent supervision or encouragement or reminders, *OR*
       (b) to get in and out of the shower or tub, *OR*
       (c) for washing difficult-to-reach areas.

☐ ☒ 3 - Participates in bathing self in shower or tub, *but* requires presence of another person throughout the bath for assistance or supervision.

☐ ☐ 4 - *Unable* to use the shower or tub and is bathed in *bed or bedside chair.*

☐ ☐ 5 - Unable to effectively participate in bathing and is totally bathed by another person.

☐   UK - Unknown

87. (M0680) Toileting: Ability to get to and from the toilet or bedside commode.

Prior   Current

☒ ☒ 0 - Able to get to and from the toilet independently with or without a device.

☐ ☐ 1 - When reminded, assisted, or supervised by another person, able to get to and from the toilet.

☐ ☐ 2 - *Unable* to get to and from the toilet but is able to use a bedside commode (with or without assistance).

☐ ☐ 3 - *Unable* to get to and from the toilet or bedside commode but is able to use a bedpan/urinal independently.

☐ ☐ 4 - Is totally dependent in toileting.

☐   UK - Unknown

(continued)

88. (M0690) Transferring: Ability to move from bed to chair, on and off toilet or commode, into and out of tub or shower, and ability to turn and position self in bed if patient is bedfast.

Prior   Current

- ☐   ☐   0 - Able to independently transfer.
- ☒   ☒   1 - Transfers with minimal human assistance or with use of an assistive device.
- ☐   ☐   2 - *Unable* to transfer self but is able to bear weight and pivot during the transfer process.
- ☐   ☐   3 - Unable to transfer self and is *unable* to bear weight or pivot when transferred by another person.
- ☐   ☐   4 - Bedfast, unable to transfer but is able to turn and position self in bed.
- ☐   ☐   5 - Bedfast, unable to transfer and is *unable* to turn and position self.
- ☐   UK - Unknown

89. (M0700) Ambulation/Locomotion: Ability to *SAFELY* walk, once in a standing position, or use a wheelchair, once in a seated position, on a variety of surfaces.

Prior   Current

- ☒   ☐   0 - Able to independently walk on even and uneven surfaces and climb stairs with or without railings (i.e., needs no human assistance or assistive device).
- ☐   ☒   1 - Requires use of a device (e.g., cane, walker) to walk alone or requires human supervision or assistance to negotiate stairs or steps or uneven surfaces.
- ☐   ☐   2 - Able to walk only with the supervision or assistance of another person at all times.
- ☐   ☐   3 - Chairfast, *unable* to ambulate but is able to wheel self independently.
- ☐   ☐   4 - Chairfast, unable to ambulate and is *unable* to wheel self.
- ☐   ☐   5 - Bedfast, unable to ambulate or be up in a chair.
- ☐   UK - Unknown

90. **(M0710) Feeding or Eating:** Ability to feed self meals and snacks. **Note:** This refers only to the process of *eating, chewing,* and *swallowing, not preparing* the food to be eaten.

Prior Current

☒   ☒   0 - Able to independently feed self.

☐   ☐   1 - Able to feed self independently but requires:
    (a) meal set-up; *OR*
    (b) intermittent assistance or supervision from another person; *OR*
    (c) a liquid, pureed or ground meat diet.

☐   ☐   2 - *Unable* to feed self and must be assisted or supervised throughout the meal/snack.

☐   ☐   3 - Able to take in nutrients orally *and* receives supplemental nutrients through a nasogastric tube or gastrostomy.

☐   ☐   4 - *Unable* to take in nutrients orally and is fed nutrients through a nasogastric tube or gastrostomy.

☐   ☐   5 - Unable to take in nutrients orally or by tube feeding.

☐   UK - Unknown

91. **(M0720) Planning and Preparing Light Meals** (e.g., cereal, sandwich) or reheat delivered meals:

Prior Current

☒   ☐   0 - (a) Able to independently plan and prepare all light meals for self or reheat delivered meals; OR
    (b) Is physically, cognitively, and mentally able to prepare light meals on a regular basis but has not routinely performed light meal preparation in the past (i.e., prior to this home care admission).

☐   ☒   1 - *Unable* to prepare light meals on a regular basis due to physical, cognitive, or mental limitations.

☐   ☐   2 - Unable to prepare any light meals or reheat any delivered meals.

☐   UK - Unknown

92. **(M0730) Transportation:** Physical and mental ability to *safely* use a car, taxi, or public transportation (bus, train, subway).

Prior Current

☐   ☐   0 - Able to independently drive a regular or adapted car; OR uses a regular or handicap-accessible public bus.

☒   ☒   1 - Able to ride in a car only when driven by another person; OR able to use a bus or handicap van only when assisted or accompanied by another person.

☐   ☐   2 - Unable to ride in a car, taxi, bus, or van, and requires transportation by ambulance.

☐   UK - Unknown

(continued)

93. (M0740) Laundry: Ability to do own laundry — to carry laundry to and from washing machine, to use washer and dryer, to wash small items by hand.

Prior Current

☐ ☐ 0 - (a) Able to independently take care of all laundry tasks; *OR*
           (b) Physically, cognitively, and mentally able to do laundry and access facilities, but has not routinely performed laundry tasks in the past (i.e., prior to this home care admission).

☒ ☐ 1 - Able to do only light laundry, such as minor hand wash or light washer loads. Due to physical, cognitive, or mental limitations, needs assistance with heavy laundry such as carrying large loads of laundry.

☐ ☒ 2 - *Unable* to do any laundry due to physical limitation or needs continual supervision and assistance due to cognitive or mental limitation.

☐   UK - Unknown

84. (M0750) Housekeeping: Ability to safely and effectively perform light housekeeping and heavier cleaning tasks.

Prior Current

☐ ☐ 0 - (a) Able to independently perform all housekeeping tasks; *OR*
           (b) Physically, cognitively, and mentally able to perform *all* housekeeping tasks but has not routinely participated in housekeeping tasks in the past (i.e., prior to this home care admission).

☐ ☐ 1 - Able to perform only *light* housekeeping (e.g., dusting, wiping kitchen counters) tasks independently.

☐ ☐ 2 - Able to perform housekeeping tasks with intermittent assistance or supervision from another person.

☐ ☐ 3 - *Unable* to consistently perform any housekeeping tasks unless assisted by another person throughout the process.

☒ ☒ 4 - Unable to effectively participate in any housekeeping tasks.

☐   UK - Unknown

95. (M0760) Shopping: Ability to plan for, select, and purchase items in a store and to carry them home or arrange delivery.

Prior Current

☐ ☐ 0 - (a) Able to plan for shopping needs and independently perform shopping tasks, including carrying packages; *OR*
           (b) Physically, cognitively, and mentally able to take care of shopping, but has not done shopping in the past (i.e., prior to this home care admission).

☐ ☐ 1 - Able to go shopping, but needs some assistance:

(a) By self is able to do only light shopping and carry small packages, but needs someone to do occasional major shopping; *OR*

(b) *Unable* to go shopping alone, but can go with someone to assist.

☒ ☒ 2 - *Unable* to go shopping, but is able to identify items needed, place orders, and arrange home delivery.

☐ ☐ 3 - Needs someone to do all shopping and errands.

☐ UK - Unknown

96. (M0770) Ability to Use Telephone: Ability to answer the phone, dial numbers, and *effectively* use the telephone to communicate.

Prior Current

☒ ☒ 0 - Able to dial numbers and answer calls appropriately and as desired.

☐ ☐ 1 - Able to use a specially adapted telephone (i.e., large numbers on the dial, teletype phone for the deaf) and call essential numbers.

☐ ☐ 2 - Able to answer the telephone and carry on a normal conversation but has difficulty with placing calls.

☐ ☐ 3 - Able to answer the telephone only some of the time or is able to carry on only a limited conversation.

☐ ☐ 4 - *Unable* to answer the telephone at all but can listen if assisted with equipment.

☐ ☐ 5 - Totally unable to use the telephone.

☐ ☐ NA - Patient does not have a telephone.

☐ UK - Unknown

MEDICATIONS

97. (M0780) Management of Oral Medications: *Patient's ability* to prepare and take all prescribed oral medications reliably and safely, including administration of the correct dosage at the appropriate times/intervals. *Excludes* injectable and I.V. medications. **(NOTE: This refers to ability, not compliance or willingness.)**

Prior Current

☒ ☒ 0 - Able to independently take the correct oral medication(s) and proper dosage(s) at the correct times.

☐ ☐ 1 - Able to take medication(s) at the correct times if:

(a) individual dosages are prepared in advance by another person; *OR*

(b) given daily reminders; *OR*

(c) someone develops a drug diary or chart.

☐ ☐ 2 - *Unable* to take medication unless administered by someone else.

☐ ☐ NA - No oral medications prescribed.

☐ UK - Unknown

(continued)

98. (M0790) Management of Inhalant/Mist Medications:
Patient's ability to prepare and take all prescribed inhalant/mist medications (nebulizers, metered dose devices) reliably and safely, including administration of the correct dosage at the appropriate times/intervals. *Excludes* **all other forms of medication (oral tablets, injectable and I.V. medications).**

Prior Current

☐   ☐   0 - Able to independently take the correct medication and proper dosage at the correct times.

☐   ☐   1 - Able to take medication at the correct times if:
(a) individual dosages are prepared in advance by another person, *OR*
(b) given daily reminders.

☐   ☐   2 - *Unable* to take medication unless administered by someone else.

☒   ☒   NA - No inhalant/mist medications prescribed.

☐   UK - Unknown

99. (M0800) Management of Injectable Medications: *Patient's ability* to prepare and take all prescribed injectable medications reliably and safely, including administration of correct dosage at the appropriate times/intervals. *Excludes* **I.V. medications.**

Prior Current

☒   ☒   0 - Able to independently take the correct medication and proper dosage at the correct times.

☐   ☐   1 - Able to take injectable medication at correct times if:
(a) individual syringes are prepared in advance by another person, OR
(b) given daily reminders.

☐   ☐   2 - Unable to take injectable medications unless administered by someone else.

☐   ☐   NA - No injectable medications prescribed.

☐   UK - Unknown

EQUIPMENT MANAGEMENT

100. (M0810) Patient Management of Equipment (includes *ONLY* oxygen, I.V./infusion therapy, enteral/parenteral nutrition equipment or supplies): *Patient's ability* to set up, monitor and change equipment reliably, and safely add appropriate fluids or medication, clean/store/dispose of equipment or supplies using proper technique. **(NOTE: This refers to ability, not compliance or willingness.)**

☐   0 - Patient manages all tasks related to equipment completely independently.

☐ 1 - If someone else sets up equipment (i.e., fills portable oxygen tank, provides patient with prepared solutions), patient is able to manage all other aspects of equipment.

☐ 2 - Patient requires considerable assistance from another person to manage equipment, but independently completes portions of the task.

☐ 3 - Patient is only able to monitor equipment (e.g., liter flow, fluid in bag) and must call someone else to manage the equipment.

☐ 4 - Patient is completely dependent on someone else to manage all equipment.

☒ NA - No equipment of this type used in care [If NA, go to *M0825*]

101. **(M0820) Caregiver Management of Equipment** (includes *ONLY* oxygen, I.V./infusion equipment, enteral/parenteral nutrition, ventilator therapy equipment or supplies): *Caregiver's ability* to set up, monitor, and change equipment reliably and safely, add appropriate fluids or medication, clean/store/dispose of equipment or supplies using proper technique. **(NOTE: This refers to ability, not compliance or willingness.)**

☐ 0 - Caregiver manages all tasks related to equipment completely independently.

☐ 1 - If someone else sets up equipment, caregiver is able to manage all other aspects.

☐ 2 - Caregiver requires considerable assistance from another person to manage equipment, but independently completes significant portions of task.

☐ 3 - Caregiver is only able to complete small portions of task (e.g., administer nebulizer treatment, clean/store/dispose of equipment or supplies).

☐ 4 - Caregiver is completely dependent on someone else to manage all equipment.

☐ NA - No caregiver

☐ UK - Unknown

THERAPY NEED

102. **(M0825) Therapy Need:** Does the care plan of the Medicare payment period for which this assessment will define a case mix group indicate a need for therapy (physical, occupational, or speech therapy) that meets the threshold for a Medicare high-therapy case mix group?

☒ 0 - No

☐ 1 - Yes

☐ NA - Not applicable

(continued)

EQUIPMENT AND SUPPLIES

Equipment needs (check appropriate box)

Has	Needs	
☐	☐	Oxygen/Respiratory Equip.
☐	☐	Wheelchair
☐	☐	Hospital Bed
☒	☐	Other (specify) _Walker_

Supplies needed and comments regarding equipment needs

Financial problems/needs

SAFETY

Safety measures recommended to protect patient from injury

_NA_

Emergency plans

Wife will call 911 for emergency care if needed

CONCLUSIONS

Conclusions/impressions and skilled interventions performed this visit

Wound care performed per care plan. Initiated
teaching regarding wound care signs & symptoms
of wound infection and emergency measures.

Date of assessment _1/2/07_

Signature of Assessor _Holly Dougherty, RN, BSN_

- Document physical changes that need to be made in the patient's home for him to receive proper care. Help his family find the resources to implement them.
- Describe the primary caregiver, including whether he lives with the patient, their relationship, his age and physical ability, and his willingness to help the patient. The patient's well-being may depend on this person's abilities.
- Show in your documentation how you made the most of the patient's strengths and resources. Strengths include support systems, good health habits and coping behaviors, a safe and healthful environment, and financial security. Resources include the physician, pharmacy, and medical equipment supplier.
- Show in your documentation that you identified the patient's weaknesses and the actions you took to assist the patient in overcoming these weaknesses.

PROGRESS NOTES

For each patient visit, write a progress note that documents:
- changes in the patient's condition
- skilled nursing interventions performed that are related to the care plan
- patient's responses to the services provided
- an event or incident in the home that would affect the treatment plan
- vital signs and systemic assessment
- patient and home-caregiver education (includes written instructional materials and brochures as well as the patient's response to the instruction and any return demonstrations)
- communication with other team members since the previous visit
- discharge plans
- time you arrived at and left the home.

To document safely and efficiently on progress notes:
- Document all events in chronological order.
- Avoid addendums.
- Provide a heading for each entry, such as "Nursing progress note," because many members of the health care team use the progress notes.

NURSING SUMMARIES

As a home health care nurse, you must compile a summary of the patient's progress (and discharge from home health care, when appropriate). You must also submit a patient progress report to the attending physician and to the reimburser to confirm the need for continuing services.

When writing these summaries, include:
- current problems, treatments, medications, interventions, and instructions
- home health care provided by other health care professionals, such as physical therapists, speech pathologists, occupational therapists, social workers, and home health care aides
- reason for any change in services
- patient outcomes and responses—both physical and emotional—to services provided.

PATIENT OR CAREGIVER TEACHING

Correct documentation will help justify to your agency and to third-party

(Text continues on page 345.)

INTERDISCIPLINARY CARE PLAN

The care plan is individualized for each patient. An example of this form is shown here.

Patient name: _Mary Long_

Primary nurse: _N. Smith, RN_

PROBLEM	GOAL	APPROACH	
Atrial fibrillation (1/3/01)	Maintain optimal cardiac output	1. Meds as ordered 2. Monitor vs, inc. apical rhythm and rate 3. observe for chest pain, dyspnea, palpitations, anxiety, etc.	
Heart failure (1/12/01)	1. Maintain fluid and electrolyte balance 2. Promote optimal gas exchange.	1. Meds as ordered 2. Nebulizer as ordered 3. Draw labs as ordered 4. I & O daily 5. Monitor edema 6. ✔ for SOB, dyspnea, congestion (lung sounds) 7. amb. as tol 8. semi Fowler's when sitting	
Gastrostomy tube insertion (1/13/01)	1. Maintain optimal nutritional status 2. Prevent skin break-down	1. Magnacal 80 ml/hr 2. Follow G-tube protocol, including site care & oral hygiene 3. Weekly weights 4. I&O daily 5. ✔ for N/V, diarrhea	

Intervention Codes

(please circle all that apply)

A1. Skilled observation
A2. Foley insertion
A3. Bladder installation
A4. Irrigation care (wd. dsg.)
A5. Irrigation decub. care - meds.
A6. Venipuncture
A7. Restorative nursing
A8. Postcataract care
A9. Bowel/Bladder training

A10. Chest physical
 (incl. postural drainage)
A11. Administer vit. B_{12}
A12. Prepare/Administer insulin
A13. Administer other
A14. Administer I.V.
A15. Teach ostomy care
A16. Teach nasogastric feeding
A17. Reposition nasogastric feeding tube
A18. Teach gastrostomy
A19. Teach parenteral nutrition

	Init. cert. period: _____
	Recert. period _____
	Init. cert. period: _____

INITIAL CERT.	RECERT. #1	RECERT. #2
GOAL MET? Y N INIT.:_____	GOAL MET? Y N INIT.:_____	GOAL MET? Y N INIT.:_____
GOAL MET? Y N INIT.:_____	GOAL MET? Y N INIT.:_____	GOAL MET? Y N INIT.:_____
GOAL MET? Y N INIT.:_____	GOAL MET? Y N INIT.:_____	GOAL MET? Y N INIT.:_____

A20. Teach care of trach.
A21. Administer care of trach.
A22. Teach inhalation Rx
A23. Administer inhalation Rx
A24. Teach administration of injections
A25. Teach diabetic care
A26. Disimpaction/enema
A27. Other
    Foot care (diabetic)
    Teach diet
    Teach disease process
    Teach use of O_2

    Instruct re: Medication child
A28. Wound care/dsg - closed
A29. Decubitus care - simple
A30. Teach care of indwelling catheter
A31. Management and evaluation of patient care plan
A32. Teaching and training (other)

CERTIFICATION OF INSTRUCTION

The model patient-teaching form here shows what was taught to a home-care patient on I.V. therapy. This type of form will help you document your teaching sessions clearly and completely.

CONTENT (check all that apply; fill in blanks as indicated)

1. ☐ Reason for therapy

2. Drug/Solution

   ☐ Dose
   ☐ Schedule
   ☐ Label accuracy
   ☐ Storage
   ☐ Container integrity

3. Aseptic technique

   ☐ Handwashing
   ☐ Prepping caps/connections
   ☐ Tubing/cap/needs
   ☐ Needleless adaptor changes

4. Access device maintenance

   Type/Name: _____
   ☒ Device / Site Inspection
   ☐ Site care/Dsg. changes
   ☐ Catheter clamping
   ☒ Maintaining patency
      ☒ Saline flushing
      ☐ Heparin locking
      ☐ Fdg. Tube /declogging
      ☐ Self insertion of device

5. Drug preparation

   ☒ Premixed containers
   ☐ Compounding
   ☐ Piggyback lipids
   ☐ Client additives

6. Method of administration

   ☐ Gravity
   ☒ Pump (name): _IVAC pump_
   ☐ Continuous   ☒ Intermittent
   ☐ Cycle/Taper:

7. Administration technique

   ☒ Pump rate/calibration
   ☐ Priming tubing   ☐ Filter
   ☐ Filling syringe
   ☐ Loading pump
   ☒ Access device hookup/disconnect

8. Potential complications/Adverse effects

   ☐ Patient drug information sheet reviewed
   ☒ Pump alarms/troubleshooting

   ☒ Phlebitis/infiltration
   ☐ Clotting/dislodgment
   ☒ Infection
   ☐ Air embolus
   ☐ Breakage/cracking
   ☐ Electrolyte imbalance
   ☐ Fluid balance
   ☐ Glucose intolerance
   ☐ Aspiration
   ☐ N / V / D / Cramping
   ☐ Other: _____
   _____

9. Self monitoring:

   ☐ Weight   ☒ Temperature   ☐ P   ☐ PB
   ☐ Urine S & A   ☐ Fingersticks
   ☐ Other: _____

10. Supply handling/disposal

    ☒ Disposal of sharps/supplies
    ☐ Narcotics
    ☒ Cleaning pump
    ☐ Changing batteries
    ☐ Blood/fluid precautions
    ☐ Chemo/spill precautions

11. Information given to client re:

    ☐ Pharmacy counseling
    ☐ Advance directives
    ☐ Inventory checks _____
    ☐ Deliveries
    ☒ 24-hour on-call staff _____
    ☒ Reimbursement _____
    ☐ Service complaints _____

12. Safety/Disaster plan

    ☐ Back up pump batteries _____
    ☒ Emergency room use _____
    ☐ Electrical _____
    ☒ Disaster _____
    ☐ Other: _____
    _____

13. Written instructions

    ☒ Yes ☐ No   If no, why _____
    _____
    _____
    _____

CERTIFICATION OF INSTRUCTION (CONTINUED)

☐ Client or caregiver demonstrates or verbalizes competency to perform home infusion therapy.

COMMENTS: _Wife incorrectly changed pump battery. Procedure reviewed. Wife then demonstrated correct procedure. Wife also concerned about frequency of dressing changes. Access site nonreddened and not edematous. Protocol reviewed. Patient states he is satisfied to wait until scheduled dressing change tomorrow._

Theory/Skill reviewed/Return demonstration completed:

Chris Basner, RN   _1-21-01_

Signature of RN Educator   **Date**

CERTIFICATION OF INSTRUCTION

I agree that I have been instructed as described above and understand that the above functions will be performed in the home by myself and caregiver, outside a hospital or medically supervised environment.

Robert Burns   _1-21-01_

Client/caregiver signature   **Date**

---

payers that visits to teach the patient or caregiver were necessary. When documenting your patient or caregiver teaching, follow these guidelines:

● Learn about the patient's and family's needs, resources, and support systems to help you outline a basic plan for teaching.

● Remember that teaching is usually an ongoing process requiring more than one visit. Until the patient becomes independent, your documentation will help other nurses continue the teaching and identify additional areas where teaching is needed. (See *Certification of instruction*.)

● Keep a list of teaching and reference materials supplied to the patient or caregiver.

● Document modifications made to accommodate the patient's or caregiver's literacy skills and native language.

● If the patient isn't physically or mentally able to perform the skills himself and no caregiver is available, report this in your documentation. Never leave a patient alone to perform a procedure until he can express understanding of it and perform it competently.

● Call equipment by the same names used on the packages and in teaching literature.

● Provide a glossary of terms, and label machines to match your instructions.

● Make sure that the patient can identify devices when speaking on the telephone.

• Document all teaching materials given to the patient, and keep copies in your records.

• Videotape your instructions and leave the tape in the home if more than one caregiver will be providing care.

• Make sure that the patient signs a teaching documentation record, which indicates that he accepts responsibility for learning self-care activities.

RECERTIFICATION

To ensure continued home health care services, you'll have to prove that the patient still requires home health care. Medicare and many managed care plans certify an initial 60-day period during which your agency can receive reimbursement for the patient's home health care. When the 60-day period is over, the insurer may certify an additional 60 days, called the *recertification period*.

When filling out recertification paperwork, make sure that your documentation requesting recertification clearly supports the patient's need for continued care within the insurer's guidelines:

• Compile a clinical summary of care, and send it to the patient's physician and then to the insurer.

• For Medicare, submit a new care plan on Form 485. This form must include data as amended by verbal order since the start of care.

• When you document the primary diagnosis, it must reflect the patient's current needs, not the original reason for the home health care.

DISCHARGE SUMMARY

You'll prepare a discharge summary:

• to obtain the physician's approval to discharge a patient

• for notifying reimbursers that services have been terminated

• for officially closing the case.

When preparing this summary, document:

• time frame covered

• services provided

• names and titles of assigned staff

• third-party payer and whether the patient is eligible for future payment (he may have exhausted his annual benefits)

• clinical and psychosocial conditions of the patient at discharge

• recommendations for further care

• caregiver involvement in care

• interruptions in home care such as readmission to the hospital

• referral to community agencies

• OASIS discharge information

• patient's response to and comprehension of patient-teaching efforts

• outcomes attained

• current medication list.

COMMUNITY REFERRALS

Local community resources, such as a free mobile health care unit or services to provide emotional support, can help maintain and promote your patients' health and well-being. Whenever you make a referral for community services, document your actions and the reasons for the referral.

Documentation guidelines

When completing documentation for your home care patient, follow these guidelines:

- Update the record with changes in the patient's condition or care plan, and document that you reported changes to the physician and other members of the interdisciplinary team. *Remember:* Medicare and Medicaid won't reimburse for skilled services implemented but not ordered by the physician.
- Make sure that all documentation is accurate. Accuracy ensures proper reimbursement and prevents the appearance of fraud.
- State in your documentation that the patient is homebound, and provide the reason for this. An example of a valid reason for being homebound is dyspnea on minimal activity; an invalid reason would be not having a car.
- If an emergency arises in the home during your presence, accompany the patient to the hospital or emergency department, and stay with him until another professional caregiver takes over. Be sure to document all assessments and interventions performed for the patient until you're relieved. Also document the date and time of transfer and the name of the caregiver who assumes responsibility for the patient.
- Make sure documentation reflects consistent adherence to the care plan by all caregivers involved.
- Whenever possible, use flow sheets and checklists to document vital signs, intake and output measurements, and nutritional data.
- Encourage the patient or home-caregiver to complete forms when appropriate. Doing so involves the patient and his family in the patient's progress and increases their feeling of control.
- At least once per week, remove completed documentation materials that have been left in the patient's home. This prevents volumes of paper from piling up or becoming misplaced and makes documentation available for review by the agency supervisor.

NANDA-I TAXONOMY II

COMPARING
DOCUMENTATION SYSTEMS

SELECTED REFERENCES

INDEX

NANDA-I TAXONOMY II

◆

The following is a list of the 2005-2006 current nursing diagnosis classifications according to their domains.

Domain: Health promotion
- Effective therapeutic regimen management
- Health-seeking behaviors (specify)
- Impaired home maintenance
- Ineffective community therapeutic regimen management
- Ineffective family therapeutic regimen management
- Ineffective health maintenance
- Ineffective therapeutic regimen management
- Readiness for enhanced management of therapeutic regimen
- Readiness for enhanced nutrition

Domain: Nutrition
- Deficient fluid volume
- Excess fluid volume
- Imbalanced nutrition: Less than body requirements
- Imbalanced nutrition: More than body requirements
- Impaired swallowing
- Ineffective infant feeding pattern
- Readiness for enhanced fluid balance
- Risk for deficient fluid volume
- Risk for imbalanced fluid volume
- Risk for imbalanced nutrition: More than body requirements

Domain: Elimination/Exchange
- Bowel incontinence
- Constipation
- Diarrhea
- Functional urinary incontinence
- Impaired gas exchange
- Impaired urinary elimination
- Perceived constipation
- Readiness for enhanced urinary elimination
- Reflex urinary incontinence
- Risk for constipation
- Risk for urge urinary incontinence
- Stress urinary incontinence
- Total urinary incontinence
- Urge urinary incontinence
- Urinary retention

Domain: Activity/Rest
- Activity intolerance
- Bathing or hygiene self-care deficit
- Decreased cardiac output
- Deficient diversional activity
- Delayed surgical recovery
- Dressing or grooming self-care deficit

- Dysfunctional ventilatory weaning response
- Energy field disturbance
- Fatigue
- Feeding self-care deficit
- Impaired bed mobility
- Impaired physical mobility
- Impaired spontaneous ventilation
- Impaired transfer ability
- Impaired walking
- Impaired wheelchair mobility
- Ineffective breathing pattern
- Ineffective tissue perfusion (specify type: renal, cerebral, cardiopulmonary, gastrointestinal, peripheral)
- Insomnia
- Readiness for enhanced sleep
- Risk for activity intolerance
- Risk for disuse syndrome
- Sedentary lifestyle
- Sleep deprivation
- Toileting self-care deficit

Domain: Perception/Cognition
- Acute confusion
- Chronic confusion
- Deficient knowledge (specify)
- Disturbed sensory perception (specify: visual, auditory, kinesthetic, gustatory, tactile, olfactory)
- Disturbed thought processes
- Impaired environmental interpretation syndrome
- Impaired memory
- Impaired verbal communication
- Readiness for enhanced communication
- Readiness for enhanced knowledge (specify)
- Unilateral neglect
- Wandering

Domain: Self-perception
- Chronic low self-esteem
- Disturbed body image
- Disturbed personal identity

- Hopelessness
- Powerlessness
- Readiness for enhanced self-concept
- Risk for loneliness
- Risk for powerlessness
- Risk for situational low self-esteem
- Situational low self-esteem

Domain: Role relationships
- Caregiver role strain
- Dysfunctional family processes: Alcoholism
- Effective breast-feeding
- Impaired parenting
- Impaired social interaction
- Ineffective breast-feeding
- Ineffective role performance
- Interrupted breast-feeding
- Interrupted family processes
- Parental role conflict
- Readiness for enhanced family processes
- Readiness for enhanced parenting
- Risk for caregiver role strain
- Risk for impaired parent/infant/child attachment
- Risk for impaired parenting

Domain: Sexuality
- Ineffective sexuality patterns
- Sexual dysfunction

Domain: Coping/Stress tolerance
- Anxiety
- Autonomic dysreflexia
- Chronic sorrow
- Complicated grieving
- Compromised family coping
- Death anxiety
- Decreased intracranial adaptive capacity
- Defensive coping
- Disabled family coping
- Disorganized infant behavior

- Fear
- Grieving
- Ineffective community coping
- Ineffective coping
- Ineffective denial
- Posttrauma syndrome
- Rape-trauma syndrome
- Rape-trauma syndrome: Compound reaction
- Rape-trauma syndrome: Silent reaction
- Readiness for enhanced community coping
- Readiness for enhanced coping
- Readiness for enhanced family coping
- Readiness for enhanced organized infant behavior
- Relocation stress syndrome
- Risk for autonomic dysreflexia
- Risk for complicated grieving
- Risk for disorganized infant behavior
- Risk for posttrauma syndrome
- Risk for relocation stress syndrome
- Risk prone health behavior

Domain: Life principles
- Decisional conflict (specify)
- Impaired religiosity
- Noncompliance (specify)
- Readiness for enhanced religiosity
- Readiness for enhanced spiritual well-being
- Risk for impaired religiosity
- Risk for spiritual distress
- Spiritual distress

Domain: Safety/Protection
- Hyperthermia
- Hypothermia
- Impaired dentition
- Impaired oral mucous membrane
- Impaired skin integrity
- Impaired tissue integrity
- Ineffective airway clearance

- Ineffective protection
- Ineffective thermoregulation
- Latex allergy response
- Risk for aspiration
- Risk for falls
- Risk for imbalanced body temperature
- Risk for impaired skin integrity
- Risk for infection
- Risk for injury
- Risk for latex allergy response
- Risk for other-directed violence
- Risk for perioperative-positioning injury
- Risk for peripheral neurovascular dysfunction
- Risk for poisoning
- Risk for self-directed violence
- Risk for self-mutilation
- Risk for sudden infant death syndrome
- Risk for suffocation
- Risk for suicide
- Risk for trauma
- Self-mutilation

Domain: Comfort
- Acute pain
- Chronic pain
- Nausea
- Social isolation

Domain: Growth/Development
- Adult failure to thrive
- Delayed growth and development
- Risk for delayed development
- Risk for disproportionate growth

NEW Nursing diagnoses
Contamination
Moral distress
Overflow urinary incontinence
Readiness for enhanced comfort
Readiness for enhanced decision making
Readiness for enhanced hope

Readiness for enhanced immunization status
Readiness for enhanced power
Readiness for enhance self-care
Risk for acute confusion
Risk for compromised human dignity
Risk for contamination
Risk for impaired liver function
Risk for unstable glucose level
Stress overload

COMPARING DOCUMENTATION SYSTEMS

◆

This table compares elements of the different documentation systems used today. Note that the second column provides information on which systems work best in which settings.

SYSTEM	USEFUL SETTINGS	PARTS OF RECORD
Narrative	◆ Acute care ◆ Long-term care ◆ Home care ◆ Ambulatory care	◆ Progress notes ◆ Flow sheets to supplement care plan
POMR Problem-oriented medical record	◆ Acute care ◆ Long-term care ◆ Home care ◆ Rehabilitation ◆ Mental health facilities	◆ Database ◆ Care plan ◆ Problem list ◆ Progress notes ◆ Discharge summary
PIE Problem-intervention-evaluation	◆ Acute care	◆ Assessment flow sheets ◆ Progress notes ◆ Problem list
FOCUS charting	◆ Acute care ◆ Long-term care	◆ Progress notes ◆ Flow sheets ◆ Checklists
CBE Charting by exception	◆ Acute care ◆ Long-term care	◆ Care plan ◆ Flow sheets, including patient-teaching records and patient discharge notes ◆ Graphic record ◆ Progress notes

Assessment	Care plan	Outcomes and evaluation	Progress notes format
◆ Initial: history and admission form ◆ Ongoing: progress notes	◆ Care plan	◆ Progress notes ◆ Discharge summaries	◆ Narration at time of entry
◆ Initial: database and care plan ◆ Ongoing: progress notes	◆ Database ◆ Nursing care plan based on problem list	◆ Progress notes (section E of SOAPIE and SOAPIER)	◆ SOAP, SOAPIE, or SOAPIER
◆ Initial: assessment form ◆ Ongoing: assessment form every shift	◆ None; included in progress notes (section P)	◆ Progress notes (section E)	◆ Problem ◆ Intervention ◆ Evaluation
◆ Initial: patient history and admission assessment ◆ Ongoing: assessment form	◆ Nursing care plan based on problems or nursing diagnoses	◆ Progress notes (section R)	◆ Data ◆ Action ◆ Response
◆ Initial: database assessment sheet ◆ Ongoing: nursing and medical order flow sheets	◆ Nursing care plan based on nursing diagnoses	◆ Progress notes (section E)	◆ SOAPIE or SOAPIER

System	Useful settings	Parts of record
FACT Flow sheet, assessment, concise, timely	◆ Acute care ◆ Long-term care	◆ Assessment sheet ◆ Flow sheets ◆ Progress notes
Core (with data, action, and evaluation—or DAE)	◆ Acute care ◆ Long-term care	◆ Kardex ◆ Flow sheets ◆ Progress notes
Computerized	◆ Acute care ◆ Long-term care ◆ Home care ◆ Ambulatory care	◆ Progress notes ◆ Flow sheets ◆ Nursing care plan ◆ Database ◆ Teaching plan

ASSESSMENT	CARE PLAN	OUTCOMES AND EVALUATION	PROGRESS NOTES FORMAT
◆ Initial: baseline assessment ◆ Ongoing: flow sheets and progress notes	◆ Nursing care plan based on nursing diagnoses	◆ Flow sheets (section R)	◆ Data ◆ Action ◆ Response
◆ Initial: baseline assessment ◆ Ongoing: progress notes	◆ Care plan	◆ Progress notes (section E)	◆ Data ◆ Action ◆ Evaluation
◆ Initial: baseline assessment ◆ Ongoing: progress notes	◆ Database ◆ Care plan	◆ Outcome-based care plan	◆ Evaluative statements ◆ Expected outcomes ◆ Learning outcomes

SELECTED
REFERENCES

◆───────◆

Brown, G. "Wound Documentation: Managing Risk," *Advances in Skin & Wound Care* 19(3):155-65, April 2006.

Charting Made Incredibly Easy, 3rd ed. Philadelphia: Lippincott Williams & Wilkins, 2006.

ChartSmart: An A-to-Z Guide to Better Nursing Documentation, 2nd ed. Philadelphia: Lippincott Williams & Wilkins, 2007.

Comeaux, K., et al. "Improve PRN Effectiveness Documentation," *Nursing Management* 37(9):58, September 2006.

Hall, L.C., and James, P.L. "Utilization of the Vista Information System Improves Documentation and Cost Savings: AP93," *Transfusion* 46 Supplement 9:201A, September 2006.

Langowski, C. "The Times They are a Changing: Effects of Online Nursing Documentation Systems," *Quality Management in Health Care* 14(2):121-25, April-June 2005.

Lawhorne, J D. "Implementation of a Documentation System of Evidence-Based Processes for the Insertion of Central Venous Catheters," *American Journal of Infection Control* 34(5):E120, June 2006.

Leisner, B.A., and Wonch, D.E. "How Documentation Outcomes Guide the Way: A Patient Health Education Electronic Medical Record Experience in a Large Health Care Network," *Quality Management in Health Care* 15(3):171-83, July-September 2006.

Monroe, K.W., et al. "Helmet Use Documentation Preinjury and Postinjury Documentation Sheet: 3:00 pm-110," *Pediatric Emergency Care* 22(9):682, September 2006.

Mosby's Surefire Documentation: How, What, and When Nurses Need To Document, 2nd ed. St. Louis: Mosby–Year Book, Inc., 2007.

Silfen, E. "Documentation and Coding of ED Patient Encounters: An Evaluation of the Accuracy of an Electronic Medical Record," *American Journal of Emergency Medicine* 24(6):664-78, October 2006.

Smith, K., et al. "Evaluating the Impact of Computerized Clinical Documentation," *CIN: Computers, Informatics, Nursing* 23(3):132-38, May-June 2005.

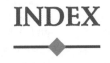

INDEX

i refers to an illustration; t refers to a table.

i refers to an illustration; t refers to a table.

i refers to an illustration; t refers to a table.

i refers to an illustration; t refers to a table.

i refers to an illustration; t refers to a table.

i refers to an illustration; t refers to a table.

i refers to an illustration; t refers to a table.

Hypotension, 54-55
Hypoxemia, 55-56

I

Implementation, 131-134
  computers and, 181
  as nursing process step, 83i
Incident report, 74-75
  completing, 141, 142-143i, 143
  facility policies on document-
    ing, 162
  functions of, 75
  review of, 76i
Incidents, 74-81
Individually developed care plan, 118,
  120-121i
Infection control, 33
Infections
  reportable, 33, 34
  reporting, to infection control
    department, 33
Information from other departments, 67
Informed consent, 144, 146-147
  elements of, 147
  in emergency situation, 235
  legal requirements for, 144, 146
  nursing responsibilities for, 147
  witnessing, 144, 148-159i
Informed refusal, 147, 149
Initial assessment
  categorizing data in, 89, 91
  collecting relevant information
    for, 88-89
  documenting, 95, 96-104i, 105,
    105i, 106i, 107, 108-109i,
    109-110
  general observations in, 90-91
  health history in, 91
  incomplete, 109-110

Initial assessment *(continued)*
  Joint Commission on the Accredita-
    tion of Healthcare Organizations
    requirements for, 94-95
  in long-term care, 286-288
  physical examination in, 91, 93-94
  relating, to nursing diagnoses, 112,
    113-114i, 114
Ink requirements for documentation, 83
Intake and output monitoring, 37, 42
  patients who require, 37
  record of, 44-45i
  simplifying documentation of, 42
Integrated admission database form,
  96-104i
Integumentary system, initial assessment of, 94
Interdepartmental communication,
  67-69
Interdisciplinary admission form,
  96-104i
Interdisciplinary care plan in home
  health care, 308, 341, 342-343i
Interdisciplinary communication,
  67-69
Intermediate care facility, level of care
  in, 277
Intermittent mandatory ventilation, 26
International Council of Nurses code
  of ethics, 146
Interventions
  documenting, 131-134
  guidelines for selecting, 117
  performing, 134
  types of, 134
Intervention statements, guidelines
  for, 117
Interview techniques, 92-93
Intracerebral hemorrhage, 56-57

---

i refers to an illustration; t refers to a table.

i refers to an illustration; t refers to a table.

i refers to an illustration; t refers to a table.

i refers to an illustration; t refers to a table.

i refers to an illustration; t refers to a table.

i refers to an illustration; t refers to a table.

i refers to an illustration; t refers to a table.

i refers to an illustration; t refers to a table.

i refers to an illustration; t refers to a table.

Urethral suppositories, documenting
administration of, 8
Urgent conditions, 237

V
Vaginal suppositories, documenting
administration of, 8
Venipuncture, multiple attempts
of, 10
Verbal orders, 71
Verification process, preoperative,
checklist for, 18, 19i, 20
Violent patient
mobilizing staff for, 168
responding to, 168-169
Vision of patient, general
observation of, 90
Visual analog pain scale, 36i
Voice-activated computer
systems, 183
Voice pagers, patient confidentiality
and, 178t

WXYZ
Withdrawal of arterial blood, 29
Wound assessment, 43
flow sheet for, 46-47i
Wound care procedures, post-
operative, 20-21
Written orders, 69
Wrong-site surgery, preventing, 18

i refers to an illustration; t refers to a table.